EKG Plain and Simple

From Rhythm Strips to 12-Leads

Karen M. Ellis, RN, CCRN

Touro Infirmary and Delgado Community College, New Orleans

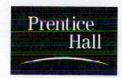
Prentice
Hall

Upper Saddle River, New Jersey 07458

Library of Congress Cataloging-in-Publication Data

Ellis, Karen.
　　EKG plain and simple : from rhythm strips to 12-leads / Karen Ellis.
　　　p. ; cm.
　　Includes index.
　　ISBN 0-13-019745-9
　　1. Electrocardiography.　I. Title.
　　[DNLM: 1. Electrocardiography. WG 140 E465e 2002]
　　RC683.5.E5 E442 2002
　　616.1'207547–dc21

　　　　　　　　　　　　　　　2001036200

Publisher: Julie Alexander

Executive Assistant & Supervisor: Regina Bruno

Acquisitions Editor: Mark Cohen

Editorial Assistant: Melissa Kerian

Managing Editor: Patrick Walsh

Production Management/Composition

　　Electronic Art Creation: North Market Street Graphics

Production Editor: Christine Furry

Interior Design: North Market Street Graphics

Director of Manufacturing and Production: Bruce Johnson

Manufacturing Buyer: Ilene Sanford

Creative Director: Cheryl Asherman

Design Coordinator: Maria Guglielmo

Marketing Manager: David Hough

Printer/Binder: Banta Company, Harrisonburg, VA

Cover Design: Joseph DePinho

Notice: The author and the publisher of this book have taken care to make certain that the equipment and schedules of treatment are correct and compatible with the standards generally accepted at the time of publication. Nevertheless, as new information becomes available, changes in treatment and in the use of equipment and procedures become necessary. The reader is advised to consult carefully the instruction and information material included in each piece of equipment or device before administration. Students are warned that the use of any techniques must be authorized by their medical advisor, where appropriate, in accordance with local laws and regulations. The publisher disclaims any liability, loss, injury, or damage incurred as a consequence, directly or indirectly, of the use and application of any of the contents of this book.

Pearson Education LTD.
Pearson Education Australia PTY, Limited
Pearson Education Singapore, Pte. Ltd
Pearson Education North Asia Ltd
Pearson Education Canada, Ltd.
Pearson Educación de Mexico, S.A. de C.V.
Pearson Education–Japan
Pearson Education Malaysia, Pte. Ltd

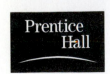

10　9　8

ISBN 0-13-019745-9

Contents

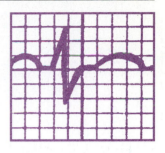

PART II: ADVANCED CONCEPTS

Introduction

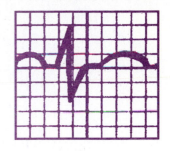

Don't you just groan at the thought of buying yet another cold, formal textbook, the kind that imparts important information, but in such a tedious way that you're lucky if you can stay awake long enough to learn anything? Well, this isn't one of those books. This text is very informal. It's written in a conversational style so that you feel you're sitting with a favorite instructor who's teaching you one-on-one. Before you know it, you've learned concepts and skills and haven't snored even once. You may have even chuckled a time or two, as there is occasional humor in this text. Humor? In a textbook? Sure. Think about your favorite instructors. Chances are they're your favorite because they knew how and when to use humor to illustrate a point. And I'll bet you still remember what they taught you. If something makes you laugh, you'll remember it. That being said, however, do not get the impression that this is not a serious textbook on electrocardiography. It is.

This text assumes no prior knowledge about electrocardiography or about the heart in general. It takes the student from square one and builds knowledge from the bottom up, pyramid style. At the base of the pyramid is cardiac anatomy and physiology—not enough to be intimidating, but just enough so that the concepts about electrocardiography have a solid foundation. Cardiac anatomy and physiology are covered in Part I of the text.

Also in Part I is information about the cardiac conduction system, leads, EKG waves and complexes, and lots of practice exercises to hone your newly learned skills. At the end of Part I is arrhythmia interpretation. Basic rhythms, their causes, clinical implications, and treatment are covered. Rhythm summary sheets and algorithms (flowcharts) help you learn rhythm interpretation, and quizzes at the end of chapters help you evaluate your comprehension of the material. There is an entire chapter of rhythm strips to interpret.

A word about the rhythm strips. Some strips have a dotted-line grid pattern in the background and others have a more solid-line grid. This is because different EKG machines print out differently. It's important to be able to interpret rhythm strips with all types of backgrounds. Also, unlike some EKG textbooks that use computer-generated rhythm strips and thus have picture-perfect strips, this text, with few exceptions, uses strips from real patients. Therefore, a few strips have nurses' writing on them or interpretive data from the EKG monitor. Also, a few strips may be a bit faded. Do not let this distract you. *Each one of these strips has something to teach you.*

Also in Part I is a brief chapter on coronary artery disease. Since electrocardiography deals with a population of individuals with cardiac problems, it makes sense not just to be adept at interpreting their rhythm strips and EKGs, but also to be knowledgeable about their disease process and symptoms. It's important to see the person beneath the EKG.

Part II is higher up the pyramid. It covers 12-lead EKG analysis, cardiac medications, intraventricular conduction defects (IVCDs), pacemakers, and diagnostic electrocardiography. There are algorithms to help in IVCD and MI recognition. You'll learn to recognize whether a patient is having a heart attack, which part of the heart is damaged, which blood vessel is involved, and which medications are used to treat it. There is an entire chapter of 12-lead EKGs to evaluate. At the end of Part II is a chapter of scenarios providing rhythm strips and/or 12-lead EKGs along with a clinical situation and asking pertinent questions to challenge you to assess the situation and decide on an intervention. This chapter helps to pull everything together. It's the apex of the pyramid.

This text is a complete guide to electrocardiography, from the basics to the more advanced concepts. It's appropriate for allied health students, nurses or nursing students, medical students or residents, and emergency medical technicians and paramedics. Though intended for beginners, it's also an excellent reference for those experienced practitioners seeking a good review.

So enough talk already. Let's get started!

Karen Ellis

Acknowledgments

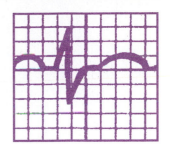

In the past year and a half, the following people have been instrumental in helping this project reach completion. I owe them all a debt of gratitude.

To my husband Lee Ellis, without whom this book would not have been published. A publisher's rep called to try to persuade Lee, who has a Ph.D. in biology, to write a book, and Lee casually mentioned that his wife had written an EKG book. Things took off from there. Lee almost single-handedly has done everything to keep our house running so I could concentrate on this effort, and on almost a daily basis he has saved my computer from being thrown down the stairs in my fits of frustration (I am personally convinced my computer hates me). He would smirk at me because he knew the computer was fine—*I* was screwing up. (I was *pretending* to mess up on the computer just so he could feel superior. Isn't it amazing what women will do for their husbands?) I love you, Lee, and truth be told, I married you because of your smirk. If that smirk goes, you're outta here, buddy. . . .

To my sons Jason, Mark, and Matthew, who knew that Mom could always be found in the computer room, and who didn't groan too loudly at the idea of frequent take-out dinners while I obsessed over this book. Jason and Mark were my comic relief, Jason because of his outfits that I swear were borrowed from a 1970s TV cop show, and Mark for folding his arms just so, showing off his *huge* biceps and grinning at me as I stare at this once scrawny kid who's now becoming a man. And my little guy Matthew is my solace. He lights the room, and my heart, with his smile. I love you, guys.

To my sister Sandra Schraibman, who, though she was positive I'd never finish this book until the *next* millenium (ha!), was cheering me on throughout this whole process. Sandra and I are all that's left of our original family, and over the past few years I've come to realize how lucky I am to have her. She has a way of cracking me up whenever I'm taking myself too seriously (that can be *very* annoying) and of galvanizing me into action when I become a slug (now that's *really* annoying). In other words, she's the best sister I could possibly have. So thank you, Sandra. Now get up off the floor. You can't be *that* shocked that I said nice stuff. . . .

To my parents, Sybil and Edward Milner, who have passed away, but whose pride in me was and still is the wind beneath my wings. I miss you.

To my cousin Irene Milliman, who didn't hear from me for prolonged stretches while I worked on this book. See, Irene, I really *was* writing a book. . . . Thank you for your patience.

To Theresa Hollins, telemetry technician extraordinaire at Touro Infirmary in New Orleans, for enthusiastically helping me out on my nightly "strip searches" by collecting hundreds of rhythm strips for me over the past several years. Theresa is always asking for my opinion on rhythm strips when she knows darn well she's almost never wrong. Theresa, thank you, thank you, thank you. This absolutely could not have been done without your help.

To Denis Lockler and Gilda Harrison, my fellow supervisors at Touro, for juggling their schedules, often at the last minute, so I could have days off to meet my deadlines. I owe you both, big-time.

To Jackie Hogan, Beverly Maxwell, Bobbie Clark, Pat Whitley, Anthony Whitfield, Sheila Francois, and all the nursing directors for putting up with my mood swings as this project neared completion. Y'all have been wonderful. Thanks so much.

To Irene Shute, ER nurse at Touro Infirmary, who many a night has greeted me with, "You've *got* to see this," as she whips out a cool EKG. I love it when Irene says, "So whaddaya think *this* is?" Thanks, Reenie.

To Anita Go, Malou Ramos, Tom Corvers, and Julie Eichhorn, who have provided me with many great rhythm strips and/or 12-lead EKGs. Thank you.

To my EKG students at Delgado Community College in New Orleans, for helping me learn how to teach and helping me keep a sense of humor. And for asking me questions I *never* would have thought of. Thanks, guys. Oh, by the way, you're having a pop test tomorrow. . . .

To my EKG buddy Nancy Williams, RN, formerly of Touro Infirmary in New Orleans but now somewhere in Oklahoma, for inspiring me to learn more about EKGs. I was always envious of Nancy's skill at reading EKGs. She and I used to have a good-natured competition going when we worked CCU together. Whenever we would disagree on an EKG or rhythm, we would both race to the textbooks to prove the other wrong. On those *extremely rare* occasions when Nancy was right, she would break out into an impromptu tap dance across CCU. I must now tell the truth. I *pretended* to be wrong those times just so she'd do the tap dance. Nancy, thank you for inspiring and challenging me.

To all the other folks at Touro Infirmary for keeping me on my toes by constantly presenting me with proof that there are exceptions to every rule in EKG interpretation. Just when you think you know something, someone shows you something that sends you back to the drawing board. . . .

To Debbie Patterson, Barbara Krawiec, Mark Cohen, and Melissa Kerian at Prentice-Hall, thank you for your faith and guidance, and for taking a chance on an unknown author.

Thank you all.

Love,

Karen

Reviewers

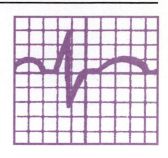

Sue Archer, RNC
Health Occupations Instructor
Mingo Job Corps CCC
Puxico, Missouri

Cheryl Cassis, MSN, RN
Associate Degree Nursing Department Chair
Belmont Technical College
St. Clairsville, Ohio

Maureen Cochran, Ph.D., RN
Suffolk University
Stoneham, Massachusetts

Sherry Haizlip, RNC, MSN
Clinical Manager-Learning Center
Medical Center of Georgia
Macon, Georgia

Melissa Holley Lowe, RN
Columbus State Community College
Columbus, Ohio

Gary Kastello, Ph.D.
Assistant Professor
Department of Health and Human Performance
Winona State University
Winona, Minnesota

Diane M. Klieger, RN, MBA, CMA
Medical Assisting Program Director
Pinellas Technical Education Centers
St. Petersburg, Florida

Carol Lockwood, RN
Putnam North Westchester Boces
Yorktown Heights, New York

James B. Miller, EMT-P
US Army EMT Program Manager
US Army Academy of Health Sciences
Fort Sam Houston, Texas

Leslie Quinn, Ph.D.
Assistant Professor
Department of Biology
Wheeling Jesuit University
Wheeling, West Virginia

Lance Villers, MA, NREMTP
University of Texas Health Science Center at San Antonio
Department of Emergency Medical Technology
San Antonio, Texas

Melissa Yopp, BSN, MSN, JD
School of Nursing
The University of Memphis
Memphis, Tennessee

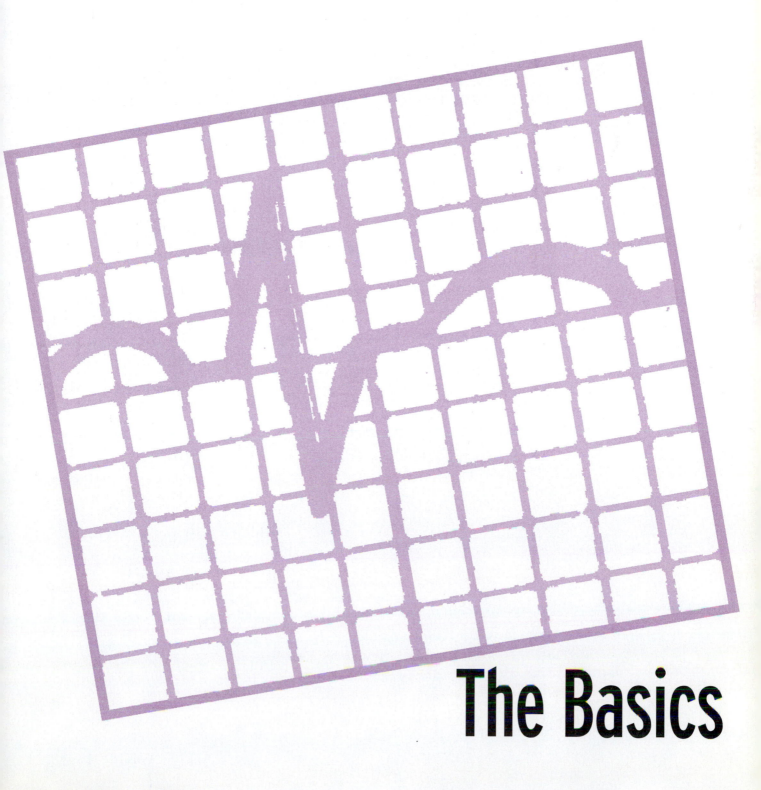

PART ONE

The Basics

Anatomy of the Heart

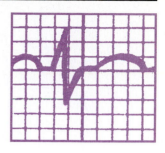

Chapter 1 Objectives

Upon completion of this chapter, the student will be able to:

- State the location of the heart and its normal size.
- Name the walls and layers of the heart.
- Name all the structures of the heart.
- Track the flow of blood through the heart.
- State the oxygen saturation of the heart's chambers.
- Describe the function and location of the heart valves.
- Describe the relationship of the valves to heart sounds.
- List the great vessels and the chamber into which they empty or from which they arise.
- Track the flow of blood through the systemic circulation.
- Name some systemic arteries and veins and the organ they supply/drain.
- Describe the function of coronary arteries.
- Differentiate between the two kinds of cardiac cells.
- Describe the sympathetic and parasympathetic nervous system.
- Describe the *fight-or-flight* and *rest-and-digest* responses.

Chapter 1 Outline

I.   Introduction

II.   Layers of the heart
   A. Pericardium, epicardium, myocardium, endocardium

III.   Heart chambers
   A. Right atrium, right ventricle, left atrium, left ventricle
   B. Septum

IV.   Heart valves
   A. Pulmonic, aortic, tricuspid, mitral
   B. Heart sounds

V.   Great vessels
   A. Superior vena cava, inferior vena cava, pulmonary artery, aorta, pulmonary veins

VI.   Track of blood flow through the heart

VII.   Track of blood flow through the systemic circulation

Chapter 1 Glossary

Apex: The pointy part of the heart where it rests on the diaphragm.

Autonomic nervous system: The nervous system controlling involuntary biological functions.

Base: The top of the heart; the area from which the great vessels emerge.

Capillaries: The smallest blood vessels in the body; nutrient and gas exchange takes place here.

Chordae tendoneae: Tendinous cords that attach to the AV valves to prevent them from everting.

Diastole: The phase of the cardiac cycle in which the heart fills with blood.

Endocardium: The innermost layer of the heart.

Epicardium: Layer of the heart that is the same as the visceral pericardium.

Mediastinum: The cavity between the lungs in which the heart is located.

Myocardium: The muscular layer of the heart.

Parietal: Referring to the wall of a body cavity.

Pericardium: The sac that encloses the heart.

Pulmonary: Pertaining to the lungs.

Semilunar: Half-moon-shaped. Refers to the aortic and pulmonic valves.

Septum: The fibrous tissue that separates the heart into right and left sides.

Syncope: Fainting spell.

Systemic: Pertaining to the whole body system.

Systole: The phase of the cardiac cycle in which the heart contracts and expels its blood.

Thoracic: Referring to the chest cavity.

Visceral: Referring to an organ itself.

Introduction

The function of the heart, a muscular organ about the size of a man's closed fist, is to pump enough blood to meet the body's metabolic needs. To accomplish this, the heart beats 60 to 100 times per minute and circulates 4 to 8 liters of blood per minute. Thus each day the average person's heart beats approximately 90,000 times and pumps out about 6,000 liters of blood. With stress, exertion, or certain pathological conditions, these numbers can quadruple.

The heart is located in the **thoracic (chest) cavity,** between the lungs in a cavity called the **mediastinum,** above the diaphragm, behind the **sternum** (breastbone), and in front of the spine. It is entirely surrounded by bony structures for protection. This bony cage also serves as a means to revive the stricken heart, as the external chest compressions of CPR compress the heart between the sternum and spine and squeeze blood out until the heart's function can be restored.

The top of the heart is the **base,** where the great vessels emerge. The bottom of the heart is the **apex,** the pointy part that rests on the diaphragm. The heart lies at an angle in the chest, with the bottom pointing to the left.

Layers of the Heart

The heart has four layers:

I.   **Pericardium.** This is the double-walled sac that encloses the heart. Think of it as the film on a hard-boiled egg. It serves as support and protection.
   A. **Visceral pericardium.** The visceral pericardium is the thin, serous inner layer of the pericardium that's continuous with the outer layer of the heart itself.
   B. **Parietal pericardium.** This is the tougher outer layer of pericardium that anchors the heart to the diaphragm and great vessels.

II. **Epicardium.** Another name for visceral pericardium.

III. **Myocardium.** The thickest layer, the myocardium is made of pure muscle and does the work of contracting. It is the part that's damaged during a heart attack.

IV. **Endocardium.** The thin innermost layer that lines the heart's chambers and folds back onto itself to form the heart valves, the endocardium is watertight to prevent leakage of blood out into the other layers. The cardiac conduction system is found in this layer.

A small amount of fluid is found between the layers of the pericardium. This **pericardial fluid** minimizes friction of these layers as they rub against each other with every heartbeat. See Figure 1-1.

Heart Chambers

The heart has four chambers:

- **Right atrium.** A receiving chamber for deoxygenated blood (blood that's had some oxygen removed by the body's tissues) returning to the heart from the body, the right atrium has an oxygen (O_2) saturation of only 60 to 75%. The blood in this chamber has so little oxygen, its color is bluish black. Carbon dioxide (CO_2) concentration is high.

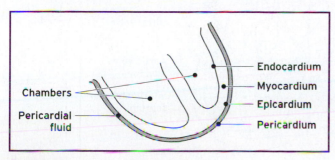

Figure 1-1   Layers of the heart.

- **Right ventricle.** The right ventricle pumps the blood to the lungs for a fresh supply of oxygen. O_2 saturation is 60 to 75%. Again, the blood is bluish black in color. CO_2 concentration is high.

- **Left atrium.** This is a receiving chamber for the blood returning to the heart from the lungs. O_2 saturation is now about 100%. The blood is full of oxygen and is now bright red in color. CO_2 concentration is extremely low, as it was removed by the lungs.

- **Left ventricle.** The left ventricle's job is to pump blood out to the entire body. It is the major pumping chamber of the heart. O_2 saturation is about 100%. Again, the blood is bright red in color. CO_2 concentration is minimal.

The atria's job is to deliver blood to the ventricles that lie directly below them. Since this is a very short trip and minimal contraction is needed to transport this blood to the ventricles, the atria are thin-walled, low-pressure chambers.

The ventricles, on the other hand, are higher-pressure chambers because they must contract more forcefully to deliver their blood into the pulmonary system and the systemic circulation. Since the trip from the right ventricle to the lungs is a short trip and pulmonary pressures are normally low, the right ventricle's pressure is relatively low (though higher than the atrial pressures), and its muscle bulk is relatively thin. The left ventricle generates the highest pressures, as it not only must pump the blood the farthest, it also must pump against great resistance–the blood pressure. For this reason, the left ventricle has three times the muscle bulk of the right ventricle and plays the prominent role in the heart's function.

The heart is divided into right and left sides by the **septum,** a muscular band of tissue. The septum separating the atria is called the **interatrial septum.** The septum separating the ventricles is called the **interventricular septum.** See Figure 1-2.

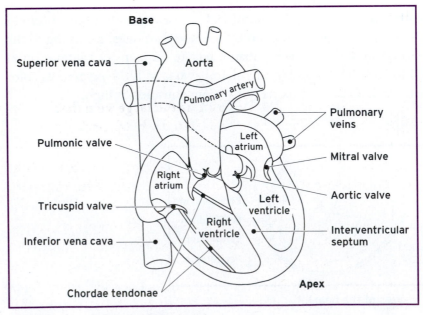

Figure 1-2   Anatomy of the heart.

Heart Valves

The heart has four valves to prevent backflow of blood:

Semilunar valves separate a ventricle from an artery and have three half-moon-shaped cusps. The term *semilunar* means half-moon. There are two semilunar valves:

- **Pulmonic.** This valve is located between the right ventricle and the pulmonary artery.

- **Aortic.** The aortic valve is located between the left ventricle and the aorta.

Atrioventricular (AV) valves are located between an atrium and a ventricle. They are supported by **chordae tendoneae** (tendonous cords), which are attached to papillary muscles and anchor the valve cusps to keep the closed AV valves from flopping backward and allowing backflow of blood. There are two AV valves:

- **Tricuspid.** Located between the right atrium and ventricle, this valve has three cusps.

- **Mitral.** The mitral valve, also called the *bicuspid valve,* is located between the left atrium and ventricle. It has two cusps.

Valves work based purely on changes in pressure. For example, the tricuspid and mitral valves open when the atrium's pressure is higher than the ventricle's. Blood then flows down from atrium to ventricle. The aortic and pulmonic valves open when the pressure in the ventricles exceeds that in the aorta and pulmonary artery. Blood then flows up into those arteries.

Valve closure is responsible for the sounds made by the beating heart. The normal lub-dub of the heart is made not by blood flowing through the heart, but by the closing of the heart's valves. S_1, the first heart sound, reflects closure of the mitral and tricuspid valves. S_2, the second heart sound, reflects closure of the aortic and pulmonic valves. Between S_1 and S_2, the heart beats and expels its blood (called **systole**). Between S_2 and the next S_1, the heart rests and fills with blood (called **diastole**). Each heartbeat has an S_1 and S_2. Note the valves on Figure 1-2.

Great Vessels

Attached to the heart at its base are the five great vessels:

- **Superior vena cava (SVC).** The SVC is the large vein that returns deoxygenated blood to the right atrium from the head, neck, and upper chest and arms.

- **Inferior vena cava (IVC).** The IVC is the large vein that returns deoxygenated blood to the right atrium from the lower chest, abdomen, and legs.

- **Pulmonary artery.** This is the large artery that takes deoxygenated blood from the right ventricle to the lungs to load up on oxygen and unload carbon dioxide. It is the *only* artery that carries deoxygenated blood.

- **Pulmonary veins.** These are large veins that return the oxygenated blood from the lungs to the left atrium. They are the *only* veins that carry oxygenated blood.

- **Aorta.** The largest artery in the body, the aorta takes oxygenated blood from the left ventricle to the systemic circulation to feed all the organs of the body.

Note the great vessels on Figure 1-2.

Blood Flow through the Heart

Now let's track a single blood cell as it travels through the heart:

Superior or inferior vena cava ➜➜ right atrium ➜➜ tricuspid valve ➜➜ right ventricle

⬇⬇

left atrium ⬅⬅ pulmonary veins ⬅⬅ lungs ⬅⬅ pulmonary artery ⬅⬅ pulmonic valve

⬇⬇

mitral valve ➜➜ left ventricle ➜➜ aortic valve ➜➜ aorta ➜➜ body (systemic circulation)

- The cell enters the heart via either the **superior** or **inferior vena cava.**
- It then enters the **right atrium.**
- Next it travels through the **tricuspid valve**
- into the **right ventricle.**
- Then it passes through the **pulmonic valve**
- into the **pulmonary artery,**
- then into the **lungs** for oxygen/carbon dioxide exchange.
- It is then sent through the **pulmonary veins**
- to the **left atrium.**
- Then it travels through the **mitral valve**
- into the **left ventricle.**
- It passes through the **aortic valve**
- into the **aorta**
- and out to the **body (systemic circulation).**

Blood Flow through the Systemic Circulation

Now let's track the blood's course throughout the systemic circulation:

Aorta ➜➜ arteries ➜➜ arterioles ➜➜ capillaries ➜➜ venules ➜➜ veins ➜➜ vena cava

- Oxygenated blood leaves the **aorta**
- and enters **arteries,**
- which narrow into **arterioles**
- and empty into each organ's **capillary bed,** where nutrient and oxygen extraction occurs.
- Then, on the other side of the capillary bed, this now-deoxygenated blood enters narrow **venules,**

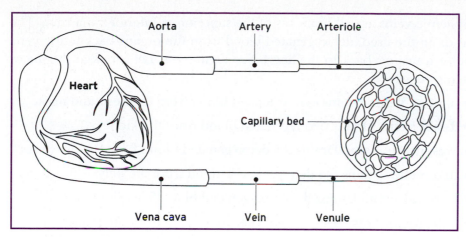

Figure 1-3   Systemic circulation.

- which widen into **veins**
- and then return to the **vena cava** for transport back to the heart. Then the cycle repeats.

See Figure 1-3.

Systemic Vasculature

Systemic arteries are all branches of the aorta, which is *the* major artery in the body. Arteries carry oxygenated blood from the aorta to the various organ systems. See Figure 1-4. Let's look at the major systemic arteries:

- **Carotid artery.** Carries oxygenated blood to the head and neck.
- **Renal artery.** Carries oxygenated blood to the kidneys.
- **Mesenteric artery.** Carries oxygenated blood to the intestines.
- **Iliac artery.** Carries oxygenated blood to the pelvis.
- **Femoral artery.** Carries oxygenated blood to the legs.
- **Subclavian artery.** Carries oxygenated blood to the arms.
- **Brachiocephalic artery.** Branches off into the subclavian and right common carotid arteries.

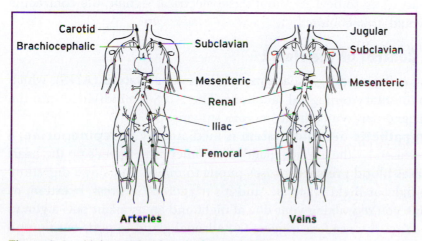

Figure 1-4   Major systemic arteries and veins.

Systemic veins are all branches of the superior or inferior vena cava. The veins drain the used, deoxygenated blood from the organs back to the vena cava for transport back to the heart. See Figure 1-4. Let's look at the major systemic veins:

- **Jugular vein.** Drains deoxygenated blood from the head and neck.
- **Renal vein.** Drains deoxygenated blood from the kidneys.
- **Mesenteric vein.** Drains the deoxygenated blood from the intestines.
- **Iliac vein.** Drains the deoxygenated blood from the pelvis.
- **Femoral vein.** Drains the deoxygenated blood from the legs.
- **Subclavian vein.** Drains deoxygenated blood from the arms.
- **Brachiocephalic vein.** Branches off into the right subclavian and right external jugular veins.

Coronary Arteries

The heart must not only meet the needs of the body, it has its own needs. Since the heart is primarily made of muscle, it requires considerable nourishment, and with the endocardium being watertight, none of the blood in the chambers can get to the myocardium to nourish it. So it has its own circulation—the **coronary arteries**—to do that. Once the myocardium has been fed by the coronary arteries, the deoxygenated blood is returned to the right atrium by the **coronary veins.** Coronary circulation is covered in Chapter 2.

Heart Cells

The heart has two kinds of cells:

- **Contractile cells** cause the heart muscle to contract, resulting in a heartbeat. Proteins called **actin** and **myosin** filaments slide between each other, causing the cell to shorten (contract) or elongate (relax). When the heart cell is relaxed, the actin and myosin are side by side. When it contracts, the actin and myosin *interdigitate,* meaning they slide into each other, making the cell shorter (contracted).
- **Conduction system cells** create and conduct electrical signals to tell the heart when to beat. Without these electrical signals, the contractile cells would *never* contract.

Nervous Control of the Heart

The heart is influenced by the **autonomic nervous system (ANS),** which controls involuntary biological functions. The ANS is subdivided into the sympathetic and parasympathetic nervous systems.

The **sympathetic nervous system** is mediated by **norepinephrine,** a chemical released by the adrenal gland. Norepinephrine speeds up the heart rate, increases blood pressure, causes pupils to dilate, and slows digestion. This is the fight-or-flight response, and it's triggered by stress, exertion, or fear. Imagine you're walking your dog at night and an assailant puts a gun to your head. Your intense fear triggers the adrenal gland to pour out norepinephrine. Your heart rate and blood pressure shoot up. Your pupils dilate to let in more light so you can see the danger and the escape path better. Digestion slows down as the body shunts blood away from nonvital areas. (Is it essential to be digesting your pizza when your life is at stake? The pizza can wait.) So the body puts digestion on hold and shunts blood to vital organs, such as the brain to help you think more clearly and to the muscles to help you fight or flee.

The **parasympathetic nervous system** is mediated by **acetylcholine,** a chemical secreted as a result of stimulation of the **vagus nerve,** a nerve that travels from the brain to the heart and other areas. It slows the heart rate, decreases blood pressure, and enhances digestion. This is the rest-and-digest response. Parasympathetic stimulation can be caused by any action that closes the **glottis,** the flap over the top of the **trachea** (the windpipe). Breath holding and straining to have a bowel movement are two actions that can cause the heart rate to slow down. It is not uncommon for paramedics to be summoned to the scene of a person found unconscious in the bathroom. Straining at stool causes vagal stimulation, which causes the heart rate to slow down. If the heart rate slows enough, **syncope** (fainting) can result. In extreme cases, the heart can stop, requiring CPR and other resuscitative efforts.

Though the heart is influenced by the autonomic nervous system, it can also, in certain extreme circumstances, function for a time without any input from this system. For example, a heart that is removed from a donor in preparation for transplant is no longer in communication with the body, yet it continues to beat on its own for a while. This is possible because of the heart's conduction system cells, which create and conduct impulses to tell the heart to beat.

In a nutshell, the sympathetic nervous system is the accelerator and the parasympathetic nervous system is the brakes.

Practice Quiz

1. The function of the heart is to _____

   _____

2. Name the four layers of the heart. _____

   _____

   _____

   _____

3. Name the four chambers of the heart. _____

   _____

   _____

   _____

4. Name the four heart valves. _____

   _____

5. The purpose of the heart valves is to _____

   _____

6. Name the five great vessels of the heart. _____

_____

_____

_____

7. The job of the coronary arteries is to _____

8. The two kinds of heart cells are _____

_____

9. The division of the autonomic nervous system that's concerned with the fight-or-flight response is _____

_____

10. The division of the autonomic nervous system that functions as the brakes is _____

_____

Practice Quiz Answers

1. The function of the heart is to **pump enough blood to meet the body's metabolic needs.**

2. The four layers of the heart are the **endocardium, myocardium, epicardium,** and **pericardium.**

3. The four chambers of the heart are the **right atrium, left atrium, right ventricle,** and **left ventricle.**

4. The four heart valves are the **tricuspid, mitral, pulmonic,** and **aortic valves.**

5. The purpose of the heart valves is to **prevent backflow of blood.**

6. The five great vessels are the **aorta, pulmonary artery, pulmonary veins, superior vena cava,** and **inferior vena cava.**

7. The job of the coronary arteries is to **provide nourishment to the heart muscle.**

8. The two kinds of heart cells are the **contractile cells** and the **conduction system cells.**

9. The division of the autonomic nervous system concerned with the fight-or-flight response is the **sympathetic nervous system.**

10. The division of the autonomic nervous system that functions as the brakes is the **parasympathetic nervous system.**

Coronary Circulation

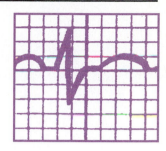

Chapter 2 Objectives

Upon completion of this chapter, the student will be able to:

- Describe the structure from which the coronary arteries arise.
- Name the three main coronary arteries and the areas of the heart they supply.
- Describe what right-dominant and left-dominant mean.
- Explain the impact of having a coronary artery configuration that is different from the norm.
- Name the three layers of the myocardium.
- Describe when and how the myocardium is fed by the coronary arteries.
- Name the main coronary veins and the areas of the heart they drain.

Chapter 2 Outline

I. Introduction
   A. Purpose, location of origin
II. Three main coronary arteries
   A. Left anterior descending coronary artery, right coronary artery, circumflex coronary artery
III. Three areas of the myocardium
   A. Subepicardium, myocardium, subendocardium
IV. Coronary veins
   A. Great cardiac vein, middle cardiac vein, coronary sinus
V. Practice quiz
VI. Practice quiz answers

Chapter 2 Glossary

Anterior: The front side.

Lateral: On the side.

Posterior: The back side.

Subendocardium: The myocardial layer just beneath the endocardium.

Subepicardium: The myocardial layer just beneath the epicardium.

Introduction

Coronary arteries provide blood supply to the myocardium and the conduction system. They arise from the base of the aorta at a place called the **aortic sinuses of Valsalva.** They course along the epicardial surface of the heart, then dive into the myocardium to provide its blood supply.

Coronary Arteries

There are three main coronary arteries (see Figure 2-1):

- **Left anterior descending (LAD).** The LAD is a branch off the **left main coronary artery.** The LAD supplies blood to the anterior wall of the left ventricle.

- **Circumflex.** The circumflex, also a branch of the left main coronary artery, feeds the lateral wall of the left ventricle. Since the LAD and the circumflex coronary arteries are branches off the left main coronary artery, blockage of the left main itself would knock out flow to both these branches. That produces a huge heart attack sometimes referred to as the *widow-maker.*

- **Right coronary artery (RCA).** The RCA feeds the right ventricle and the inferior wall of the left ventricle. In about 70% of people, the RCA gives rise to a branch, the **posterior descending artery (PDA),** that feeds the posterior wall of the heart. These people are called *right-dominant.* However, in some people the PDA arises from the circumflex artery, which is part of the left coronary artery system. These people are called *left-dominant.*

Table 2-1 shows the areas supplied by the three main coronary arteries.

Some people have coronary artery configurations different from the norm. For example, some people are born with a very short LAD, but have a very long PDA that reaches up from the back of the heart to the front to feed the areas that the short LAD can't reach. As long as the myocardium gets its blood supply, the abnormal coronary artery configuration is not a problem.

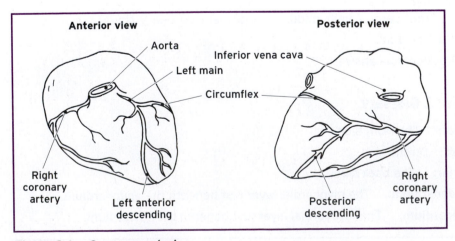

Figure 2-1   Coronary arteries.

Table 2-1 Areas Supplied by the Coronary Arteries

CORONARY ARTERY	AREAS SUPPLIED
Right coronary artery (RCA)	• Sinus node in 55% of people • AV node in 90% of people • Bundle of His • Posterior fascicle (branch) of the left bundle branch • Posterior third of the septum • Right atrial and ventricular walls • Inferior wall of the left ventricle
Left anterior descending (LAD)	• Anterior two-thirds of the septum • Right bundle branch • Anterior fascicle of the left bundle branch • Anterior wall of the left ventricle • Lower segment of the AV junction
Circumflex	• Sinus node in 45% of people • Posterior fascicle of the left bundle branch • Lateral wall of the left ventricle

Myocardium

The heart muscle (**myocardium**) is divided into three areas:

- **Subepicardium.** The subepicardium is the myocardial layer closest to the epicardium. It's the outermost layer of the myocardium.

- **Myocardium.** This is the middle layer.

- **Subendocardium.** The subendocardium is the innermost layer of the myocardium, just beneath the endocardium. It's the most vulnerable layer of the myocardium because it's the deepest layer and therefore farthest away from a blood supply.

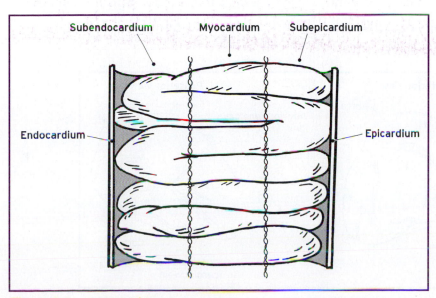

Figure 2-2 Layers of the myocardium.

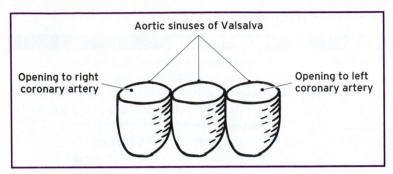

Figure 2-3   Aortic valve and openings to coronary arteries.

The first area to be fed by the coronary arteries is the subepicardium. The last to be fed is the subendocardium. In Figure 2-2, the myocardium is viewed longitudinally.

During systole, the heart sends blood out to the body, but not to its own coronary circulation. Only in diastole is the heart able to feed itself. Why is that? During systole, blood pours out of the left ventricle through the aorta. Some of this blood collects in the aortic sinuses of Valsalva, the three cusps that make up the aortic valve. Located in the right and left sinuses are the openings to the right and left coronary arteries. Blood cannot enter the coronary arteries during systole because the heart muscle is contracting and essentially squeezing the coronary arteries shut. During diastole, the heart muscle stops contracting and the blood that's collected in the aortic sinuses drains into the coronary arteries and feeds the myocardium. See the aortic valve in Figure 2-3.

Coronary Veins

The job of the coronary veins is to return the deoxygenated blood from the myocardium to the right atrium, just as all deoxygenated blood returns to the right atrium. There are three major coronary veins (see Figure 2-4):

- **Great cardiac vein.** This vein drains the anterior aspect of the heart.
- **Middle cardiac vein.** This vein drains the posterior heart.

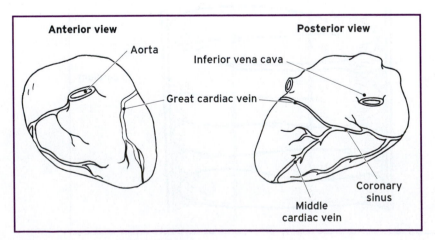

Figure 2-4   Coronary veins.

- **Coronary sinus.** This is a large vein that collects the blood from the great cardiac vein and the middle cardiac vein and returns this blood to the right atrium.

Practice Quiz

1. Name the three main coronary arteries. _____

   _____

   _____

2. Name the three areas of the myocardium. _____

   _____

   _____

3. The heart feeds its own muscle during which phase of the cardiac cycle?

   _____

4. In 90% of people, the AV node is fed by which coronary artery?

   _____

5. Name the three major cardiac veins. _____

   _____

   _____

Practice Quiz Answers

1. The three main coronary arteries are the **LAD,** the **RCA,** and the **circumflex.**
2. The three areas of the myocardium are the **subendocardium,** the **myocardium,** and the **subepicardium.**
3. The heart feeds its own muscle during **diastole.**
4. In 90% of people, the AV node is fed by the **RCA.**
5. The three major cardiac veins are the **great cardiac vein,** the **middle cardiac vein,** and the **coronary sinus.**

Coronary Artery Disease

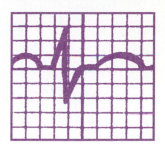

Chapter 3 Objectives

Upon completion of this chapter, the student will be able to:

- Explain the difference between angina and an MI.
- Explain the physiologic events that cause chest pain to develop.
- List the symptoms of a heart attack.
- Explain how denial can prevent the person from seeking treatment in a timely manner.
- Name three treatments for coronary artery disease.
- Explain CABG.
- Explain balloon angioplasty.
- Explain how thrombolytics are helpful during an MI.
- Describe nitroglycerin's effect on the coronary arteries.

Chapter 3 Outline

I.   Introduction
II.   Angina
III.   Myocardial infarction
IV.   Symptoms of a heart attack
        A. Pain, shortness of breath, pallor, sweating, feeling of impending doom, nausea and vomiting
V.   Treatment of coronary artery disease
        A. Medications, coronary artery bypass graft, balloon angioplasty, thrombolytics
VI.   Practice quiz
VII.   Practice quiz answers

Chapter 3 Glossary

Anaerobic: Without oxygen.

Angina: Chest pain caused by a decrease in myocardial blood flow.

Angioplasty: An invasive procedure in which a small balloon is used to open narrowed arteries.

Atheroma: Fatty plaque that builds up on the walls of arteries, narrowing their lumen (internal diameter).

Denial: The tendency of patients to think that what they are experiencing is something much less serious than it really is.

Myocardial infarction: Heart attack.

Neuropathy: Condition that causes a decrease in sensation, especially pain, in susceptible individuals.

Plaque: Fatty deposits on the walls of arteries; also called *atheroma.*

Silent MI: A heart attack not accompanied by the usual symptoms.

Stent: A mesh device introduced into coronary arteries to prevent their reocclusion after balloon angioplasty.

Thrombolytic: Clot-dissolving.

Introduction

Coronary artery disease is a condition in which the coronary arteries are narrowed by a lifelong buildup of fatty deposits called **atheroma** or **plaque** on their inner walls. Over time, this plaque absorbs calcium from the bloodstream and hardens–hence the expression, "hardening of the arteries." Coronary artery disease can lead to angina or a heart attack.

Angina

Angina is a reversible condition brought about by a mismatch between myocardial blood supply and demand. Due to narrowing of the coronary arteries, there is inadequate blood flow to the myocardium just at a time when the myocardium is demanding more because of stress or exertion. At rest, the amount of blood that can get through this narrowed area is enough to perfuse (nourish) the heart. But with stress or exertion, the heart works harder and requires more blood flow and more oxygen. The narrowed coronary arteries simply cannot deliver enough blood to meet the demand. If the heart does not get enough oxygen, it tries to do without–it goes **anaerobic.** As a by-product of anaerobic metabolism, **lactic acid** builds up in the myocardium. This causes angina pain. After the stress or exertion that was causing the problem stops, the heart's demand for blood and oxygen decreases, and the amount of blood that can get through is again enough. The lactic acid is washed away, causing the pain to go away. No myocardial damage occurs.

In Figure 3-1, the heart is under stress or exertion. Inadequate coronary blood flow occurs, and angina pain results. In Figure 3-2, the heart is at rest. There is adequate blood flow. The pain eases.

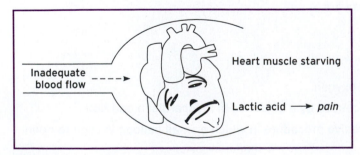

Figure 3-1 Inadequate blood flow.

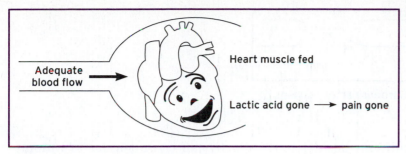

Figure 3-2   Adequate blood flow.

Myocardial Infarction

Myocardial Infarction (MI) is a heart attack. This is caused by a complete interruption of blood flow to a section of heart muscle. In 90% of heart attacks, a blood clot is completely obstructing (blocking) the flow of blood through a coronary artery. The heart muscle in that area then dies. Heart attacks are not reversible. Once heart tissue dies, it does not regenerate—it simply forms scar tissue. See Figure 3-3.

Angina or an MI can also be caused by coronary artery spasm. See Figure 3-4.

Symptoms of a Heart Attack

- **Pain** in any of these areas—the chest, neck, arm, jaw, upper back—usually described as a "squeezing sensation," "an elephant on the chest," "heaviness," "tightness," or "pressure." Some heart attack victims never have pain at all. This is especially true with diabetics, who may have **neuropathy,** decreased pain nerve transmission.

- **Shortness of breath**

- **Pallor**

- **Sweating**

- **Feeling of impending doom**

- **Nausea/vomiting**

Any or all of these symptoms may be seen during a heart attack. Some people, unfortunately, have no symptoms that alert them to a heart problem, and their MI is diagnosed later during a routine physical exam. This is a **silent MI.** The lack of symptoms prevents timely intervention to minimize heart damage.

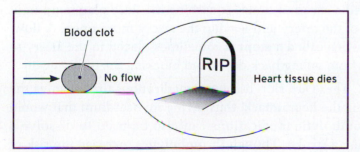

Figure 3-3   Myocardial infarction.

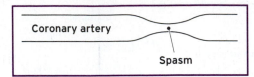

Figure 3-4   Coronary artery spasm.

Many conditions besides heart attacks can cause similar symptoms—ulcers, blood clots in the lung, inflammation of the pericardial sac or the lining of the lung. It is often difficult to know what the problem is without having a battery of tests done at the hospital. The EKG is instrumental in helping diagnose heart attacks. Dead heart muscle does not conduct electrical impulses, so the EKG, which is a printout of the heart's electrical impulses, will look different during and after a heart attack. Angina may cause a temporary change in the EKG, but this usually returns to normal when the circulation is restored. A major concern with heart attacks is **denial,** the tendency of heart attack victims to think that what they're feeling is indigestion, gas, a pulled muscle—anything but a heart attack. This denial prevents them from seeking medical help in a timely fashion and can result in greater heart damage than if they'd come to the hospital sooner.

Treatment of Coronary Artery Disease

- **Medications. Nitroglycerin** is a standard medication given to cardiac patients. It causes the coronary arteries to dilate (open wider), thus improving coronary blood flow and washing out the lactic acid that's causing chest pain. **Heparin** is an anticoagulant (blood thinner) that prevents the formation of blood clots that could cause or extend a heart attack. Other medications are aimed at decreasing the heart's workload or improving its pumping ability.

- **Coronary artery bypass graft.** This is traditional bypass surgery. Contrary to popular belief, it is not open-heart surgery. The coronary arteries lie on the epicardium in plain view of the surgeon. The heart does not have to be opened in order to accomplish bypass. A piece of vein from the leg or an artery to the breast is attached to the aorta and connected to the coronary artery just past the blocked area. This provides a detour for the blood to get around the blockage and feed the myocardium.

- **Balloon angioplasty.** In this procedure, a small tube with a balloon at its tip is introduced into the narrowed section of coronary artery. The balloon is inflated a series of times, squashing the fatty plaque up tight against the wall of the artery and leaving the artery more open. A flow-through mesh device called a **stent** is sometimes placed in the artery to keep the plaque from falling back down and blocking the artery again.

- **Thrombolytics.** These are clot-dissolving medications that dissolve the blood clot causing the heart attack, thus saving myocardium that would have died. Thrombolytic medications can also be used to dissolve a blood clot causing a stroke. Though thrombolytics increase the risk of bleeding, they have been remarkably successful at saving lives of heart attack and stroke victims.

Practice Quiz

1. A reversible condition brought about by a mismatch between supply and demand to the myocardium and caused by narrowed coronary arteries is

   _____

2. Death of heart muscle tissue caused by a complete interruption of blood flow to a particular area is called _____

3. Name five symptoms of a myocardial infarction. _____

   _____

   _____

   _____

   _____

4. What effect does nitroglycerin have on the coronary arteries?

   _____

5. What do thrombolytics do? _____

   _____

Practice Quiz Answers

1. A reversible condition brought about by a mismatch between supply and demand to the myocardium and caused by narrowed coronary arteries is **angina.**

2. Death of heart muscle tissue caused by a complete interruption of blood flow to a particular area is called a **myocardial infarction.**

3. Symptoms of a myocardial infarction are **chest pain, shortness of breath, pallor, sweating, feeling of impending doom,** and **nausea/ vomiting** (pick any five).

4. **Nitroglycerin causes the coronary arteries to dilate.**

5. **Thrombolytics dissolve blood clots.**

Cardiac Physiology

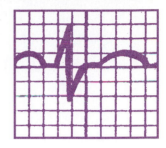

Chapter 4 Objectives

Upon completion of this chapter, the student will be able to:

- State what occurs in each phase of the cardiac cycle.
- Relate the effects of diastole and systole to the EKG.
- Define *blood pressure.*
- State what is normal blood pressure and what constitutes hypertension and hypotension.
- Define *pulse pressure.*
- Define *MAP* and state its significance.
- Define *cardiac output.*
- Write the equation for cardiac output.
- Describe how a rapid heart rate affects cardiac output.
- Describe why well-conditioned athletes have heart rates slower than normal.
- Define *peripheral vascular resistance.*
- Define *preload.*
- Define *contractility* and explain its effects on preload.
- Define *afterload* and explain its effects on cardiac output.
- Describe the role of chemoreceptors and baroreceptors.
- Define *compliance.*

Chapter 4 Outline

I.   Introduction
II. Diastole
     A. Rapid filling phase, diastasis, atrial kick
III. Effects of diastole on the EKG
IV. Systole
     A. Isovolumetric contraction, ventricular ejection, protodiastole, isovolumetric relaxation
V.   Effects of systole on the EKG
VI. Pressures
VII. Control mechanisms
     A. Blood pressure
     B. Cardiac output

Chapter 4 Glossary

Afterload: The pressure against which the heart must pump in order to expel its blood.

Baroreceptors: Receptors inside arterial walls that sense changes in blood pressure.

Blood pressure: The pressure exerted on the arterial walls by the circulating blood.

Cardiac output: The amount of blood expelled by the heart each minute.

Chemoreceptors: Receptors in arterial walls that sense changes in pH and oxygenation status.

Compliance: The ability of a heart chamber, in particular the left ventricle, to expand to accommodate the influx of blood.

Contractility: The ability of a cardiac cell to contract and do work.

Depolarization: The wave of electrical current that changes the resting negatively charged cardiac cell to a positively charged one.

Diastolic pressure: The pressure in the arteries during diastole.

Ejection: Pushing out of blood.

Heart rate: The number of times the heart beats in one minute.

Homeostasis: Balance. Refers to the body's ability to compensate for change.

Hypertension: Elevated blood pressure.

Hypotension: Low blood pressure.

Ischemic: Oxygen deprivation.

Isovolumetric: Keeping the same volume.

Mean arterial pressure: The average pressure in the aorta during the cardiac cycle.

Perfusion pressure: The pressure required to perfuse an organ or tissue with required nutrients.

Peripheral vascular resistance: A measure of the friction the circulating blood encounters after it leaves the heart and flows through the arteries.

Preload: The pressure in the left ventricle at the end of diastole, when its volume is greatest.

Pulse pressure: The mathematical difference between the systolic and diastolic pressures.

Starling's law: The law that states that, up to a point, increased preload will increase the force of contractility.

Stroke volume: The volume of blood expelled by the heart with each beat.

Systolic pressure: The pressure in the arteries during systole.

Introduction

The **cardiac cycle** refers to the mechanical events that occur to pump blood. There are two phases to the cardiac cycle–**systole** and **diastole.** During systole the ventricles contract and expel their blood. During diastole the ventricles relax and fill. Each of these phases has several phases of its own. See Figures 4-1 and 4-2.

Diastole

- **Rapid-filling phase.** This is the first phase of diastole. The atria, having received blood from the superior and inferior venae cavae as well as the coronary sinus, are full of blood and therefore have high pressure. The ventricles, having just expelled their blood into the pulmonary artery and the aorta, are essentially empty and have lower pressure. This difference in pressure causes the AV valves to pop open and the atrial blood to flow down to the ventricles. (Fluid moves from high pressure to low pressure.) Imagine the atria as a sponge. When the sponge is saturated with water, the water pours out in a steady stream at first.

- **Diastasis.** In the second phase of diastole, the pressure in the atria and ventricles starts to equalize as the ventricles fill and the atria empty, so blood flow slows. As the sponge becomes emptier, the flow slows to a trickle.

- **Atrial kick.** This is the last phase of diastole. The atria are essentially empty, but there is still a little blood to deliver to the ventricle. Since the sponge is almost empty of water, what must be done to get the last little bit of water out of it? Right, the sponge must be squeezed. The atria therefore contract, squeezing in on themselves and propelling the remainder of blood into the ventricles. The pressure in the ventricles at the end of this phase is high, as the ventricles are now full. Atrial pressure is low, as the atria are essentially empty. The AV valve leaflets, which have been hanging down in the ventricle in their open position, are pushed upward by the higher ventricular volume and its sharply rising pressure until they slam shut, ending diastole. S_1 is heard at this time. Atrial kick provides 15 to 30% of ventricular filling and is a very important phase.

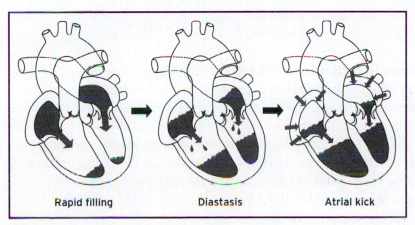

Rapid filling   Diastasis   Atrial kick

Figure 4-1   Phases of diastole.

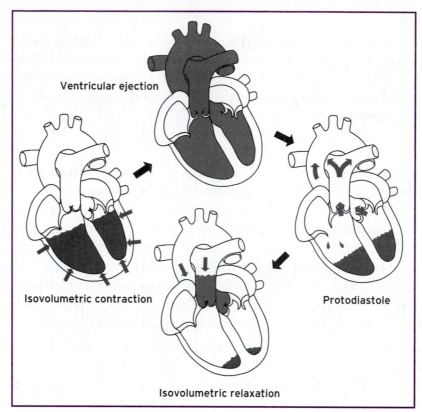

Figure 4-2 Phases of systole.

Some heart rhythm abnormalities cause a loss of the atrial kick by causing the atria to wiggle instead of contract. This causes an automatic decrease in cardiac output.

Effects of Diastole on the EKG

The first two phases of diastole are not manifested on the EKG. The final phase, atrial kick, is. Atrial contraction occurs as a result of **atrial depolarization** (the delivery of an electrical stimulus to the atria). In order for atrial kick to occur, the atria must first have been depolarized. No tissue in the heart will contract until it has been depolarized. On the EKG, this atrial depolarization is seen as a **P wave.** Chapter 5 will cover this electrophysiology in depth. The EKG reflects only the heart's electrical activity, not its mechanical functioning.

Systole

- **Isovolumetric contraction.** This is the first phase of systole. The ventricles are full, but the pressure in them is not high enough to exceed the blood pressure and pop the semilunar valves open. Since the ventricles cannot increase their pressure by adding more volume (they're as full as they're going to get), they squeeze down on themselves, forcing their muscular walls inward, thereby putting pressure on the blood inside and causing the ventricular pressure to rise sharply. No blood flow occurs during this phase because all the valves are closed. This phase results in the greatest consumption of myocardial oxygen.

- **Ventricular ejection.** The second phase of systole. With the ventricular pressures now high enough, the semilunar valves pop open and blood pours out of the ventricles into the pulmonary artery and the aorta. Half the blood empties quickly and the rest a little slower.

- **Protodiastole.** The third phase of systole. Ventricular contraction continues, but blood flow slows as the ventricular pressure drops (since the ventricle is becoming empty) and the aortic and pulmonary arterial pressures rise (because they are filling with blood from the ventricles). Pressures are equalizing between the ventricles and the aorta and pulmonary artery.

- **Isovolumetric relaxation.** The final phase of systole. Ventricular pressure is low because the blood has essentially been pumped out. The ventricles relax, causing the pressure to drop further. The aorta and pulmonary artery have higher pressures now, as they are full of blood. Since there is no longer any forward pressure from the ventricles to propel this blood further into the aorta and pulmonary artery, some of the blood in these arteries starts to flow back toward the aortic and pulmonic valves. This back pressure causes the valve leaflets, which had been pushed up into the aorta and pulmonary arteries in their open position, to slam shut, ending systole. S_2 is heard now.

Effects of Systole on the EKG

Once the atria have delivered their blood to the ventricles, the ventricles are depolarized and a **QRS complex** is written on the EKG. Ventricular contraction then follows. Remember, depolarization is necessary before any heart tissue can contract.

Pressures

- **Blood pressure (BP).** The pressure exerted on the walls of the arteries by the circulating blood, blood pressure is recorded as the **systolic pressure** (the pressure in the arteries during ventricular contraction) over the **diastolic pressure** (the pressure in the arteries during ventricular relaxation). Normal blood pressure is in the range of 90/50 to 140/90. **Hypertension,** high blood pressure, is a blood pressure greater than 140/90. **Hypotension,** low blood pressure, is a blood pressure less than 90/50. Blood pressure is measured in millimeters of mercury (mmHg). Blood pressure measurements are usually done at the **brachial artery** in the bend of the elbow.

- **Pulse pressure (PP).** This is the mathematical difference between the systolic and diastolic pressures: PP = SBP − DBP. For a blood pressure of 90/50, for example, the pulse pressure would be 90 − 50 = 40. Pulse pressure will narrow or widen with certain pathological conditions, so it is important to know the baseline reading.

- **Mean arterial pressure (MAP).** This is the average pressure in the aorta during the cardiac cycle. MAP is the mathematical sum of the diastolic blood pressure plus ⅓ of the pulse pressure: MAP = DBP + ⅓PP. For a blood pressure of 90/50, for example, the calculation would be as follows:

$$\text{MAP} = 50 + \tfrac{1}{3}(90 - 50)$$
$$= 50 + \tfrac{1}{3}(40)$$
$$= 50 + 13.3$$
$$= 63.3 \text{ (round off to 63)}$$

MAP is significant because it is an indicator of **perfusion pressure** (the arterial pressure required by an organ's capillary bed in order to saturate its tissues with the required amount of blood and oxygen). If the MAP is too low, the perfusion pressure will not be adequate and the organ can become **ischemic** (oxygen-deprived). For example, the heart requires an MAP of about 60 mmHg to enable adequate perfusion of myocardial cells. If a person has a blood pressure of 70/40, that would provide an MAP of 50, which would be too low for adequate coronary perfusion. Angina or an MI could result.

- **Cardiac pressures.** These are the pressures inside the heart's chambers. You'll recall that the right side of the heart is a low-pressure side and the left is a high-pressure side. **Mean pressures** are those measured with the AV valves open, so the pressures equalize between atria and ventricles. See Figure 4-3.

Control Mechanisms

The goal of the body is **homeostasis,** or balance. When one function or action of the body changes, there must be an equal but opposite reaction in order to maintain balance. Like a seesaw, when one end goes up, the other end goes down. That keeps the seesaw board straight and level. Let's look at the control mechanisms that regulate the following.

Blood Pressure

Blood pressure is controlled by many factors, some of which are listed here:

- **Blood volume.** The more blood in the arteries, the greater the pressure on the walls of those arteries. Bottom line: Increased blood volume causes increased BP, and decreased blood volume causes decreased BP.

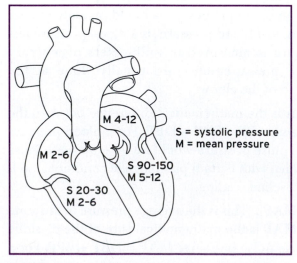

Figure 4-3 Cardiac pressures, measured in mmHg.

- **Cardiac output.** Low cardiac output provides less blood to the arteries; therefore arterial pressure is lower. Bottom line: Low cardiac output results in low BP, and high cardiac output results in a higher BP.

- **Kidney function.** The kidneys are responsible for excreting excess fluid from the body. The greater the circulating blood volume, the greater the BP, and the greater the amount of urine excreted by the kidneys in an attempt to lower this BP. Decreased blood volume causes decreased urine excretion, as the kidneys reabsorb the fluid to try to elevate the low BP. Bottom line: Poorly functioning kidneys are unable to excrete enough fluid and thus tend to cause a higher BP. Properly functioning kidneys promote a more normal BP.

- **Arterial elasticity.** Arterial walls are elastic in order to accommodate the changing blood volume circulating within. If this blood volume falls, the arterial walls sense the decrease in pressure inside and constrict down against the blood inside, causing the arterial pressure to rise. If the blood volume rises, the arteries dilate to accommodate this extra volume, and the pressure drops. Bottom line: Arterial constriction leads to higher BP, and arterial dilatation leads to lower BP. Pathological conditions such as arteriosclerosis, or hardening of the arteries, cause the arteries to lose their ability to stretch. This results in elevated BP.

- **Heart rate.** Extremely fast or slow heart rates can result in decreased cardiac output, which can lower the BP.

- **Body surface area.** The heavier a person is, the more small blood vessels are required to perfuse those extra tissues with blood and oxygen and the higher the resistance to the flow of blood by these small vessels. Bottom line: The heavier a person is, the greater the likelihood of high BP. Weight loss can lower the BP.

Cardiac Output

Cardiac output is the amount of blood pumped out by the heart every minute. It is controlled by two factors:

- **Heart rate.** Heart rate is the number of times the heart beats every minute. A heart rate that is too fast or too slow can cause decreased cardiac output.

- **Stroke volume.** Stroke volume is the amount of blood pumped out by the heart with each beat. Decreased stroke volume will decrease the cardiac output if the heart rate does not change to compensate.

Cardiac output is calculated by multiplying the heart rate by the stroke volume. The equation is $CO = HR \times SV$. If the heart rate is 100 beats per minute and the stroke volume is 30 cc (about an ounce), the cardiac output would be $100 \times 30 = 3,000$ cc, or about 3 liters per minute. In other words, if your heart beats 100 times every minute and pumps out 30 cc with each beat, it would pump out 3,000 cc per minute. That's the cardiac output.

A change in either the heart rate or the stroke volume will necessitate a change in the other to maintain the same cardiac output. For example, if the heart rate falls in half, the stroke volume must double in order to maintain the same cardiac output. Likewise, if the stroke volume changes, the heart rate must also change to compensate. Let's look at some examples of this:

- Well-conditioned athletes typically have heart rates slower than normal. This is because the exercise has increased their heart size and therefore the stroke volume is increased. Since the heart pumps out more than the normal amount with each beat, it doesn't need to beat as often.

- On the other hand, a person who has just suffered a heart attack has a lower stroke volume since some of the myocardium has been damaged, so the heart rate must speed up to maintain the same cardiac output as before the heart attack.

- A person who develops a very rapid heart rate will have a decrease in stroke volume, causing the cardiac output to drop. The fast heart rate results in decreased time for the ventricles to fill up with blood, so the stroke volume drops and the cardiac output drops. Up to a certain point, an increased heart rate can increase the cardiac output. After that point is exceeded, however, the cardiac output falls.

Peripheral Vascular Resistance (PVR)

PVR is the measure of the friction the circulating blood encounters after it leaves the heart and flows through the arteries. The greater the friction, the greater the PVR. The less the friction, the lower the PVR. PVR is also called **systemic vascular resistance (SVR).**

Preload

This is the pressure in the left ventricle at the end of diastole, when the ventricular volume is highest. Factors affecting preload are the following:

- **Blood volume.** The greater the circulating blood volume, the greater the amount of blood filling the left ventricle and the higher the preload. The lower the blood volume, the less blood there is in the left ventricle at the end of diastole and the lower the preload.

- **Contractility.** With normal contractility, there is always some blood remaining in the left ventricle at the end of systole. (The heart never pumps out *all* of its blood.) If the force of contraction increases, the preload will decrease. This is because the left ventricle will have pumped out more blood than it usually does in systole, so there is less than the normal amount of blood left in the ventricle after systole. As a result, there is less than the normal amount of blood in the left ventricle after the next diastole, when it's the fullest. Likewise, the weaker the contraction, the more blood there is left in the ventricle at the end of systole (because the weakened ventricle can't pump as much out); then during diastole more blood is dumped on top of that, causing an increase in preload. Bottom line: An increase in contractility causes a decrease in preload. A decrease in contractility causes an increase in preload.

Afterload

This is the resistance the heart has to overcome in order to expel its blood through the semilunar valves. It is reflected clinically by SVR (PVR). Increased afterload increases cardiac workload and can decrease cardiac output. A decrease in afterload can increase cardiac output. Bottom line: If the heart has to overcome great resistance in order to expel its blood, it is likely that less blood will be expelled, thus decreasing cardiac output. If the resistance is low, the amount pumped out will be greater, thus raising cardiac output.

Baroreceptors

Baroreceptors are specialized tissues in the arterial walls that sense changes in blood pressure. In response, they signal the autonomic nervous system to constrict or dilate the arteries to increase or decrease the blood pressure. For example, say you lost a lot of blood in an accident. Your blood pressure would drop because there is less blood inside your arteries. The baroreceptors would sense this drop in BP and would stimulate the sympathetic nervous system to pour out norepinephrine to constrict your arteries, thereby increasing your BP.

Chemoreceptors

Chemoreceptors sense changes in oxygen level, carbon dioxide level, and pH of the blood. They then cause changes in heart rate and respiratory depth and rate in order to return the abnormal levels of these chemicals to their normal values. Say you were very short of breath because of a blood clot in your lung. Your blood oxygen level has fallen below normal levels. The chemoreceptors would sense this decrease in oxygen level and would cause your heart rate to speed up in order to pump the oxygen around faster. Also your respirations would become deeper and faster in order to take in more oxygen.

Compliance

This is the ability of the ventricle to stretch to accommodate the influx of blood from the atrium. A compliant ventricle stretches easily. A noncompliant ventricle is stiff and resists filling. Noncompliance increases cardiac workload and can thus decrease cardiac output by decreasing preload and stroke volume. One cause of noncompliance is poor myocardial blood flow, which decreases oxygen delivery to the ventricle and decreases the ventricle's ability to stretch.

Contractility

Contractility refers to the heart's ability to squeeze its blood out. **Starling's law** states that, up to a point, increased preload will result in increased force of contraction. Increased preload causes increased stretch of myocardial fibers, which in turn causes those fibers to snap back and contract more forcefully. However, if the fibers are overstretched, they can no longer snap back. Instead, they become floppy and incapable of effective contraction. Cardiac output can then drop. Imagine the elastic on a new pair of underwear. Its elastic is so strong, you can stretch it and it will snap back and slingshot across the room. But gain a few (hundred) pounds and this now-overstretched elastic is so floppy that it doesn't snap back anymore. It lies in a heap on the floor. Bottom line: Up to a certain point, increased preload causes increased contractility. After the point of no return, however, increased preload will only overburden the heart and cause decreased contractility.

Practice Quiz

1. List the three phases of diastole. _____
   _____
   _____

2. List the four phases of systole. _____
   _____
   _____
   _____

3. What is blood pressure? _____

4. Write the equation for pulse pressure. _____

5. Write the equation for mean arterial pressure (MAP). _____

6. Write the equation for cardiac output. _____

7. Starling's law states that _____
   _____

8. Define preload. _____

9. Define afterload. _____
   _____

10. Baroreceptors sense changes in _____

Practice Quiz Answers

1. The three phases of diastole are **rapid filling, diastasis,** and **atrial kick.**

2. The four phases of systole are **isovolumetric contraction, ventricular ejection, protodiastole,** and **isovolumetric relaxation.**

3. **Blood pressure is the measurement of the pressure exerted on the walls of the arteries by the circulating blood.**

4. **PP = SBP − DBP.**

5. **MAP = DBP + ⅓PP.**

6. **CO = HR × SV.**

7. Starling's law states that, **up to a certain point, an increase in preload will cause an increase in the force of contractility, but overstretch of the cardiac fibers will result in decreased contractility.**

8. **Preload is the amount of blood in the left ventricle at the end of diastole.**

9. **Afterload is the pressure the heart has to expel its blood against.**

10. Baroreceptors sense changes in **pressure.**

Electrophysiology

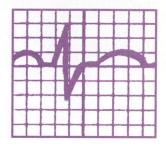

Chapter 5 Objectives

Upon completion of this chapter, the student will be able to:

- Define the terms *polarized, depolarization,* and *repolarization* and relate them to contraction and relaxation.
- Describe and label the phases of the action potential.
- Define *transmembrane potential.*
- Draw and explain the P wave, QRS complex, T wave, and U wave.
- Explain where the PR and ST segments are.
- Define the *absolute* and *relative refractory periods* and the implications of each.
- Be able to label, on a rhythm strip, all the waves and complexes.
- Explain the difference between a three-channel recorder and a single-channel recorder.
- Explain the delineations of EKG paper. How many seconds is a small block and big block? How many small blocks in one minute? How many big blocks in a minute?
- On a rhythm strip, determine if the PR, QRS, and QT intervals are normal or abnormal.
- Name the waves in a variety of QRS complexes.

Chapter 5 Outline

Chapter 5 Glossary

Amplitude: The height of the waves and complexes on the EKG.

Baseline: The line from which the EKG waves and complexes take off. Also called the *isoelectric line.*

Depolarization: The wave of electrical current that changes the resting negatively charged cardiac cell into a positively charged one. Depolarization should result in cardiac muscle contraction.

Intervals: Measurements of time between EKG waves and complexes.

Isoelectric line: Literally means "line with same electricity." It is also called the *baseline.*

Plateau: A leveling off.

Polarized: Possessing an electrical charge.

P wave: The EKG wave reflecting atrial depolarization.

QRS complex: The EKG complex representing ventricular depolarization.

Refractory: Resistant to.

Repolarization: The wave of electrical current that returns the cardiac cell to its resting electrically negative state. Repolarization should result in cardiac muscle relaxation.

T_a wave: The usually unseen wave that reflects atrial repolarization.

Transmembrane potential: The electrical charge at the cell membrane.

T wave: The EKG wave that represents ventricular repolarization.

U wave: A small wave sometimes seen on the EKG. It follows the T wave and reflects late ventricular repolarization.

Introduction

Cardiac cells at rest are electrically negative on the inside as compared to the outside. Movement of charged particles (**ions**) of sodium and potassium into and out of the cell cause changes which can be picked up by sensors on the skin and printed out as an EKG.

Depolarization and Repolarization

The negatively charged resting cardiac cell is called **polarized.** When the cell is stimulated by an electrical impulse, sodium rushes into the cell and potassium leaks out, causing the cell to become positively charged. This is called **depolarization.** During cell recovery, ions shift back to their original places and return the cell to its negative charge. This is called **repolarization.** See Figure 5-1.

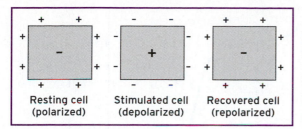

Figure 5-1 Depolarization and repolarization.

Depolarization and repolarization are electrical events. Contraction and relaxation are mechanical events. Depolarization should result in muscle contraction. Repolarization should result in muscle relaxation. *Electrical precedes mechanical.* There can be no heartbeat (a mechanical event) without first having had depolarization (the electrical stimulus). This is like a vacuum cleaner. Its job is to suck up dirt, but it cannot do its job without being plugged into an electrical source first.

Does plugging in that vacuum cleaner guarantee it will work? No. It could have a mechanical malfunction that prevents it from working. So can the heart. The electrical and mechanical systems are two separate systems. Either one (or both) can malfunction. Electrical malfunctions show up on the EKG. Mechanical malfunctions show up clinically.

Are you lost? Imagine this scenario: A man has a heart attack that damages a large portion of his myocardium. His heart's electrical system has not been damaged, so it sends out its impulses as usual. The muscle cells, however, have been so damaged that they are unable to respond to those impulses by contracting. Consequently, the EKG shows the electrical system is working, but the patient is clinically dead—no pulse, no breathing, no nothing. The vacuum cleaner was plugged in, but it was broken and couldn't do its job.

The Action Potential

Let's look at what happens to the ventricular muscle cell when it's stimulated by the conduction system impulse. See Figure 5-2. There are four phases to the action potential:

- In **phase 4,** the cardiac cell is at rest. It is negatively charged with a resting **transmembrane potential** (the electrical charge at the cell membrane) of −90 millivolts. Electrically, nothing is happening.

- In **Phase 0,** the cell is stimulated by the conduction system. Sodium rushes into the cell, potassium rushes out, and this results in a positive charge within the cell. This is called **depolarization.** You can see that at the top of phase 0, the cell's charge is above the zero mark. Phase 0 corresponds with the QRS complex of the EKG.

- **Phases 1** and 2 are **early repolarization.** Calcium is released in these two phases, resulting in ventricular contraction. Phases 1 and 2 correspond with the ST segment of the EKG. Phase 2 is called the **plateau phase,** because the waveform levels off here.

- **Phase 3** is **rapid repolarization.** Sodium and potassium return to their normal places, thus returning the cell to its resting negative charge. Phase 3 corresponds with the T wave of the EKG. The cell relaxes.

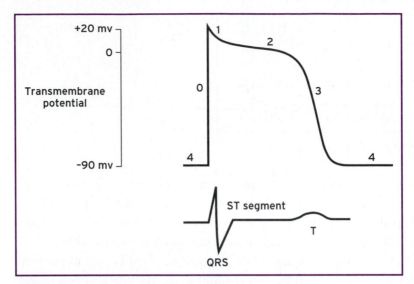

Figure 5-2   Action potential.

EKG Waves and Complexes

Depolarization and repolarization of the atria and ventricles result in waves and complexes on the EKG paper. Let's examine these waveforms. See Figure 5-3.

- **P wave.** Represents atrial depolarization. The normal P is small, rounded, and upright, but many things can alter the P wave shape.

- **T_a wave.** Represents atrial repolarization—usually not seen, as it occurs at the same time as the QRS complex.

- **QRS complex.** Represents ventricular depolarization. The normal QRS is spiked in appearance, consisting of one or more deflections from the baseline. The QRS complex is the most easily identified structure on the EKG tracing. Its shape can vary.

- **T wave.** Represents ventricular repolarization. The normal T wave is broad and rounded. If there is a QRS complex, there *must* be a T wave after it. Many things can alter the T wave shape.

- **U wave.** Represents late repolarization and is not normally seen. If present, the U wave follows the T wave. It should be shallow and rounded, the same deflection as the T wave (i.e., if the T wave is upright, the U wave should be also).

Each P-QRS-T sequence is one heartbeat. The flat lines between the P

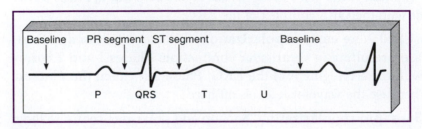

Figure 5-3   EKG waves and complexes.

wave and the QRS and between the QRS and T wave are called the **PR segment** and the **ST segment,** respectively. During these segments, no electrical activity is occurring. The flat line between the T wave of one beat and the P wave of the next beat is called the **baseline** or **isoelectric line.** The baseline is the line from which the waves and complexes take off.

Atrial contraction occurs during the P wave and the PR segment. Ventricular contraction occurs during the QRS and the ST segment. It's like this: The atria depolarize and a P wave is written on the EKG paper. Following this, the atria contract, filling the ventricles with blood. Then the ventricles depolarize, causing a QRS complex on the EKG paper. The ventricles then contract. The EKG waves and complexes tell us something electrical is happening. Flat lines indicate that no electrical activity is occurring.

Refractory Periods

The word **refractory** means "resistant to." Let's look at the periods when the cardiac cell resists responding to another impulse. See Figure 5-4.

- **Absolute.** The cell cannot accept another impulse because it's still dealing with the last one. Absolutely no stimulus, no matter how strong, will result in another depolarization during this time.

- **Relative.** A strong stimulus will result in depolarization.

- **Supernormal period.** Even a weak stimulus will cause depolarization. The cardiac cell during this period is hyper, and it doesn't take much to set it off and running. In fact, stimulation at this time often results in very fast, dangerous rhythms.

Waves and Complexes Identification Practice

Following are strips on which to practice identifying P waves, QRS complexes, and T waves. You'll recall that P waves are normally upright, but they can also be inverted (upside down) or biphasic (up *and* down). P waves usually precede the QRS complex, so find the QRS and then look for the P wave. Some rhythms have more than one P wave and others have no P at all. Write the letter *P* over each P wave you see.

The QRS complex is the most easily identified structure on the strip because of its spiked appearance. Write *QRS* over each QRS complex.

T waves are normally upright, but can also be inverted or biphasic. Wherever there is a QRS complex, there must be a T wave. Write a *T* over each T wave.

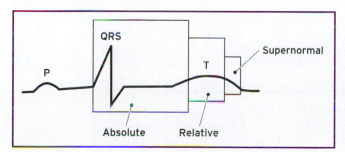

Figure 5-4 Refractory periods.

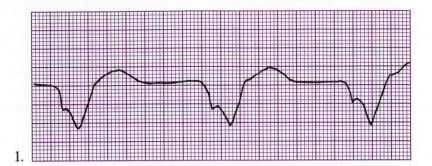

1.

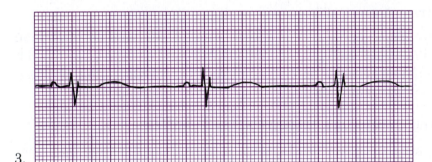

2.

3.

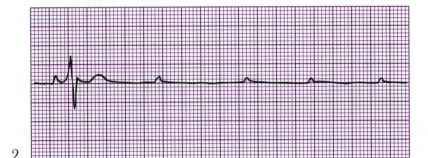

4.

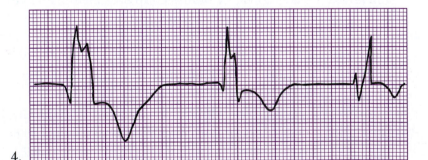

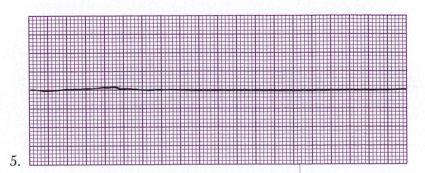

5.

Answers to Waves and Complexes Practice

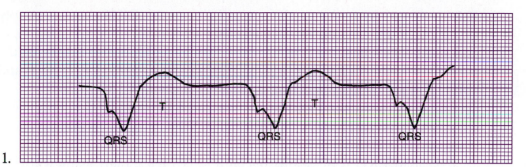

1.

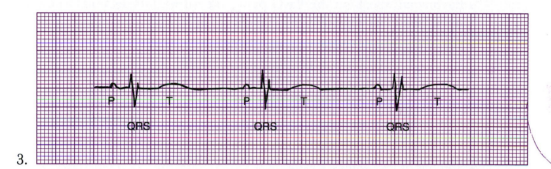

2.

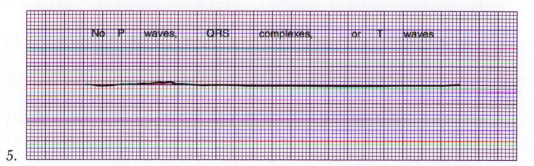

3.

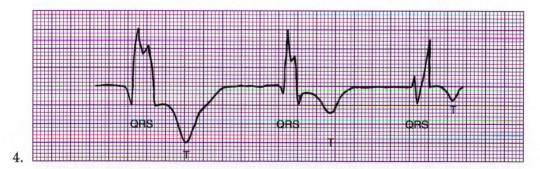

4.

5.

EKG Paper

Before we go any further, let's look at EKG paper. EKG paper is simply graph paper divided into small blocks that are 1 millimeter (mm) in height and width. Dark lines are present every fifth block to further subdivide the paper both vertically and horizontally. Measurements of the EKG waves and complexes are done by counting these blocks. Counting horizontally measures time, or **intervals.** Intervals are measured in seconds. Counting vertically measures **amplitude,** or the height of the complexes. Amplitude is measured in millimeters.

A 12-lead EKG is done on special 8 × 11 inch paper, using a **three-channel recorder** that prints a simultaneous view of three leads at a time in sequence until all 12 leads are recorded.

Rhythm strips are recorded on small rolls of special paper about 3 inches wide and several hundred feet in length. A 6- to 12-second strip is usually obtained, and the paper is cut to the desired length afterward. Rhythm strip paper often has lines at the top of the paper at 1- to 3-second intervals. Rhythm strips are run on **single-channel recorders,** which print out only one lead at a time.

Let's look at the EKG paper delineations:

- Each small block on the EKG paper measures 0.04 second (from one small line to the next).
- Five small blocks equals one big block.
- One big block equals 0.20 second.
- 25 small blocks equals 1 second.
- Five big blocks equals 1 second.
- 1,500 small blocks equals 1 minute.
- 300 big blocks equals 1 minute.

No matter whether the EKG paper is 12-lead size or rhythm strip size, the delineations will be the same.

Some EKG machines print out on paper with dotted lines in place of solid lines. As on the other kind of paper, every fifth dotted line is darker to subdivide the paper.

Figure 5-5 is an example of rhythm strip paper. **Identifying data,** such as name, date, time, and room number, and **interpretive data,** such as heart rate, are printed at the top of the paper.

See Figure 5-6 for a 12-lead EKG. Note the lead markings in Figure 5-6. Leads are arranged in four columns of three leads. Leads I, II, and III are in the first column, then aVR, aVL, and aVF in the second column, V_1 to V_3 in the third column, and V_4 to V_6 in the last column. At the very bottom of the paper is a page-wide rhythm strip, usually of either lead II or V_1.

Intervals

Now let's look at **intervals,** the measurement of time between the P-QRS-T waves and complexes. The heart's current normally starts in the right atrium, then spreads through both atria and down to the ventricles. Interval meas-

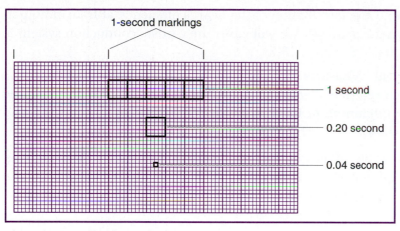

Figure 5-5   Rhythm strip paper.

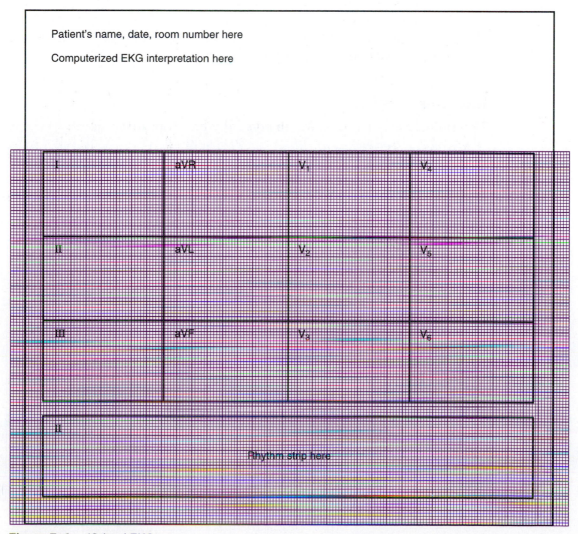

Figure 5-6   12-lead EKG.

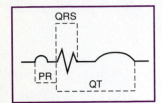

Figure 5-7   Intervals.

urements enable a determination of the heart's efficiency at transmitting its impulses down the pathway. We will cover the cardiac conduction system in detail in Chapter 6. See Figure 5-7.

- **PR interval.** Measures the time it takes for the impulse to get from the atria to the ventricles. Normal PR interval is 0.12 to 0.20 s. It's measured from the beginning of the P wave to the beginning of the QRS and includes the P wave and the PR segment.

- **QRS interval.** Measures the time it takes to depolarize the ventricles. Normal QRS interval is less than 0.12 s, usually between 0.06 and 0.10 s. It's measured from the beginning of the QRS to the end of the QRS.

- **QT interval.** Measures depolarization and repolarization time of the ventricles. The QT interval is measured from the beginning of the QRS to the end of the T wave and includes the QRS complex, the ST segment, and the T wave. QT interval will vary with the heart rate. At normal heart rates of 60 to 100, the QT interval should be less than or equal to one-half the distance between successive QRS complexes (called the **R-R interval**). To quickly determine if the QT is prolonged, draw a line midway between QRS complexes. If the T wave ends at or before this line, the QT is normal. If it ends after the line, it is prolonged and can lead to lethal arrhythmias.

Intervals Practice

Determine the intervals on the enlarged rhythm strips that follow.

PR interval. Count the number of small blocks between the beginning of the P and the beginning of the QRS. Multiply by 0.04 second.

QRS interval. Count the number of small blocks between the beginning and end of the QRS complex. Multiply by 0.04 second.

QT interval. Count the number of small blocks between the beginning of the QRS and the end of the T wave. Multiply by 0.04 second.

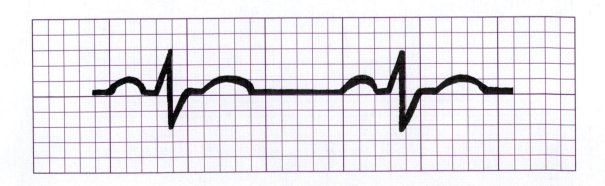

1. PR _____   QRS _____   QT _____

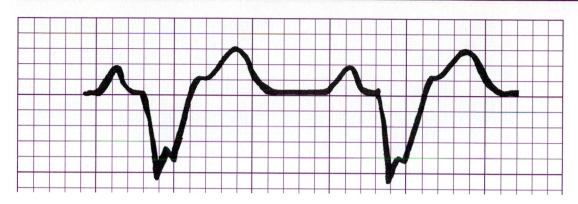

2. PR _____ QRS _____ QT _____

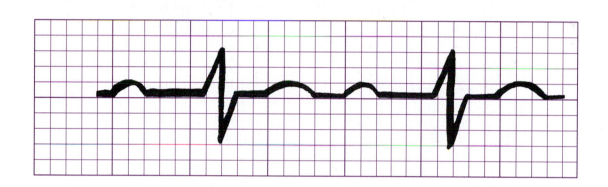

3. PR _____ QRS _____ QT _____

Answers

1. PR 0.12, QRS 0.08, QT 0.24.
2. PR 0.12, QRS 0.14, QT 0.32.
3. PR 0.24, QRS 0.08, QT 0.28.

Now let's practice intervals on normal-size EKG paper.

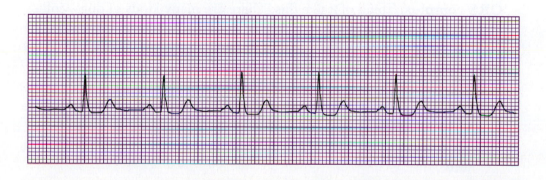

1. PR _____ QRS _____ QT _____

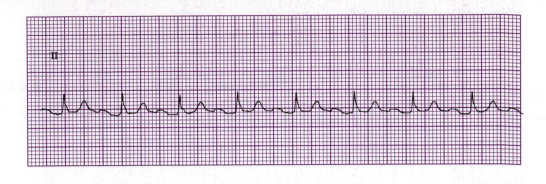

2. PR _____ QRS _____ QT _____

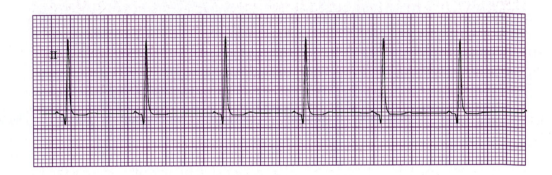

3. PR _____ QRS _____ QT _____

Answers

1. PR 0.20, QRS 0.08, QT 0.36.
2. PR 0.22, QRS 0.08, QT 0.32.
3. PR 0.08, QRS 0.12, QT 0.36.

QRS Nomenclature

The QRS complex is composed of waves that have different names–Q, R, and S–but no matter what waves it's composed of, it's still referred to as the **QRS complex.** Think of it like this: There are many kinds of dogs–collies, boxers, terriers, and so forth–but they're still dogs. Likewise, the QRS complex can have different names, but it's still a QRS complex. Let's look at the waves that can make up the QRS complex.

- A **Q wave** is a negative deflection that occurs before a positive deflection. There can be only one Q wave, and it must be the first wave of the QRS complex.

- An **R wave** is any positive deflection. There can be more than one R wave.

- An **S wave** is a negative deflection that follows an R wave. There can be more than one.

- A **QS wave** is a negative deflection with no positive deflection at all.

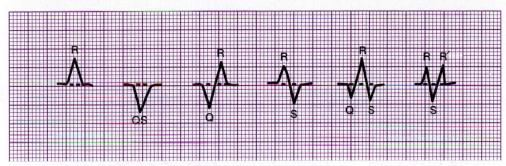

Figure 5-8   Examples of QRS complexes.

- A second R wave is written **R′**, called "R prime." A third R wave is **R″**, called "R prime prime." S waves can also have primes. There is no limit to the number of primes.

As in the alphabet, Q comes before R and S comes after R. See Figure 5-8. The dotted line indicates the baseline. Any wave in the QRS complex that goes above the baseline is an R wave; any wave going below the baseline is either a Q or an S wave.

QRS Nomenclature Practice

Name the waves in the following QRS complexes:

1. _____   2. _____   3. _____

4. _____   5. _____   6. _____

Now draw the following:

1. RSR′   2. QRS   3. QS

4. QR   5. RS   6. R

Answers to QRS Nomenclature Practice

Answers to "Name the waves"

1. R.
2. QS. This cannot be called a Q or an S because there is no R wave to precede or follow, so the QRS complex that is completely negative is called QS.
3. QR.
4. RS.
5. QRS.
6. RSR'.

Answers to "Draw the QRS complexes"

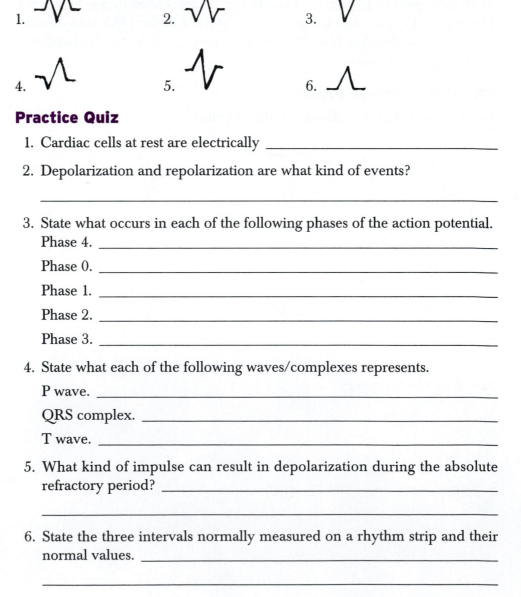

1. 2. 3. 4. 5. 6.

Practice Quiz

1. Cardiac cells at rest are electrically _____

2. Depolarization and repolarization are what kind of events?

   _____

3. State what occurs in each of the following phases of the action potential.
   Phase 4. _____
   Phase 0. _____
   Phase 1. _____
   Phase 2. _____
   Phase 3. _____

4. State what each of the following waves/complexes represents.
   P wave. _____
   QRS complex. _____
   T wave. _____

5. What kind of impulse can result in depolarization during the absolute refractory period? _____

   _____

6. State the three intervals normally measured on a rhythm strip and their normal values. _____

   _____

   _____

7. Is a Q wave a positive deflection or a negative deflection?

   _____

8. What kind of deflection is an R wave? _____

9. Amplitude is measured by counting the number of blocks in which direction—horizontally or vertically? _____

10. Intervals are measured by counting the number of blocks in which direction—horizontally or vertically? _____

Practice Quiz Answers

1. Cardiac cells at rest are electrically **negative.**

2. Depolarization and repolarization are **electrical events.**

3. Phase 4. **The cardiac cell is at rest.**
   Phase 0. **Depolarization occurs when sodium rushes into the cell.**
   Phase 1. **Early repolarization. Calcium is released.**
   Phase 2. **The plateau phase of early repolarization. Calcium is released.**
   Phase 3. **Rapid repolarization. Sodium rushes out of the cell.**

4. The P wave represents **atrial depolarization.**
   The QRS complex represents **ventricular depolarization.**
   The T wave represents **ventricular repolarization.**

5. **No impulse can result in depolarization during the absolute refractory period.**

6. **PR interval—normal 0.12 to 0.20 s.**

   QRS interval—normal <0.12 s.

   QT interval—normal <½ the R-R interval.

7. The Q wave is a **negative deflection.**

8. The R wave is a **positive deflection.**

9. Amplitude is measured by counting the number of blocks **vertically.**

10. Intervals are measured by counting the number of blocks **horizontally.**

The Cardiac Conduction System

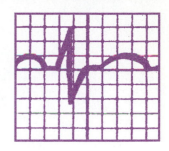

Chapter 6 Objectives

Upon completion of this chapter, the student will be able to:

- Define *pacemaker.*
- List the different pacemakers of the heart and their inherent rates.
- Track the cardiac impulse from the sinus node through the conduction system.
- Define the four characteristics of cardiac cells.
- Describe the difference between *escape* and *usurpation.*
- Draw the little hearts and arrows to indicate conduction in situations such as the ventricle escaping due to failure of the higher pacemakers.
- Label a rhythm strip as being representative of either escape or usurpation.
- Define *arrhythmia.*
- Tell what happens in each of the following scenarios:
  When the sinus node fails
  When the sinus node and atria both fail
  When the sinus node, atria, and AV node all fail

Chapter 6 Outline

I.   Introduction
II.   Conduction pathway through the heart
III. Characteristics of cardiac cells
IV.   Inherent rates of the pacemaker cells
V.   Conduction variations
      A. Normal conduction
      B. Sinus fails, AV node escapes
      C. All higher pacemakers fail, ventricle escapes
      D. Block in conduction, AV node escapes
VI.   Practice quiz
VII. Practice quiz answers

Chapter 6 Glossary

Automaticity: The ability of a cardiac cell to initiate an impulse without outside stimulation.

Conductivity: The ability of a cardiac cell to pass an impulse along to neighboring cells.

Contractility: The ability of a cardiac cell to contract and do work.

Escape: A safety mechanism in which a lower pacemaker fires at its slower inherent rate when the faster, predominant pacemaker fails.

Excitability: The ability of a cardiac cell to depolarize when stimulated.

Inherent: Preset, automatic heart rate of the pacemaker cells. This is the rate at which the pacemaker cells will fire if not acted on by outside stimuli to speed up or slow down.

Pacemaker: The intrinsic or artificial focus that propagates or initiates the cardiac impulse.

Usurpation: The act of stealing control away from another.

Introduction

The conduction system is a pathway of specialized cells whose job is to create and conduct the electrical impulses that tell the heart when to pump. The area of the conduction system that initiates the impulses is called the **pacemaker.** See Figure 6-1.

Conduction Pathway

Let's look at the conduction pathway through the heart:

Sinus node →→ **interatrial tracts** →→ **atrium** →→ **AV node**

↘ ↘

ventricle ←← **Purkinje fibers** ←← **bundle branches** ←← **bundle of His**

- The impulse originates in the **sinus node,** located in the upper right atrium just beneath the opening of the superior vena cava. The sinus node is the heart's normal pacemaker.

- From here it travels through the **interatrial tracts** (also called **internodal tracts**). These special conductive highways carry the impulses through the atria to

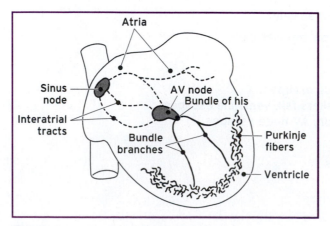

Figure 6-1 Cardiac conduction system.

- the **atrial tissue.** The atria then depolarize, and a P wave is written on the EKG.
- The impulse travels to the **AV node,** a specialized group of cells located just to the right of the septum in the lower right atrium. The AV node slows impulse transmission a little, allowing the newly depolarized atria to propel their blood into the ventricles.
- Then the impulse travels through the **bundle of His,** located just beneath the AV node, to
- the **left** and **right bundle branches,** the main highways to the ventricles.
- Then the impulse is propelled through the **Purkinje fibers.**
- Finally, the impulse arrives at the **ventricle** itself, causing it to depolarize. A QRS complex is written on the EKG paper.

Cardiac Cells

Cardiac cells have several characteristics:

- **Automaticity** The ability to create an impulse without outside stimulation.
- **Conductivity** The ability to pass this impulse along to neighboring cells.
- **Excitability** The ability to respond to this stimulus by depolarizing.
- **Contractility** The ability to contract and do work.

The first three characteristics are electrical. The last is mechanical.

Though the sinus node is the normal pacemaker of the heart, other cardiac cells can become the pacemaker if the sinus node fails. Let's look at that a little closer.

Inherent (Escape) Rates of the Pacemaker Cells

- Sinus node: 60 to 100 beats per minute
- Atria: 60 to 80 beats per minute
- AV node: 40 to 60 beats per minute
- Ventricle: 20 to 40 beats per minute

The sinus node, you'll note, has the fastest inherent rate of all the potential pacemaker cells. This means that, barring any outside stimuli that speed it up or slow it down, the sinus node will fire at its rate of 60 to 100 beats per minute. The lower pacemakers (atrium, AV node, and ventricle) have slower inherent rates, each one having a slower rate than the one above it.

The fastest pacemaker at any given moment is the one in control. Thus the lower pacemakers are inhibited, or restrained, from firing as long as some other pacemaker is faster. The lower pacemakers serve as a backup in case of conduction failure from above. The only thing that inhibits those pacemakers from escaping (taking over as the pacemaker at their slower inherent rate) is if they have been depolarized by a faster impulse. If that faster impulse never

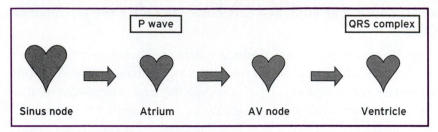

Figure 6-2   Normal conduction.

arrives, the next pacemaker in line will assume that *it* is now the fastest and should escape its restraints to become the new pacemaker.

Conduction Variations

Normal conduction of cardiac impulses is dependent on the health of each part of the conduction system. Failure of any part of the system necessitates a variation in conduction. Let's look at several conductive possibilities. See Figure 6-2.

In Figure 6-2, the sinus node fires out its impulse. When the impulse depolarizes the atrium, a P wave is written. The impulse then travels to the AV node, then to the ventricle. A QRS is written when the ventricle is depolarized.

If the sinus node fails, however, one of the lower pacemakers will escape its restraints and take over at its slower inherent rate, thus becoming the heart's new pacemaker. If the atrium escapes, it fires at its rate of 60 to 80 beats per minute. If the AV node escapes, it will fire at a rate of 40 to 60. If the ventricle takes over, the rate will be 20 to 40. Needless to say, if the ventricle has to kick in as the pacemaker, it is a grave situation, since it means that all the pacemakers above it have failed. Remember—no pacemaker can escape unless it's the fastest at that particular time.

Though the atrium is the pacemaker next in line below the sinus node and theoretically should be the one to take over if the sinus node fails, *it is very uncommon for the atrium to fire at its escape rate.* The atria like to fire rapidly, not slowly, so in fact *the AV node is the pacemaker that most often escapes when the sinus node fails.*

In Figure 6-3, the sinus node has failed. Since the atria don't like to escape, the AV node is now the fastest escape pacemaker. It creates an impulse and sends it forward toward the ventricle and backward toward the atria, providing the P and the QRS.

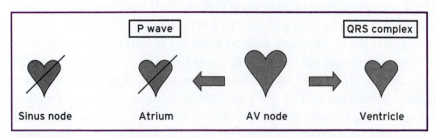

Figure 6-3   Sinus fails. AV node escapes.

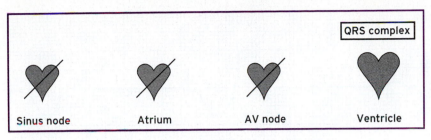

Figure 6-4   All higher pacemakers fail. Ventricle escapes.

In Figure 6-4, the sinus node, atrium, and AV node have all failed. The only pacemaker left is the ventricle, so it takes over as the pacemaker, providing the QRS. There is no P wave when the ventricle escapes.

What if the sinus node fires its impulse out but the impulse is blocked at some point along the conduction pathway? The first pacemaker below the block should escape and become the new pacemaker.

In Figure 6-5, the sinus node fires out its impulse, which depolarizes the atrium and writes a P wave. The impulse is then blocked between the atrium and the AV node. Since the faster sinus impulse never reaches the AV node, the AV node thinks the sinus node has failed. So it escapes, creates its own new impulse, and becomes the new pacemaker, sending the impulse down to the ventricle and backward to the atria. (Backward conduction can work even when forward conduction is blocked.) If the impulse were blocked between the AV node and the ventricle, the ventricle would become the new pacemaker.

Each of the pacemakers can fire at rates faster or slower than their inherent rates if there are outside stimuli. We've talked about escape. Let's look at an example of escape compared with usurpation.

Escape occurs when the predominant pacemaker slows dramatically (or fails completely) and a lower pacemaker takes over at its inherent rate, providing a new rhythm that is slower than the previous rhythm. *An escape beat is any beat that comes in after a pause that's longer than the normal R-R interval. Escape beats are lifesavers.*

In Figure 6-6, the normal pacemaker stops suddenly and there is a long pause, at the end of which is a beat from a lower pacemaker and then a new rhythm with a heart rate slower than before. This is escape.

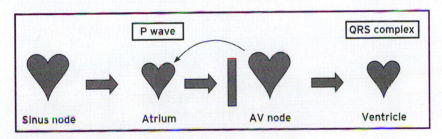

Figure 6-5   Block in conduction. AV node escapes.

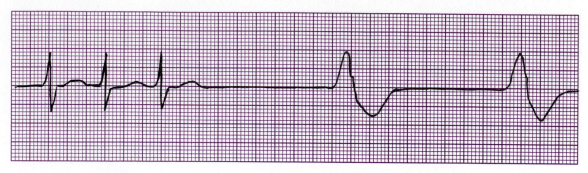

Figure 6-6 Escape.

Usurpation, which means "to take control away from," occurs when one of the lower pacemakers gets hyper and fires in at an accelerated rate, stealing control away from the predominant pacemaker. Usurpation results in a faster rhythm than before, and it starts with a beat that comes in earlier than expected.

In Figure 6-7, the controlling pacemaker is cruising along and suddenly an impulse from a lower pacemaker fires in early, takes control, and is off and running with a new, faster rhythm. This is usurpation.

Abnormalities of the conduction system can produce **arrhythmias,** abnormal heart rhythms. Though most often these conduction system problems are related to heart disease, there are also specific diseases that affect the conduction system outright. Whatever the cause, conduction system abnormalities can prove harmful or fatal if not treated appropriately.

Practice Quiz

1. List the three characteristics of heart cells. _____

   _____

   _____

2. State the inherent rates of the pacemaker cells.

   Sinus node _____

   Atrium _____

   AV node _____

   Ventricle _____

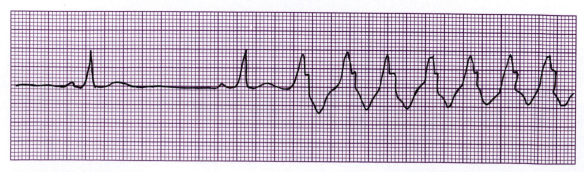

Figure 6-7 Usurpation.

3. Define *escape*. _____

_____

4. Define *usurpation*. _____

_____

5. List, in order of conduction, the eight structures of the conduction pathway through the heart. _____

_____

_____

_____

Practice Quiz Answers

1. The four characteristics of heart cells are **automaticity, conductivity, excitability,** and **contractility.**

2. The inherent rate of the sinus node is **60 to 100,** the atrium is **60 to 80,** the AV node is **40 to 60,** and the ventricle is **20 to 40.**

3. **Escape occurs when the prevailing pacemaker slows or fails and a lower pacemaker takes over as the pacemaker at a slower rate than before.**

4. **Usurpation occurs when a lower pacemaker becomes hyper and fires at an accelerated rate, stealing control away from the predominant pacemaker and providing a faster heart rate than before.**

5. The eight structures of the conduction pathway are the **sinus node,** the **interatrial tracts,** the **atrium,** the **AV node,** the **bundle of His,** the **bundle branches,** the **Purkinje fibers,** and the **ventricle.**

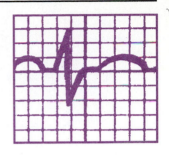

Lead Morphology and Placement

Chapter 7 Objectives

Upon completion of this chapter, the student will be able to:

- Define *electrode.*
- Describe the difference between an electrocardiograph and an electrocardiogram.
- Name the bipolar leads and state the limbs that compose them.
- Name the unipolar augmented leads.
- Explain what augmentation does to the EKG.
- Explain Einthoven's law.
- Draw and label Einthoven's triangle.
- Name the leads composing the hexiaxial diagram.
- Describe the location of the precordial leads.
- Name the two leads most commonly used for continuous monitoring in the hospital.
- Explain the electrocardiographic truths.
- Describe the normal QRS complex deflections in each of the 12 leads on an EKG.

Chapter 7 Outline

Chapter 7 Glossary

Augment: Increase.

Axilla: Armpit.

Bipolar: Having a positive and a negative pole.

Clavicle: Collarbone.

Einthoven's law: The law stating that the height of the QRS in lead I added to the height of the QRS in lead III equals the height of the QRS in lead II.

Einthoven's triangle: The triangle formed by joining leads I, II, and III at the ends.

Electrocardiogram: A printout of the electrical signals generated by the heart.

Electrocardiograph: The EKG machine.

Electrocardiography: The printing out of the electrical signals generated by the heart.

Electrodes: Adhesive patches attached to the skin to receive electrical signals from the heart.

Hexiaxial: Consisting of six lines.

Isoelectric complex: The QRS complex whose positive and negative deflections are most equal.

Lead: Another name for electrode *or* an electrocardiographic picture of the heart.

Precordial: Chest.

Telemetry: A method of remotely monitoring a patient's rhythm. The patient carries a small transmitter that relays his or her cardiac rhythm to a receiver at another location.

Triaxial: Consisting of three lines.

Unipolar: A lead consisting of only a positive pole.

Vector: An arrow depicting the direction of electrical current flow in the heart.

Introduction

Electrocardiography is the recording of the heart's electrical impulses by way of sensors, called **electrodes,** placed at various locations on the body. Willem Einthoven, inventor of the EKG machine and the "father of electrocardiography," postulated that the heart is in the center of the electrical field that it generates. He put electrodes on the arms and legs, far away from the heart. The right-leg electrode was used as a ground electrode to minimize the hazard of electric shock to the patient and to stabilize the EKG. The electrodes on the other limbs were used to create leads. A **lead** is simply an electrocardiographic picture of the heart. A 12-lead EKG provides 12 different views of the heart's electrical activity.

Why is it necessary to have 12 leads? The more leads, the better the chance of interpreting the heart's electrical activity. Have you ever waved to someone you saw from a distance, then realized when you got a better look that it wasn't who you thought it was? The more views you have, the better your chance of recognizing this person, right? Same thing with the heart. The more views of the heart's electrical activity, the better the chance of recognizing its abnormalities. So we have leads that view the heart from the side, the front, the bottom, and anterior to posterior.

The printed EKG is called an **electrocardiogram.** The EKG machine is an **electrocardiograph.**

Bipolar Leads

Bipolar leads are so named because they require a positive pole and a negative pole. The positive electrode is the one that actually "sees" the current.

- **Lead I.** Measures the current traveling between the right and left arms. The right arm is negative and the left arm is positive.

- **Lead II.** Measures the current traveling between the right arm and the left leg. The right arm is negative and the left leg is positive.

- **Lead III.** Measures the current traveling between the left arm and the left leg. The left arm is negative and the left leg is positive.

In Figure 7-1, you'll notice that in the bipolar leads the right arm is always negative and the left leg is always positive. Also note that the left arm can be positive or negative depending on which lead it is a part of. If you join leads I, II, and III at the middle, you get the **triaxial diagram** seen in Figure 7-2.

If you join Leads I, II, and III at their ends, you get a triangle called **Einthoven's triangle,** seen in Figure 7-3.

Einthoven stated that lead I + lead III = lead II. This is called **Einthoven's law.** It means that the height of the QRS in lead I added to the height of the QRS in lead III will equal the height of the QRS in lead II. In other words, lead II should have the tallest QRS of the bipolar leads. See Figure 7-4.

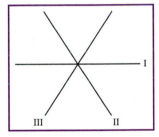

Figure 7-2 The triaxial diagram.

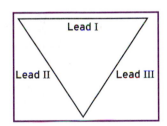

Figure 7-3 Einthoven's triangle.

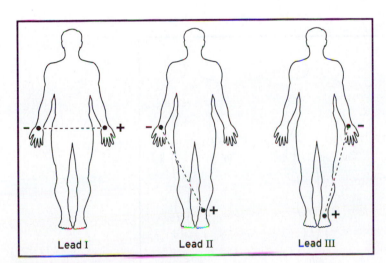

Figure 7-1 The bipolar leads.

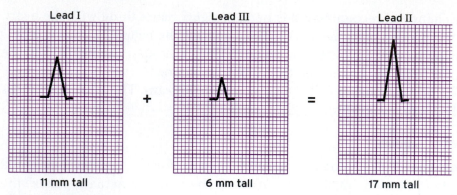

Lead I		Lead III		Lead II
11 mm tall	+	6 mm tall	=	17 mm tall

Figure 7-4   Einthoven's law.

Augmented Leads

- • aVR. Measures the current traveling toward the right arm. This is a positive electrode. The electrode is on the right arm.
- • aVL. Measures the current traveling toward the left arm. This is a positive electrode. The electrode is on the left arm.
- • aVF. Measures the current traveling toward the left foot (or leg). This is a positive electrode. The electrode is on the left leg.

See Figure 7-5. These are called **augmented leads** because they generate such small waveforms on the EKG paper that the EKG machine must augment (increase) the size of the waveforms so they'll show up on the EKG paper. These leads are also **unipolar,** meaning they require only one electrode to make the leads. In order for the EKG machine to augment the leads, it uses a midway point between the other two limbs as a negative reference point.

Both the bipolar and augmented leads are also called **frontal leads** because they look at the heart from only the front of the body.

If you join leads aVR, aVL, and aVF in the middle, you get the triaxial diagram shown in Figure 7-6.

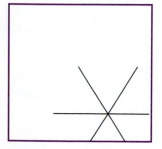

Figure 7-6   Triaxial diagram with augmented leads.

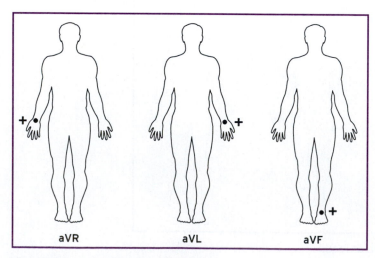

| aVR | aVL | aVF |

Figure 7-5   The augmented leads.

If all the frontal leads—I, II, III, aVR, aVL, and aVF—are joined at the center, the result looks like Figure 7-7. This **hexiaxial diagram** is used to help determine the direction of current flow in the heart.

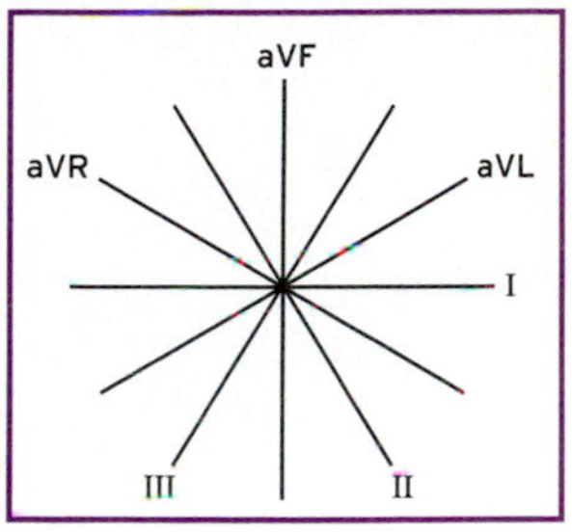

Precordial (Chest) Leads

These leads are located on the chest. They are also unipolar leads, and each one is a positive electrode. The precordial leads see a wrap-around view of the heart from the horizontal plane. These leads are named V_1, V_2, V_3, V_4, V_5, and V_6. See Figure 7-8.

Location of the precordial leads

V_1 Fourth intercostal space, right sternal border (abbreviated 4th ICS, RSB)

V_2 Fourth intercostal space, left sternal border (4th ICS, LSB)

V_3 Between V_2 and V_4

V_4 Fifth intercostal space, midclavicular line (5th ICS, MCL)

V_5 Fifth intercostal space, anterior axillary line (5th ICS, AAL)

V_6 Fifth intercostal space, midaxillary line (5th ICS, MAL)

Intercostal spaces are the spaces between the ribs. The fourth intercostal space is the space *below* the fourth rib; the fifth intercostal space is below the fifth rib, and so on. The **midclavicular line** is a line down from the middle of the clavicle (collarbone). The **anterior axillary line** is a line down from the front of the axilla (armpit). The **midaxillary line** is down from the middle of the axilla. *The space immediately below the clavicle is* not *an intercostal space.*

Continuous Monitoring

For patients in the hospital, continuous EKG monitoring may be needed. These patients are attached to either a 3-lead or a 5-lead cable, which is then attached to a remote receiver/transmitter (called **telemetry**) or to a monitor

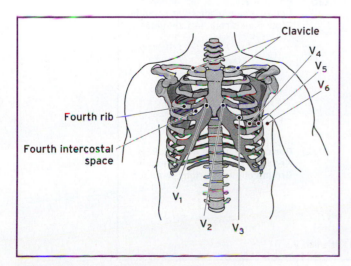

Figure 7-7 The hexiaxial diagram.

Figure 7-8 The precordial leads.

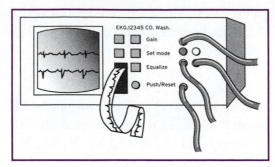

Figure 7-9   Bedside monitor.

at the bedside (see Figure 7-9). Both of these setups send the EKG display to a central terminal where the rhythms are observed and identified.

Since these patients may be on the monitor for days or longer, it is necessary to alter the placement of lead electrodes to allow for freedom of movement and to minimize artifact.

Figure 7-10 shows the two most commonly used leads for continuous monitoring. Note lead placement is on the subclavicle (collarbone) area and the chest or lower abdomen instead of on the arms, legs, and chest. Also note the ground electrode may be located somewhere other than the right leg.

Electrocardiographic Truths

- An impulse traveling toward (or parallel to) a positive electrode writes a positive complex on the EKG paper.

- An impulse traveling away from a positive electrode writes a negative complex.

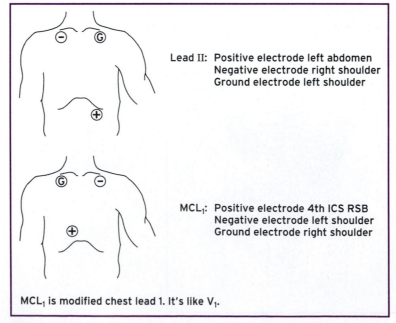

Figure 7-10   Lead placement for continuous monitoring.

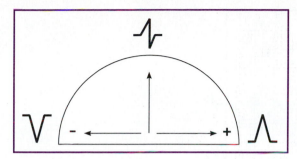

Figure 7-11   Electrocardiographic truths.

- An impulse traveling perpendicularly to the positive electrode writes an **isoelectric** complex (one that is as much positive as it is negative).
- If there is no impulse at all, there will be no complex—just a flat line.

See Figure 7-11.

Normal QRS Deflections

How should the QRS complexes in the normal EKG look? Let's look at the frontal leads:

Lead I   Should be positive.

Lead II   Should be positive.

Lead III   Should be small but mostly positive.

aVR   Should be negative.

aVL   Should be positive.

aVF   Should be positive.

Normal vector forces of the heart flow top to bottom, right to left. A **vector** is an arrow that points out the general direction of current flow. The current of the heart normally starts in the sinus node, which is in the right atrium, and terminates in the left ventricle. Figure 7-12 shows what the vector representing normal heart current looks like.

We've already said what the QRS complex in each lead should look like. Let's look at that a little more closely. In Figure 7-13 we have lead I, which

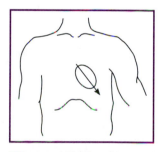

Figure 7-12 Normal vector.

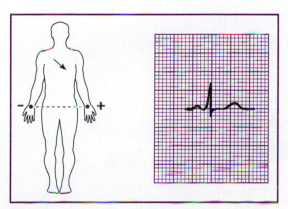

Figure 7-13   Normal QRS deflection in lead I.

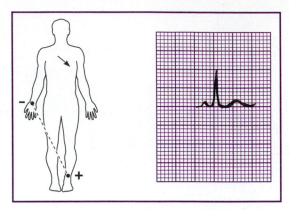

Figure 7-14   Normal QRS deflection in lead II.

joins right and left arms. The positive electrode is on the left arm. Normal current of the heart flows right to left, traveling toward the left side, where lead I's positive electrode is. This results in a positive (upward) complex in lead I.

In Figure 7-14, we have lead II, which connects the right arm and left leg. Recall the left leg is positive. Normal heart current flows top to bottom, right to left, parallel to lead II. Therefore lead II should be strongly positive.

Next is lead III, which joins left arm and left foot. The positive electrode is on the left leg. Normal current flows toward this electrode, producing a positive complex. The complex in lead III is very often small. See Figure 7-15.

In aVR, the positive electrode is on the right arm. Normal current flows right to left, away from this electrode, and aVR should therefore be negative. See Figure 7-16.

In aVL, the positive electrode is on the left arm. Normal current flows toward the left, producing a positive complex. See Figure 7-17.

In aVF, the positive electrode is on the left leg. Normal current flows toward the left leg, so aVF should have a positive complex. See Figure 7-18.

Now let's look at the precordial leads:

V_1 Should be negative.

V_2 Should be negative.

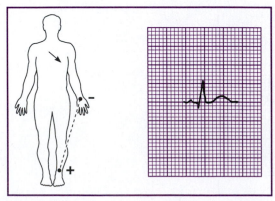

Figure 7-15   Normal QRS deflection in lead III.

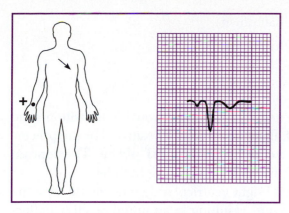

Figure 7-16   Normal QRS deflection in aVR.

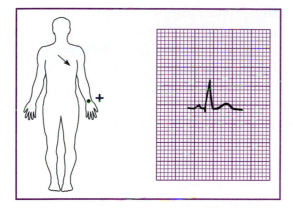

Figure 7-17   Normal QRS deflection in aVL.

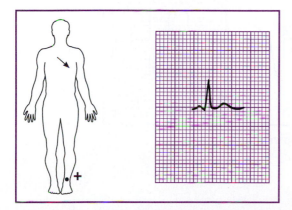

Figure 7-18   Normal QRS deflection in aVF.

V_3 Should be about half up, half down.

V_4 Should be about half up, half down.

V_5 Should be positive.

V_6 Should be positive.

The precordial leads start out negative, then go through a transition zone where they become half-and-half, then they become positive. For the precordial leads we look at current flow in the **horizontal plane.** The septum depolarizes from left to right and the ventricles from right to left.

See Figure 7-19. In V_1, septal and right ventricular depolarization send the current toward the positive electrode, resulting in an initial positive deflection. Then the current travels away from the positive electrode as it heads toward the left ventricle. Thus, V_1 should have a small R wave and a deep S wave. The complex is mostly negative, since most of the heart's current is traveling toward the left ventricle, away from the V_1 electrode.

In V_6, just the opposite occurs. Initially, the impulse is heading away from the positive electrode during septal and right ventricular depolarization, then it travels toward it during left ventricular activation. See Figure 7-20.

The other leads in between show a gradual transition from negative to positive complexes.

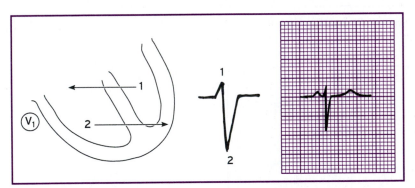

Figure 7-19   Normal QRS deflection in V_1.

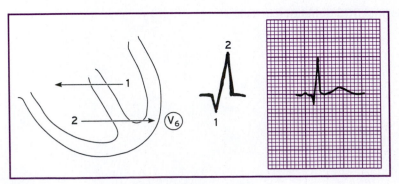

Figure 7-20   Normal QRS deflection in V_6.

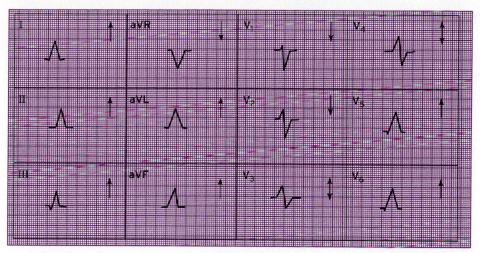

Normal 12-Lead EKG   The arrows indicate the correct deflection of the QRS complexes.

Lead Morphology Practice

Determine if the following QRS morphologies are normal. If not, tell what the abnormality is.

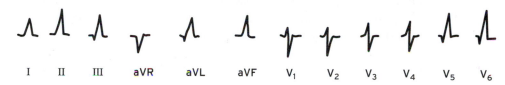

I   II   III   aVR   aVL   aVF   V₁   V₂   V₃   V₄   V₅   V₆

1. _____

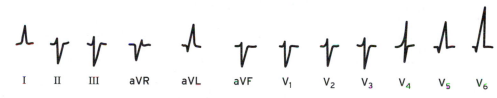

I   II   III   aVR   aVL   aVF   V₁   V₂   V₃   V₄   V₅   V₆

2. _____

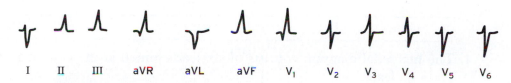

I   II   III   aVR   aVL   aVF   V₁   V₂   V₃   V₄   V₅   V₆

3. _____

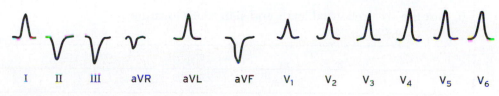

I   II   III   aVR   aVL   aVF   V₁   V₂   V₃   V₄   V₅   V₆

4. _____

Answers to Lead Morphology Practice

1. **Normal morphology.**

2. **Abnormal morphology.** Let's go lead by lead. Lead I is normal. Leads II and III are negative deflections and they should be positive; aVR is OK, as is aVL; aVF is negative and it should be positive. The precordial leads are OK.

3. **Abnormal morphology.** Lead I is negative and it should be positive. Leads II and III are OK; aVR is positive and it should *always* be negative; aVL is negative and should be positive; aVF is OK. V_1 is positive, but should be negative. V_2 is OK, more negative than positive. V_3 is positive, but should be isoelectric. V_4 is isoelectric when it should be getting more positive. V_5 and V_6 are negative when they should be positive.

4. **Abnormal morphology.** Lead I is positive, as it should be. Leads II and III are negative, but should be positive; aVR and aVL are OK; aVF is negative but should be positive. The precordial leads are all positive–this is completely abnormal.

Just by analyzing the morphology of each lead, we can get an idea of whether there is any pathology on the EKG. Three of the preceding four EKGs were abnormal in some way. As we continue further along in this text, we will learn the implications of this abnormality, and we'll learn more ways to analyze EKGs.

Practice Quiz

1. Who is Willem Einthoven? _____

2. List the three bipolar leads and the limbs they connect.

   _____

   _____

   _____

3. List the three augmented leads and the location of their positive pole.

   _____

   _____

   _____

4. The hexiaxial diagram consists of six leads joined at the center. List those six leads.

   _____

5. The precordial leads see the heart from what plane? _____

6. List the six precordial leads and state their location.

   _____

   _____

   _____

   _____

_____

_____

7. Name the two leads most commonly used for continuous monitoring.

_____

8. An impulse traveling toward a positive electrode writes a _____ complex on the EKG.

9. Should aVR have a positive QRS complex or a negative one?

_____

10. The QRS complexes in the precordial lead start out primarily

_____

Practice Quiz Answers

1. **Willem Einthoven won the Nobel Prize for inventing the EKG machine.**

2. The three bipolar leads are **leads I, II, and III. Lead I connects the right and left arms. Lead II connects the right arm and left foot. Lead III connects the left arm and left foot.**

3. The three augmented leads are as follows:

   aVR   **Positive pole is on the right arm.**

   aVL   **Positive pole is on the left arm.**

   aVF   **Positive pole is on the left foot.**

4. The six leads composing the hexiaxial diagram are **leads I, II, III, aVR, aVL,** and **aVF.**

5. The precordial leads see the heart from the **horizontal plane.**

6. The precordial leads and their locations are as follows:

   V_1 **4th ICS, RSB**

   V_2 **4th ICS, LSB**

   V_3 **Between V_2 and V_4**

   V_4 **5th ICS, MCL**

   V_5 **5th ICS, AAL**

   V_6 **5th ICS, MAL**

7. The two leads most commonly used for continuous monitoring are **leads II** and **V_1.**

8. An impulse traveling toward a positive electrode writes a **positive** complex on the EKG.

9. aVR should have a **negative** QRS complex.

10. The QRS complexes in the precordial leads start out primarily **negative.**

Technical Aspects of the EKG

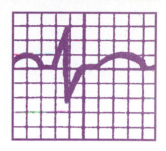

Chapter 8 Objectives

Upon completion of this chapter, the student will be able to:

- Identify the control features of an EKG machine and describe the functions of each.
- Describe what a galvanometer does.
- Differentiate between *macroshock* and *microshock*.
- Describe and identify on a rhythm strip the different kinds of artifact.
- Correctly tell how to troubleshoot artifact.
- Explain the purpose of telemetry monitoring.

Chapter 8 Outline

I.   Introduction
II.   EKG machine control features
      A. Chart speed, sensitivity control, standardization, position control, frequency response, stylus heat control
III. Electrical safety
      A. Macroshock, microshock
IV.   Artifact
      A. Somatic tremors, baseline sway, 60-cycle interference, broken recording
V.   Troubleshooting
VI.   Artifact troubleshooting practice
VII. Answers to artifact troubleshooting practice
VIII. Telemetry monitoring
IX.   Practice quiz
X.   Practice quiz answers

Chapter 8 Glossary

Artifact: Unwanted jitter or interference on the EKG tracing.

Calibration: A method of verifying the correct performance of an EKG machine.

Galvanometer: A component of an EKG machine that transforms electrical energy into mechanical energy, allowing the EKG to be printed out.

Macroshock: A large electrical shock caused by improper or faulty grounding of electrical equipment.

Microshock: A small electrical shock made possible by a conduit, such as a pacemaker, directly in the heart.

Somatic: Referring to the body.

Stylus: The pen on the EKG machine.

Troubleshooting: Determining and alleviating the cause of artifact and recording errors.

Introduction

The heart, electrically speaking, is a transmitter, and the EKG machine is a receiver. Let's look at how the EKG machine works.

The electrical impulses sent out by the heart course not only through the conduction system but also throughout the body. **Electrodes,** small adhesive patches with conductive gel on the skin side, pick up these impulses and send them through **lead wires** to a cable into the EKG machine. There an **amplifier** magnifies the signal and a **galvanometer** converts the electrical activity into mechanical energy, which in turn causes the **stylus** to record the EKG. See Figure 8-1.

Control Features

EKG machines have various control features:

- **Chart speed.** This regulates the speed at which the paper prints out. Normal speed is 25 mm/s. Changing the speed to 50 mm/s doubles the width of the waves and complexes.

- **Sensitivity control.** This regulates the height of the complexes. Normal setting is 1. Changing to 2 doubles the height of the complexes. Changing to ½ shrinks it.

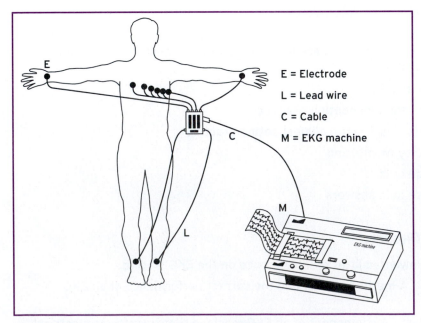

E = Electrode

L = Lead wire

C = Cable

M = EKG machine

Figure 8-1 Man attached to EKG machine.

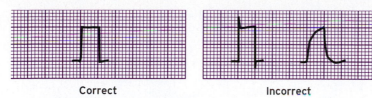

Correct   Incorrect

Figure 8-2   Calibration waves.

- **Standardization.** This checks the machine's calibration. Throwing 1 millivolt of electricity into the EKG machine should cause the stylus (the pen) to print out a square wave 10 mm high on the EKG paper. Incorrect standardization reveals a square wave that is too tall, too short, or slurred at the top or bottom. Do not use a machine that's not calibrated properly. Its printout may not be accurate. See Figure 8-2.

- **Position control.** This allows the baseline to be moved up or down on the paper.

- **Frequency response.** This filters out extraneous noise and artifact to provide a smoother tracing.

- **Stylus heat control.** This allows the stylus to write darker (hotter stylus) or lighter (cooler stylus).

Whenever any setting is changed from the norm, document this change at the top of the EKG printout. For example, if the sensitivity control is increased to 2 instead of set at the usual 1, note this. Documentation prevents misinterpretation of any EKG changes that might result from changes to the control features.

Electrical Safety

There are two kinds of electrical shock the patient can sustain from faulty equipment:

- **Macroshock.** This is a high-voltage shock that results from inadequate grounding of electrical equipment. If there is a frayed or broken wire or cord, electrical outlet damage, or other electrical malfunction, the 110 volts of electricity running through the power line can go directly to the patient, causing burns, neurologic damage, or fatal heart rhythm disturbances. The patient's dry, intact skin will offer some resistance to the electricity, but not enough to prevent injury.

- **Microshock.** This is a subtle hazard, but one that could have equally disastrous results for the patient. Microshock involves a direct path to the heart by means of a device inside or attached to it, such as a pacemaker. A small voltage exists on the outside of the metal pacemaker because of the proximity of the electrical components inside to the surrounding case. Normally a small **leakage current** is produced and carried harmlessly away by the ground wire attaching the patient's bed to the electrical socket in the room. If the ground wire is frayed, however, a small amount of current could travel into the heart and shock it from the inside. Since the inside of the body is a wet environment, there is less protection against shock. Even a small shock directed into the heart can cause injury or death.

Precaution: Check for frayed wires or components before doing an EKG.

Artifact

Artifact is unwanted interference or jitter on the EKG tracing. This makes reading the EKG difficult. There are four kinds of artifact:

- **Somatic tremors.** The word *somatic* means "body." This is a jittery pattern caused by the patient's tremors or by shaking wires. Try to help the patient relax. Cover him if he's cold. Make sure the wires are not tangled or loose. Sometimes this artifact cannot be corrected, such as in a patient with constant tremors from Parkinson's disease. In that case, make a few attempts at a readable tracing and keep the best one. At the top of the EKG, write "best effort times three attempts" or something to that effect so the physician will know this was not simply a poor tracing done by an inattentive technician. Note the shakiness of the tracing in Figure 8-3. Sometimes you can pick out the QRS complexes and sometimes not. Redo the EKG until the tracing is more easily readable.

- **Baseline sway.** This is where the baseline moves up and down on the EKG paper. It's often caused by lotion or sweat on the skin interfering with the signal reaching the machine. Sometimes it's associated with the breathing pattern. Wipe off any lotion or sweat with a towel and put a little alcohol at the electrode site to defat the skin and help the patches stick better. On Figure 8-4, note the baseline swaying upward as if someone had snagged a finger under it and pulled it upward. It's not a big problem, because the waves and complexes are all still clear.

- **60-cycle interference.** This results in a thick-looking pattern on the paper. It's caused by too many electrical things plugged in close by. Unplug as many machines as you safely can until you finish doing the EKG. Don't forget portable phones and pagers—they can cause interference also. In Figure 8-5, see how the baseline is very thick-looking? It's as if someone used a thick Magic Marker to write this baseline. Normally the baseline is much finer.

- **Broken recording.** This can be caused by a frayed or fractured wire or by a loose electrode patch or cable. Check first for loose electrodes or

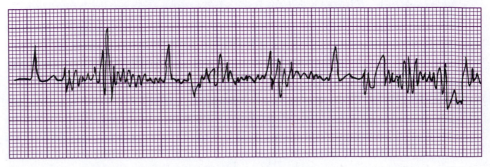

Figure 8-3 Somatic tremors artifact.

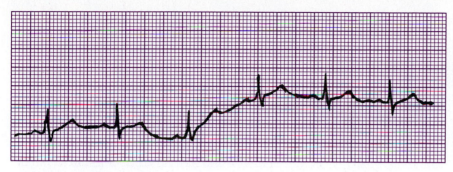

Figure 8-4   Baseline sway.

cables. If those are OK, the artifact may be from a fractured wire. If so, use a different EKG machine. Never do an EKG with a faulty machine. In Figure 8-6, note that at first the QRS complexes are easily visible, then the stylus is all over the place, going up and down trying to find the signal.

Troubleshooting

Troubleshooting involves determining and alleviating the cause of artifact and recording errors. For example, what if you only saw baseline sway in leads I, II, and aVR? Lead I connects the right and left arms, lead II is right arm and left foot, and aVR is right arm. The common lead is on the right arm. Change that electrode, and the problem should be corrected. Always note what leads the problem is in and find the common limb. Direct your corrective efforts there.

How do you know if the electrodes are properly placed? Remember the normal configuration of the leads. All the frontal leads except aVR should be positive, and the precordial leads start out negative, then eventually become positive. Say you do an EKG and the complexes are all screwed up—I is negative, aVR is positive, and the precordial leads start out positive and become negative. Obviously the lead placement is wrong. Redo the EKG with the leads correctly placed. A big clue to incorrect lead placement or lead reversal is a negative P-QRS-T in lead I. That is completely wrong unless the patient's heart is on the right side (a rare occurrence). So if you find that your lead I is completely negative, check your lead placement. The right and left arm leads were probably accidentally reversed.

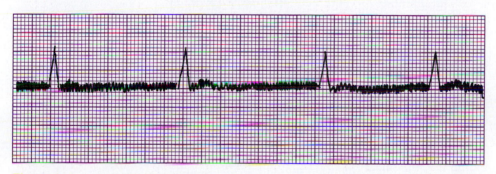

Figure 8-5   60-cycle interference.

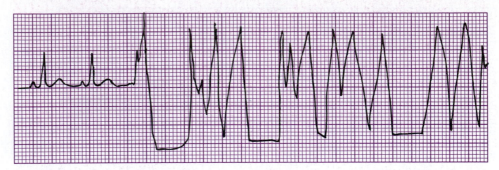

Figure 8-6 Broken recording.

Artifact Troubleshooting Practice

On these EKGs, state in which leads the artifact is found, and the necessary corrective action.

1.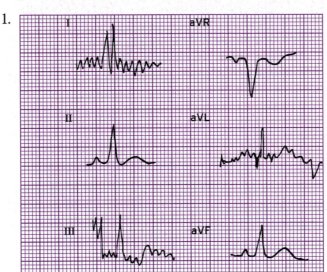

Artifact location _____

_____

Corrective action _____

_____

_____

_____

2.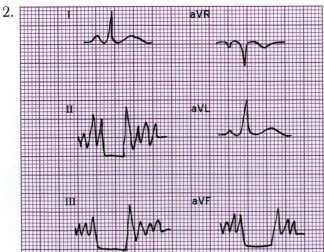

Artifact location _____

_____

Corrective action _____

_____

_____

3.

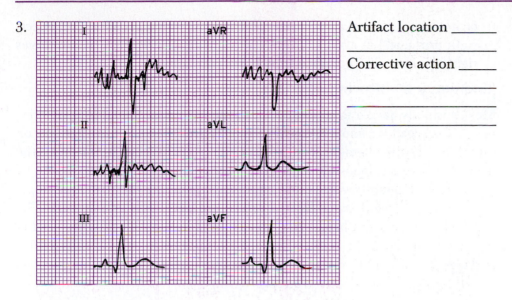

Artifact location _____
_____
Corrective action _____
_____
_____
_____

Answers to Artifact Troubleshooting Practice

1. The artifact is in leads **I, III,** and **aVL.** Corrective action is to check for and reattach or reconnect loose or disconnected electrodes or lead wires on the **left arm.** If an electrode patch is loose or missing, put on a new patch. *Never put a used patch back on. It will not stick well enough to ensure good impulse transmission.* How do we know the problem is on the left arm? Refer to Figure 8-7. What is the common limb shared by all these leads? I connects right arm and left arm. III connects left arm and left leg. aVL involves left arm only. The common limb is the left arm. Direct corrective efforts there.

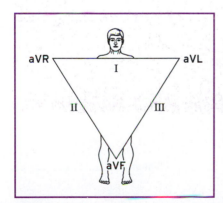

Figure 8-7 Leads.

2. The artifact is in leads **II, III,** and **aVF.** Corrective action is to check the **left leg** for loose or disconnected electrodes or lead wires and to reattach/reconnect them as necessary. What is the common limb? II connects right arm and left leg. III connects left arm and left leg. aVF involves left leg only. The common limb is the left leg.

3. The artifact is in leads **I, II,** and **aVR.** Corrective action is to check the **right arm** for loose or disconnected electrodes or lead wires and to reat-

tach/reconnect them as necessary. What is the common limb? I connects right arm and left arm. II connects right arm and left leg. III involves right arm only. The common limb is the right arm.

Telemetry Monitoring

Most hospitals have a floor dedicated to the care of patients on telemetry, which you recall is remote cardiac monitoring. Most or all of the patients on this floor are on telemetry, and the nurse or technician monitoring the telemetry desk is responsible for watching those patients' rhythms.

Patients on telemetry are often *ambulatory,* meaning they are able to get out of bed and walk around. As a result, artifact is not uncommon. The altered lead placement helps—you'll recall the 3-lead or 5-lead wires used in telemetry monitoring are all on the chest or abdomen instead of the arms and legs as with a 12-lead EKG—but artifact still occurs. Troubleshoot artifact the same way as with a 12-lead EKG.

Telemetry Monitoring Analysis

Date _____

Rate
_____
PR _____
QRS _____
QT _____
Analysis _____ Signature _____

Date _____

Rate
_____
PR _____
QRS _____
QT _____
Analysis _____ Signature _____

Date _____

Rate
_____
PR _____
QRS _____
QT _____
Analysis _____ Signature _____

Figure 8-8 Sample telemetry monitoring sheet.

Rhythm strips become part of the patient's permanent medical record, as do 12-lead EKGs. Unlike 12-lead EKGs, however, rhythm strips are small and must be mounted onto a standard-size page for inclusion in the record. The **telemetry monitoring sheet** is a special form for mounting and interpreting these rhythm strips. See a sample telemetry sheet, Figure 8-8. At the top of the form is a space for the patient's name and other identifying information.

Rhythm strips are mounted onto their slots on the form, usually by taping them from behind with double-sided tape. If tape touches the front of the strip, the rhythm beneath the tape will fade and become unreadable.

Each rhythm strip is examined for heart rate, intervals, and rhythm identification. If there are alarm limits set to alert the technician that the heart rate or rhythm has violated those settings, those alarm limits are documented as well. Most monitors are equipped with alarm limits that can be set by the technician.

Rhythm strips are obtained at intervals that vary from institution to institution, but are typically once every four to eight hours, and also in between if rhythm or rate changes occur. The goal is to provide a representative sample of the patient's rhythms throughout the day. This will enable the physician to assess the effect of treatment and to diagnose arrhythmias (rhythm abnormalities). For example, a patient is being treated with medication to slow down her very rapid heart rate. Yesterday, when the medication was started, her heart rate was 145. Today, four doses later, her heart rate is 122. Telemetry has documented that the treatment is working.

Practice Quiz

1. What is the function of the EKG machine? _____
   _____

2. Normal chart speed for running a 12-lead EKG is _____ millimeters per second.

3. What does the sensitivity control do? _____
   _____

4. How much should the stylus be deflected when 1 millivolt of electricity is thrown into the system? _____

5. Define *macroshock.* _____
   _____

6. Define *microshock.* _____
   _____

7. The first anatomic landmark to look for when placing electrodes is the _____

8. Name the four kinds of artifact. _____
   _____
   _____
   _____

9. If there is artifact in leads I, aVR, and II, toward which limb would you direct your troubleshooting efforts? _____

10. If there's artifact in II, III, and aVF, toward which limb would you direct your troubleshooting efforts? _____

Practice Quiz Answers

1. The function of the EKG machine is to **print out a representation of the electrical signals generated by the heart.**

2. Normal chart speed for running a 12-lead EKG is **25** millimeters per second.

3. The sensitivity control **adjusts the height of the waves and complexes.**

4. When 1 millivolt of electricity is thrown into the EKG machine's system, the stylus should be deflected **10 millimeters.**

5. Macroshock **is a high-voltage electrical shock that results from inadequate grounding of electrical equipment.**

6. Microshock is **a lower voltage shock that involves a conduit directly into the patient, such as a pacemaker.**

7. The first anatomic landmark to look for when placing electrodes is the **clavicle on the patient's right side.**

8. The four kinds of artifact are **somatic tremors, baseline sway, 60-cycle interference,** and **broken recording.**

9. If there is artifact in I, aVR, and II, troubleshooting efforts should be directed toward the **right arm.**

10. If there is artifact in II, III, and aVF, troubleshooting efforts should be directed toward the **left foot.**

Rhythm Regularity

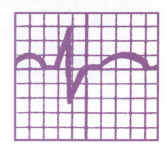

Chapter 9 Objectives

Upon completion of this chapter, the student will be able to:

- Determine the type of regularity on a variety of rhythm strips.
- Explain how to determine *atrial* versus *ventricular regularity.*
- Explain how to differentiate between the different types of regularity.

Chapter 9 Outline

Chapter 9 Glossary

R-R interval: The distance between consecutive QRS complexes.

Introduction

Rhythm regularity is concerned with the constancy of the QRS complexes. Though we can also determine **atrial regularity** by examining constancy of P waves, this chapter focuses on regularity of the QRS complexes. Why is regularity important? It can help pinpoint the type of rhythm we're interpreting. Some rhythms are quite regular, whereas others are completely unpredictable. To determine the regularity of a rhythm, compare the **R-R intervals** (the distance between consecutive QRS complexes). To compare R-Rs, count the number of little blocks between QRS complexes.

Regularity Types

There are three basic types of regularity:

1. **Regular.** Regular rhythms are those in which the R-R intervals vary by only one or two little blocks. In regular rhythms, the QRS complexes

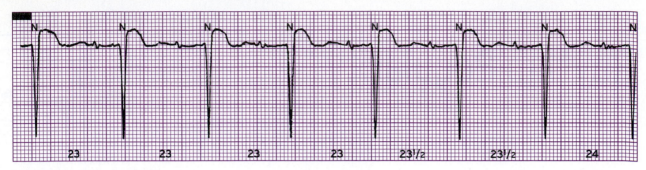

Figure 9-1 Regular rhythm.

usually look alike. Imagine these regular R-Rs as the ticking of a clock. In Figure 9-1, the R-R intervals are all 23 to 24 little blocks apart. The rhythm is regular.

2. **Regular but interrupted.** This is a regular rhythm that is interrupted by either premature beats or pauses. At first glance, these rhythms look irregular, but closer inspection reveals that only one or two beats, or a burst of several beats, make them look irregular, and that the rest of the R-R intervals are constant. The beats that interrupt this otherwise regular rhythm may look the same as the surrounding regular beats or may look quite different.

In Figure 9-2, the rhythm is regular until the sixth QRS pops in prematurely. *Premature beats* are those that arrive early, before the next normal beat is due. Typically, after a premature beat, there is a short pause, then the regular rhythm resumes. That's what happened on this strip. The R-Rs are 15 to 16 little blocks apart except where beat number 6 popped in. Think of premature beats as hiccups. Imagine you're breathing normally and suddenly you hiccup. This hiccup pops in between your normal breaths and temporarily disturbs the regularity of your breathing pattern. Afterward, your breathing returns to normal.

In Figure 9-3, the rhythm is regular until a sudden pause temporarily disturbs the regularity of the rhythm. Before and after the pause, the R-R intervals are constant—25 to 26 little blocks apart. During the pause, the R-R is 43 little blocks. Imagine these pauses are like a sudden power outage. Say you've got an electric clock ticking regularly, and suddenly, the power goes out for a few seconds, then comes back on. The outage temporarily disturbs the clock's otherwise normal, regular ticking pattern.

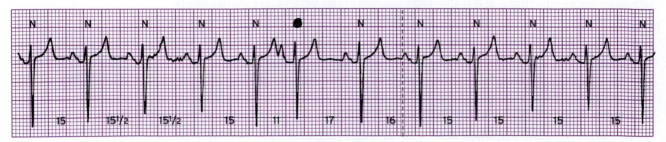

Figure 9-2 Regular rhythm interrupted by a premature beat.

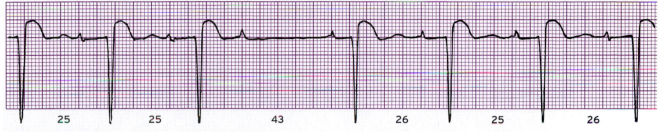

Figure 9-3   Regular rhythm interrupted by a pause.

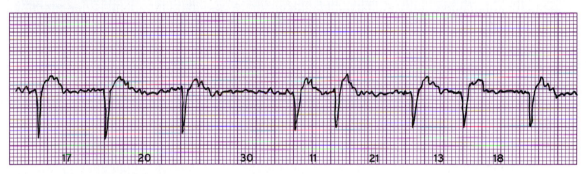

Figure 9-4   Irregular rhythm.

3. **Irregular.** Irregular rhythms are those in which the R-R intervals vary, not just because of premature beats or pauses, but because the rhythm is intrinsically irregular. R-R intervals will vary throughout the strip. Imagine these varying R-Rs as the interval of time between rain showers. Maybe it rains once a week for two weeks in a row, then it rains again in three weeks, then after a month passes, then after a week and a half, then two months. The pattern is one of irregularity—it happens when it happens.

In Figure 9-4, the R-R intervals are all over the place. Some QRS complexes are close together, others are farther apart. There is no sudden change, no regular pattern interrupted by a premature beat or pause. From beat to beat, the R-Rs vary. This is an intrinsically irregular rhythm. Do you see the difference between this rhythm and the strips of the regular but interrupted rhythms?

Can irregular rhythms ever be interrupted by premature beats or pauses? Yes, they can, but these interruptions only serve to make the underlying rhythm look even more irregular. Nothing is gained by adding this as another type of regularity.

Whenever you see a rhythm that looks irregular, look closely to make sure it's not a regular but interrupted rhythm.

Practice Strips: Regularity of Rhythms

For each of these strips, determine if it is regular, regular but interrupted, or irregular.

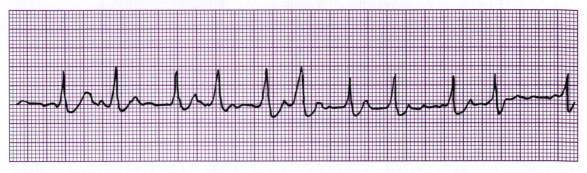

1. Answer _____

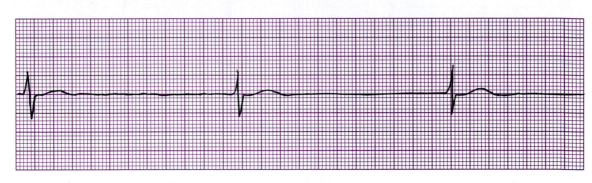

2. Answer _____

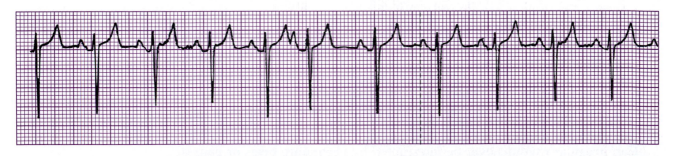

3. Answer _____

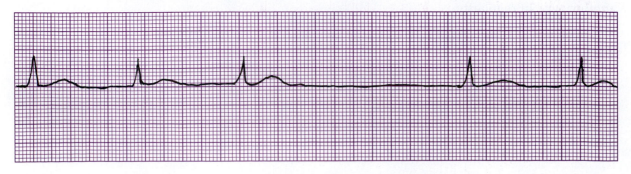

4. Answer _____

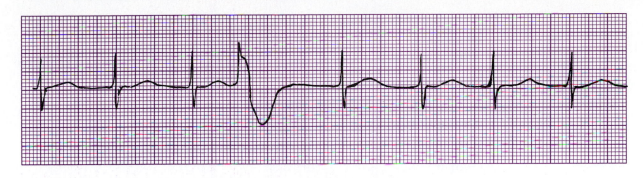

5. Answer _____

Answers to Regularity Practice Strips

1. **Irregular.** The R-R intervals are all over the place, with no hint of regularity.

2. **Regular.** The R-R intervals are all about 56 little blocks.

3. **Regular but interrupted.** This is the strip shown a few pages ago as an example of regular but interrupted rhythms. Look back if you don't recognize it.

4. **Regular but interrupted.** The R-R intervals are all 28 to 29 blocks except for the long pause that interrupts this otherwise regular rhythm.

5. **Regular but interrupted.** Again, the R-R intervals are regular before and after the premature beat (and the expected short pause after it).

Practice Quiz

1. Name the three types of regularity. _____

   _____

   _____

2. A rhythm with R-R intervals that vary throughout the strip is a _____ rhythm.

3. A rhythm that is regular except for premature beats or pauses is a _____ _____ rhythm.

4. A rhythm in which the R-R intervals vary by only one or two little blocks is a _____ rhythm.

5. Define R-R interval. _____

   _____

Practice Quiz Answers

1. The three types of regularity are **regular, regular but interrupted,** and **irregular.**

2. A rhythm with R-R intervals that vary throughout the strip is an **irregular** rhythm.

3. A rhythm that is regular except for premature beats or pauses is a **regular but interrupted** rhythm.

4. A rhythm in which the R-R intervals vary by only one or two little blocks is a **regular** rhythm.

5. R-R interval is defined as **the distance between two consecutive QRS complexes.**

Calculating Heart Rate

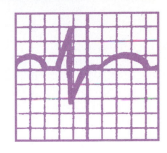

Chapter 10 Objectives

Upon completion of this chapter, the student will be able to:

- Calculate the heart rate on a variety of strips, using the different methods.
- Define *heart rate.*
- Tell how to calculate atrial rate.
- Tell what kind of heart rate to calculate for the different types of rhythm regularity.

Chapter 10 Outline

I.   Introduction
II. Methods of calculating heart rate
     A. The 6-second strip method, big block method, memory method, little block method
III. Summary of kinds of heart rate to calculate
IV. Practice strips: calculating heart rate
V.   Answers to calculating heart rate practice
VI. Practice quiz
VII. Practice quiz answers

Chapter 10 Glossary

Atrial rate: The number of P waves or other atrial waves per minute.

Heart rate: The number of QRS complexes per minute. It's the same as ventricular rate.

Mean rate: Average heart rate over one minute.

Ventricular rate: The number of QRS complexes per minute. Same as heart rate.

Introduction

Calculating heart rate involves counting the number of QRS complexes in one minute and is recorded in **beats per minute.** Heart rate is the same as **ventricular rate.** We can also determine the **atrial rate** by counting P waves, but the bottom line is this: When we calculate heart rate, we count

QRS complexes. Though the most accurate way to determine the heart rate would be to run a minute-long rhythm strip and count every QRS complex, this is extremely time-consuming and impractical. Imagine calculating the heart rate of 40 patients on a telemetry floor. It would take close to an hour—obviously not the most practical use of time. So we use other methods to calculate heart rate, and these methods all use a 6- or 12-second rhythm strip and the following premise: If the heart rate stays for the full minute as it is right now, at the end of that minute the heart rate will be so-and-so. That's a big leap of faith, since the second we print out our rhythm strip, the heart rate could change drastically from what it is on our rhythm strip. Nevertheless, the following methods have been used for years and are the next best thing to counting the whole minute's worth of QRS complexes.

Methods for Calculating Heart Rate

• **The 6-second strip method.** This is the least accurate of all the methods. Though it is considered by many experts to be the method of choice for irregular rhythms, it does not give much information and can be misleading. Using this method, count the number of QRS complexes on a 6-second rhythm strip and multiply by 10. This tells the **mean rate,** or average rate. If there are 3 QRS complexes on a 6-second strip, for example, the rate would be 30 beats per minute. (If there are 3 QRS complexes in 6 seconds, there would be 30 in 60 seconds, or 1 minute.) See Figure 10-1.

In Figure 10-1, both strips have 5 QRS complexes in 6 seconds, so both have a mean rate of 50. Though both rhythms are irregular, with QRS complexes unevenly spaced throughout the strip, strip B is much more irregular than strip A. In fact, the heart rate in strip A varies only from a rate of 40 to

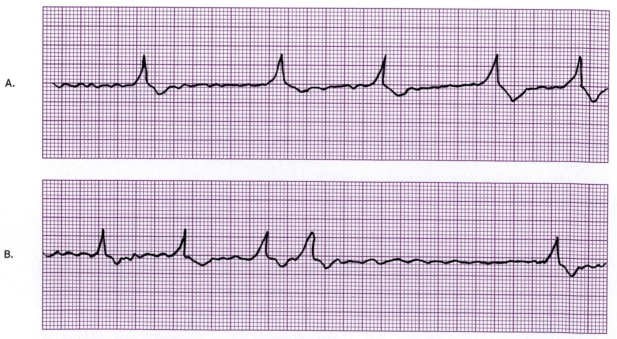

A.

B.

Figure 10-1 Two rhythms, both with mean rate of 50.

a rate of 68 beats per minute (you'll learn that soon), whereas strip B varies from a rate of 23 to 137 beats per minute. Obviously, strip B has wild heart rate swings. Saying the mean rate is 50 doesn't really provide adequate information. Since treatment for rhythm disturbances depends in large part on the heart rate, it makes more sense to provide a *range* of heart rates from the slowest to the fastest, in addition to the mean rate. If a person is being treated with medication to slow down a fast heart rate, for example, it is important to know how slow and how fast the heart rate is in order to determine the effectiveness of treatment. A mean rate alone simply does not provide this information—the heart rate range does. The heart rate range is calculated using one of the other methods. Bottom line: The mean heart rate, as determined using the 6-second strip method, should only be used along with the heart rate range. It is not adequate by itself.

- **The big block method.** If the rhythm is regular, meaning the QRS complexes are evenly spaced, count the number of big blocks between the same point in any two successive QRS complexes (usually R wave to R wave) and divide into 300, since there are 300 big blocks in one minute. If the rhythm is irregular, find the two QRS complexes that are the closest together (this will tell the fastest heart rate) and then the two that are the farthest apart (for the slowest heart rate), and count the number of big blocks between each pair. Divide each into 300. This will provide the heart rate range. For the big block method, it's easiest if you start with a QRS that falls on a dark line. So, for example, if there are three big blocks between QRS complexes, the heart rate would be 300 ÷ 3 = 100. If, when counting the big blocks, there are little blocks left over, count each little block as 0.2 and add this to the number of big blocks, then divide into 300. Where does this 0.2 come from? Each little block is one-fifth a big block, and one-fifth is the same as 0.2 when entered into your calculator. See Figure 10-2.

In Figure 10-2(a), all the QRS complexes are regular and all start on a dark line, so that makes it easy. There are two full blocks between QRS complexes, so 300 ÷ 2 = 150. The heart rate is 150 beats per minute. In Figure 10-2(b), the rhythm is irregular, so you need to indicate the heart rate range, slowest to fastest, along with the mean rate. QRS numbers 4 and 5 are the farthest apart, so we calculate the heart rate there to find the slowest heart rate. But wait. QRS numbers 4 and 5 don't start on a dark line. What do we do now? Simple. QRS number 4 starts on the second line inside a big block; do you see that? Simply go to the next block's second line (always go to the right) and that's one big block's worth. From then on, each block's second line would be another block's worth. From QRS number 4 to QRS number 5 we have eight full big blocks and two little blocks. So our calculation is 300 ÷ 8.4 = 36. Remember, the two leftover little blocks are each worth 0.2, so since we have two little blocks left over, that's 0.4 added to the number of big blocks, all divided into 300. So the slowest heart rate on this strip is 36. What's the fastest? QRS numbers 3 and 4 are the closest together, so they will indicate the fastest heart rate. QRS number 3 falls on a dark line. There are three big blocks and two little blocks between QRS numbers 3 and 4.

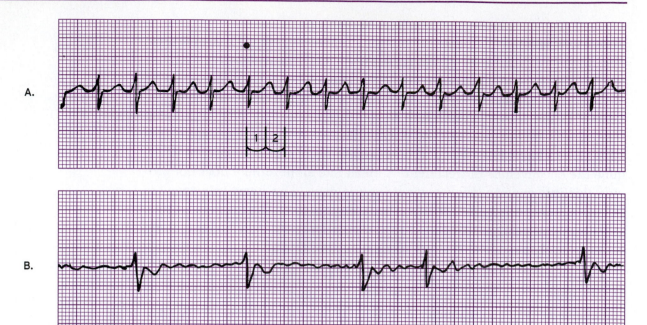

Figure 10-2 Big block method with (a) regular rhythm and (b) irregular rhythm.

The calculation is $300 \div 3.4 = 88$. Thus the heart rate range is 36 to 88, with a mean rate of 50.

- **The memory method.** This is simply the big block method with the math already done for you. This is the fastest method and is widely used in hospitals and other clinical areas. See Table 10-1. The number of big blocks between QRS complexes is divided into 300 to arrive at the answer.

Memorize the sequence 300–150–100–75–60–50–43–37–33–30. Using this memory method, what would the heart rate be if there were five big blocks between QRS complexes? One big block would be 300, two would be 150, three would be 100, four would be 75, and five would be 60. So the heart rate would be 60. *Memorize this sequence of numbers!* It will save you lots of time.

- **The little block method.** In this method, count the number of little blocks between QRS complexes and divide into 1,500, since there are

Table 10-1 Memory Method of Calculating Heart Rate

NUMBER OF BIG BLOCKS BETWEEN QRS	HEART RATE	NUMBER OF BIG BLOCKS BETWEEN QRS	HEART RATE
1	300	6	50
2	150	7	43
3	100	8	37
4	75	9	33
5	60	10	30

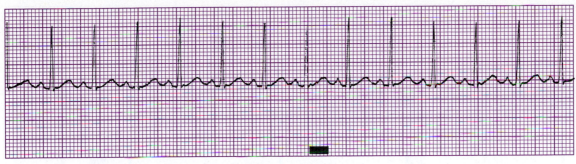

Figure 10-3 Little block method of calculating heart rate.

1,500 little blocks in one minute. By now you're thinking, "You've got to be kidding! Count those tiny blocks?!" (You may well be in bifocals by the end of this chapter.) Actually, it's not that bad. Remember each big block is made up of five little blocks. Simply count each big block as five and the leftover little blocks as one. See Figure 10-3.

In Figure 10-3, there are 11 little blocks between QRS complexes, so the calculation is 1,500 ÷ 11 = 137. You can also use this method to calculate the heart rate range in irregular rhythms.

Types of Heart Rate to Calculate

Heart rate calculation is regularity-based. The kind of heart rate you calculate will depend on the rhythm's regularity.

- **For regular rhythms,** calculate the heart rate by choosing any two successive QRS complexes and using either the big block or the little block method.

- **For irregular rhythms,** calculate the mean rate by using the 6-second strip method, then calculate the heart rate range using either the big block or the little block method.

- **For rhythms that are regular but interrupted by premature beats,** ignore the premature beats and calculate the heart rate, using either the big block or little block method, on an uninterrupted part of the strip. Premature beats do not impact the heart rate much, as they are typically followed by a short pause that at least partially, if not completely, makes up for the prematurity of the beat. See Figure 10-4.

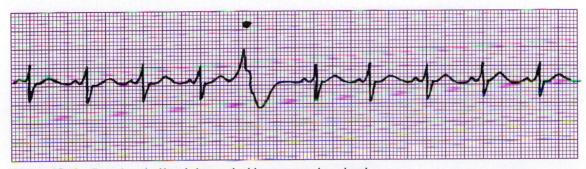

Figure 10-4 Regular rhythm interrupted by a premature beat.

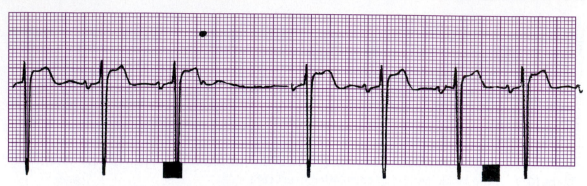

Figure 10-5 Regular rhythm interrupted by a pause.

In Figure 10-4, the fifth QRS is a premature beat. Ignore this premature beat for purposes of heart rate calculation. The heart rate is 100.

- **For rhythms that are regular but interrupted by pauses,** calculate the heart rate range slowest to fastest, along with the mean rate. Since pauses can be very lengthy, they can greatly impact the heart rate, so it's important to take them into account when calculating heart rate. See Figure 10-5.

In Figure 10-5, the regular rhythm is interrupted by a pause. Here the mean rate is 70, since there are 7 QRS complexes on this 6-second strip. There are 34 little blocks between the third and fourth QRS complexes, giving a rate of 44. There are 20 little blocks between the remainder of QRS complexes, for a heart rate of 75. The heart rate range is 44 to 75.

To sum up, see Table 10-2.

Calculating heart rate is a basic skill you will use throughout this book, and indeed throughout your work with EKGs. With practice, you will become expert at it. Now let's get to the practice.

Table 10-2 Kind of Heart Rate to Calculate for Different Types of Regularity

RHYTHM REGULARITY	KIND OF HEART RATE TO CALCULATE
Regular	One heart rate
Irregular	Range slowest to fastest, plus mean rate
Regular but interrupted by premature beats	One heart rate (ignoring premature beats)
Regular but interrupted by pauses	Range slowest to fastest, plus mean rate

Practice Strips: Calculating Heart Rate

Calculate the heart rate on these strips.

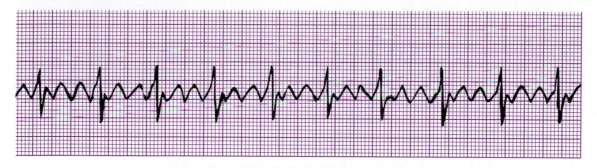

1. Heart rate _____

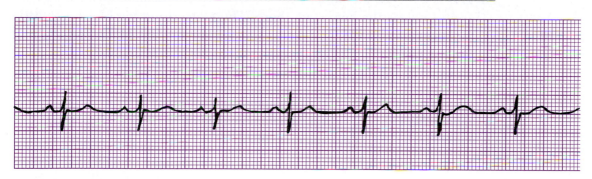

2. Heart rate _____

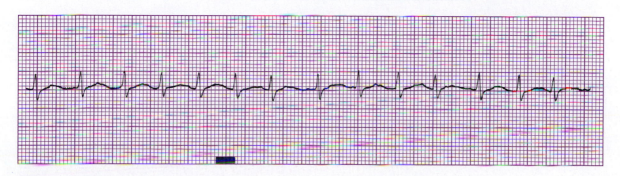

3. Heart rate _____

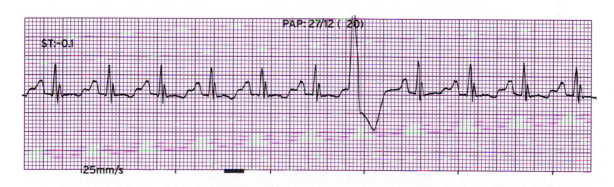

4. Heart rate _____

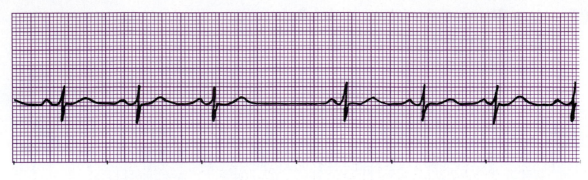

5. Heart rate _____

Answers to Calculating Heart Rate Practice

1. This is a regular rhythm, so choose any two consecutive QRS complexes and calculate the heart rate there. There are three big blocks (15 little blocks) between QRSs. Divide 300 ÷ 3 for the big block method and 1,500 ÷ 15 for the little block method. The heart rate is **100.**

2. Another regular rhythm. The heart rate is **75.**

3. This is a regular rhythm interrupted by a premature beat. We therefore ignore the premature beat for the purposes of heart rate calculation. The heart rate is **107,** as there are 14 little blocks between QRS complexes.

4. Though at first glance this rhythm appears regular, closer examination reveals that the R-R intervals vary from 9½ to 12½ little blocks apart. Since it is an irregular rhythm, we need the heart rate range along with the mean rate. The range is **about 120 to 155, with a mean rate of 140.**

5. This is a regular rhythm interrupted by a pause, so we calculate the range and the mean rate. There are 35 little blocks during the pause, and 20 little blocks between the regular QRS complexes. The heart rate range is therefore **43 to 75, with a mean rate of 70.**

Practice Quiz

1. Name the four methods for calculating heart rate. _____

   _____

   _____

   _____

2. The least accurate method of calculating heart rate is the _____

3. When using the big block method, each leftover little block counts as_____

4. When using the little block method, count the number of little blocks between QRS complexes and divide into _____

5. Write the sequence of the memory method. _____

   _____

6. With regular rhythms interrupted by premature beats, how is the heart rate calculated? _____

Practice Quiz Answers

1. The four methods for calculating heart rate are the **6-second strip method,** the **big block method,** the **little block method,** and the **memory method.**

2. The least accurate method of calculating heart rate is the **6-second strip method.**

3. When using the big block method, each leftover little block counts as **0.2.**

4. When using the little block method, count the number of little blocks between QRS complexes and divide into **1,500.**

5. The memory method is **300–150–100–75–60–50–43–37–33–30.**

6. With regular rhythms interrupted by premature beats, the heart rate is calculated by **ignoring the premature beat and calculating the heart rate on an uninterrupted portion of the strip.**

Rhythm Strip Analysis Tools

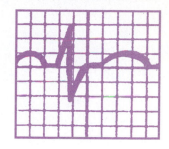

Chapter 11 Objectives

Upon completion of this chapter, the student will be able to:

- Use the five steps to correctly identify a variety of rhythms.
- Use the algorithms to correctly identify rhythms from each type (sinus, sinus interruptions, atrial, junctional, ventricular, and AV blocks).
- Use the rhythm summary sheets to find the rhythm criteria all in one place.
- Use the pictorial review to differentiate between various rhythms.

Chapter 11 Outline

I.   Introduction
II.   The five steps to rhythm interpretation
III. Algorithms for rhythm interpretation
      A. Main algorithm, sinus algorithm, sinus interruptions algorithm, atrial algorithm, junctional algorithm, ventricular algorithm, AV block algorithm
IV.   Rhythm summary sheets and pictorial review
V.   Rhythm regularity summary

Chapter 11 Glossary

Algorithm: Flowchart.

Arrhythmia: Literally means "absence of rhythm," but has become accepted to mean abnormal rhythm.

Dysrhythmia: Abnormal rhythm.

Introduction

When we analyze a rhythm strip, we are looking for pathology in the form of arrhythmias. Though the term **arrhythmia** actually means absence of rhythm, and **dysrhythmia** means abnormal rhythm, the two terms have become interchangeable over the years, and it is acceptable to use either term to refer to abnormal rhythms. This text will use the term *arrhythmia*, as that is the term most commonly used by healthcare providers.

Arrhythmias can originate in any of the heart's pacemakers. Some of these rhythms are benign, causing no problem, and others are lethal, killing almost instantly. It's important to know not just what rhythm the patient is in now, but what rhythm preceded it and what's normal for this particular patient. Every patient is an individual, and what is normal for one person may not be what the textbooks say is normal. Even so-called normal rhythms or heart rates can be cause for concern. For example, if a patient has a heart rate of 110 for two consecutive days, and it suddenly drops to 66, which is normal, it may be a sign of trouble—the patient may be at 66 on his way to 0. *Always look at the trend.* Only so much information can be obtained from a single rhythm strip. Comparing the present rhythm strip to previous ones paints a better picture of the patient's condition.

It's important to *treat the patient, not just the rhythm.* As a rule, any significant change in rhythm or heart rate should prompt an immediate assessment of the patient's condition. Two patients can have the same rhythm and heart rate, but differ drastically in their tolerance of it. If the patient has a rhythm you cannot immediately identify, but it's a change from previously, *check on the patient and come back to the strip later.* The patient's life may well depend on your prompt action.

This chapter will focus on rhythm interpretation tools—those valuable steps, **algorithms** (flowcharts), and summary sheets that will aid in differentiating one rhythm from another. The first tool, the five steps to rhythm interpretation, should be used whenever analyzing a strip. It will ask you to evaluate the criteria each rhythm meets, thus enabling you to interpret the rhythm. The algorithms section contains flowcharts that will, when used correctly, tell you exactly what the rhythm is. The rhythm summary sheets present a summary of all the rhythm criteria, along with a pictorial review, so you can turn to this section for a quick comparison of criteria. And finally, the rhythm regularity summary points out the type of regularity of each rhythm. For example, if you know the rhythm is irregular but aren't sure what rhythm it is, you can turn to this summary to determine which rhythms are irregular and which are not. This aids in the process of elimination and can illuminate the way if you're in the dark.

These tools should help in honing your rhythm interpretation skills. Do not, however, use them as an excuse not to learn each rhythm's criteria, which will be presented in upcoming chapters. Use them rather as an adjunct, a helpful source when you're stumped trying to identify a rhythm.

The Five Steps to Rhythm Interpretation

Ask the following questions for each rhythm strip:

1. Are there QRS complexes?
   - If yes, are they the same shape, or does the shape vary?
   - If no, skip to question 4.

2. Is the rhythm regular, regular but interrupted, or irregular?
   - Compare the R-R intervals.

3. What is the heart rate?
   - If the heart rate is greater than 100, the patient is said to have a **tachycardia.**
   - If the heart rate is less than 60, the patient has a **bradycardia.**

4. Are there P waves?
   - If so, what is their relationship to the QRS? In other words, are the Ps always in the same place relative to the QRS, or are the Ps in different places with each beat?
   - Are any Ps not followed by a QRS?
   - Are the Ps all the same shape, or does the shape vary?
   - Is the **P-P interval** (the distance between consecutive P waves) regular?

5. What are the PR and QRS intervals?
   - Are the intervals within normal limits, or are they too short or too long?
   - Are the intervals constant on the strip, or do they vary from beat to beat?

Algorithms for Rhythm Interpretation

In this and other chapters, you will see algorithms, or flowcharts, which are designed to help you identify rhythms or features on rhythm strips or 12-lead EKGs. In this chapter, there are seven algorithms: a main algorithm and six secondary algorithms (one for each type of rhythm—sinus, sinus interruptions, atrial, junctional, ventricular, and AV block).

Each algorithm consists of questions and answers, with arrows pointing the way to the next step. Your job is to answer the questions and follow the arrows to the final answer. Some of the algorithms are busy-looking and might cause uneasiness when first approaching them. Fear not. At most, you will have to answer only six or seven questions (and usually fewer) to find the final answer.

These algorithms will be a big help in rhythm interpretation. However, they are not foolproof. If you answer a question incorrectly, the algorithm will point you in the wrong direction. Also, like any set of rules, these are meant to be broken. There will undoubtedly be some rhythms that are not alluded to on the algorithms. Patients do not always have textbook rhythms, and as a result, their rhythms sometimes confound even the most experienced interpreter. Most basic rhythms, however, *should* be interpretable using these algorithms.

Eventually, as you become more comfortable with rhythm interpretation, you will not need these algorithms. They are just to get you started.

Main Algorithm for EKG Rhythm Interpretation

This algorithm is designed to point you to the secondary algorithms that will then pinpoint the rhythm. Here are some rules to get you started:

1. All matching upright P waves are sinus Ps until proven otherwise. Sinus rhythms have an atrial rate ≤160 at rest.

2. On rhythms with two different-shaped P waves, one of those Ps is *probably* sinus; on rhythms with three or more different-shaped Ps, one cannot be sure if *any* are sinus Ps.

Main Algorithm

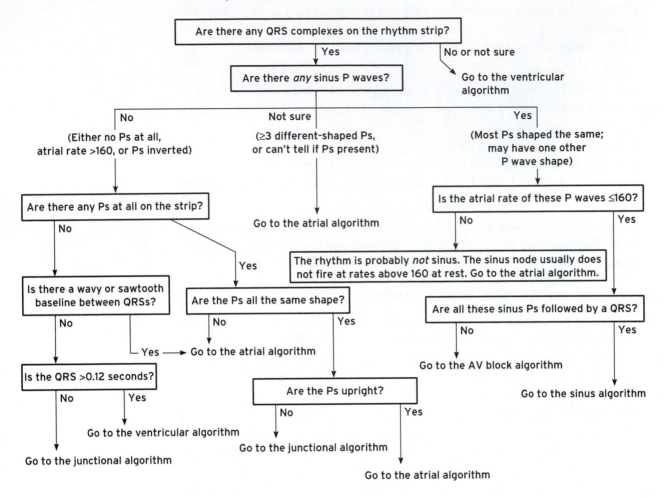

How to Use the Main Algorithm

First, you won't need this algorithm at all if you already know what kind of rhythm you're looking at (sinus, atrial, junctional, etc.). In that case, you'll go straight to the appropriate secondary algorithm. The main algorithm is most helpful when you don't know which secondary algorithm to go to.

OK, let's get started. The premise of the main algorithm is that, since most of the rhythms you will see in real life will be sinus rhythms, it makes sense to first see if the rhythm is sinus. Once that is ruled in or out, then rhythm interpretation can continue. All upright P waves shaped the same (matching) are considered to be sinus P waves until proven otherwise. What constitutes such proof? A heart rate greater than 160 with the patient at rest. Most authorities have adopted this figure as the upper limit of the sinus node at rest. See Figure 11-1.

In Figure 11-1, *are there any QRS complexes?* Yes. Follow the yes arrow to the next question.

Are there any sinus P waves? In other words, are there any matching upright P waves? Yes, in fact all the P waves look alike. So they are sinus P waves until proven otherwise. We answer yes to the first question and follow the arrow to the next question.

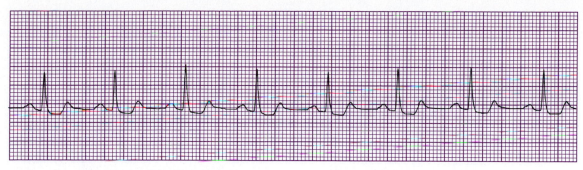

Figure 11-1 Rhythm for identification.

Is the atrial rate of these P waves less than or equal to 160? This is a double check. Remember—if the rate is greater than 160 with the patient at rest, those matching upright P waves are not sinus Ps. On our strip, the rate is about 75, so we answer yes to the question and follow the arrow.

Are all these sinus P waves followed by a QRS? Yes. We follow the arrow, and it tells us to go to the sinus algorithm. So we know the rhythm is a sinus rhythm of some sort, and we'll go to the sinus algorithm to find which of the sinus rhythms it is. Now see Figure 11-2.

Are there any QRS complexes on this strip? Yes. Follow the yes arrow to the next question.

Are there any sinus P waves on this strip? That's a good question. The P wave shapes keep changing. There are at least three different shapes. One of those shapes might be a sinus P, but we can't be sure, so we follow the not-sure arrow, which points us to the atrial algorithm. Obviously, the rhythm is not sinus—it's atrial of some sort.

One more. See Figure 11-3. *Are there any QRS complexes on this strip?* Yes. Follow the yes arrow.

Are there any sinus Ps? No, there are no Ps at all, so we follow the arrow to the next question.

Are there any Ps at all? We've already said no. Follow the arrow to the next question.

Is there a wavy or sawtooth baseline between QRS complexes? Yes, the baseline is wavy. The arrow directs us to go to the atrial algorithm. Are you getting a feel for this algorithm?

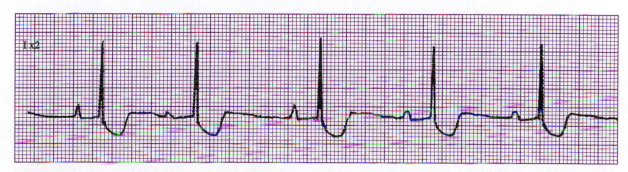

Figure 11-2 Second rhythm for identification.

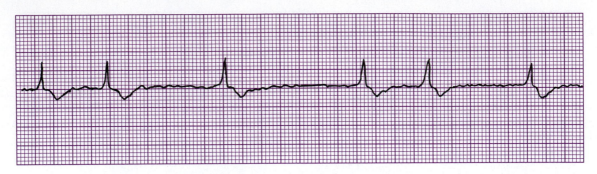

Figure 11-3 Third rhythm for identification.

Sinus Algorithm

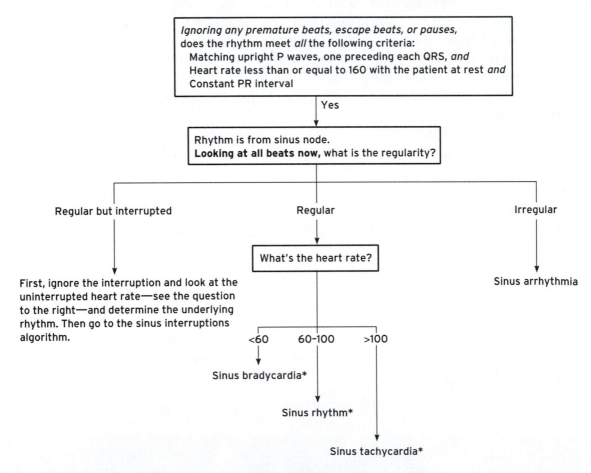

Ignoring any premature beats, escape beats, or pauses,
does the rhythm meet *all* the following criteria:
  Matching upright P waves, one preceding each QRS, *and*
  Heart rate less than or equal to 160 with the patient at rest *and*
  Constant PR interval

Yes

Rhythm is from sinus node.
Looking at all beats now, what is the regularity?

Regular but interrupted   Regular   Irregular

First, ignore the interruption and look at the uninterrupted heart rate—see the question to the right—and determine the underlying rhythm. Then go to the sinus interruptions algorithm.

What's the heart rate?

<60   60-100   >100

Sinus bradycardia*

Sinus rhythm*

Sinus tachycardia*

Sinus arrhythmia

* **If the PR interval is >0.20 s, there is an additional first-degree AV block. And if the QRS interval is ≥0.12 seconds, there is an additional bundle branch block.**

Sinus Interruptions Algorithm

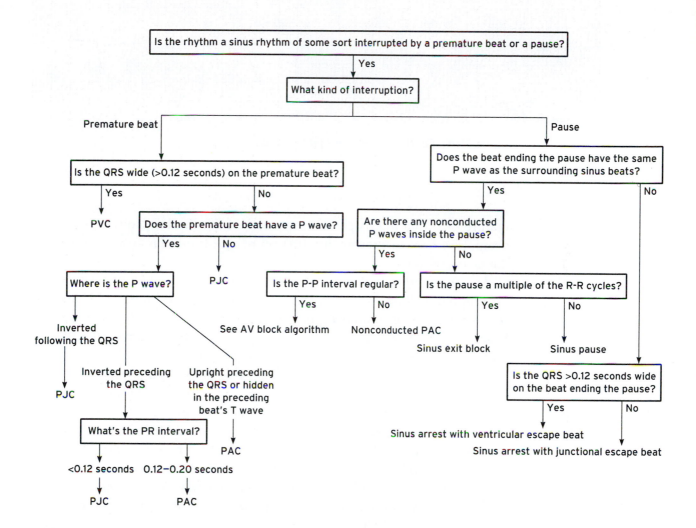

How to Use the Sinus and Sinus Interruptions Algorithms

These algorithms are not as complicated as they look. At most, you will have to answer only seven questions. Always start off with the sinus algorithm. Use the sinus interruptions algorithm only if directed to do so by the sinus algorithm. Refer to Figure 11-4.

Does the rhythm meet the criteria of matching upright P waves, one preceding each QRS complex, a heart rate less than or equal to 160 with the patient at rest, and a constant PR interval? Yes to all questions. On this strip, we have a pre-

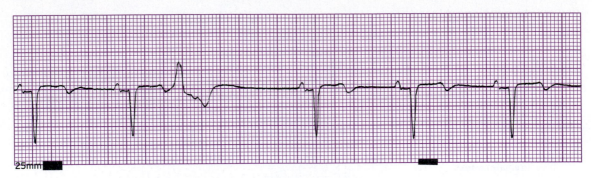

Figure 11-4 Fourth rhythm for identification.

mature beat that interrupts the regularity of the rhythm, so we ignore that premature beat to answer that first set of questions. Then we move on to the next question.

Looking at all beats now, what is the regularity? The rhythm is regular but interrupted. Follow the arrow. We are now told to determine the heart rate, so we calculate our uninterrupted heart rate to be about 58. Looking at the heart rates to the right, we see that our rhythm is sinus bradycardia. We are told to go now to the sinus interruptions algorithm.

Is the rhythm a sinus rhythm of some sort interrupted by a premature beat or a pause? Yes, it is a sinus bradycardia interrupted by a premature beat.

What kind of interruption? Follow the arrow that says "premature beat." Do you see the premature beat on the strip? It's the third QRS complex. See the normal R-R interval? Suddenly, the R-R is shorter here because of the premature beat. Follow the arrow to the next question.

Is the QRS wide (>0.12 seconds) on the premature beat? Yes, it's >0.12 seconds, so it is wide. We follow the arrow to the answer: PVC. Our rhythm is sinus bradycardia with a PVC.

Now see Figure 11-5. *Go back to the sinus algorithm again. Does Figure 11-5 meet the sinus rhythms criteria?* Yes. All the P waves match, there's one P preceding each QRS, the heart rate is less than 160, and the PR interval is constant.

What is the regularity? The rhythm is regular.

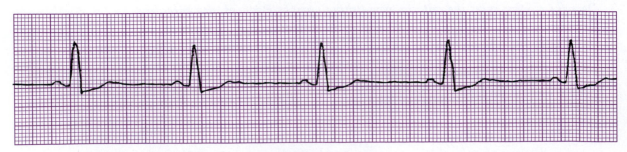

Figure 11-5 Fifth rhythm for identification.

What's the heart rate? The heart rate is about 45, so the arrow saying "<60" tells us the rhythm is *sinus bradycardia*. Note the asterisk after the term *sinus bradycardia*. The footnote tells us there is a first-degree AV block if the PR interval is >0.20 and a bundle branch block if the QRS interval is ≥0.12 seconds. The PR interval on this strip is about 0.16 seconds, so there is no first-degree AV block. The QRS interval is 0.12 to 0.14 seconds, however, so there *is* an additional bundle branch block (BBB). The rhythm is therefore sinus bradycardia with a bundle branch block. In Chapter 22, you will learn how to determine the type of BBB.

Atrial Algorithm

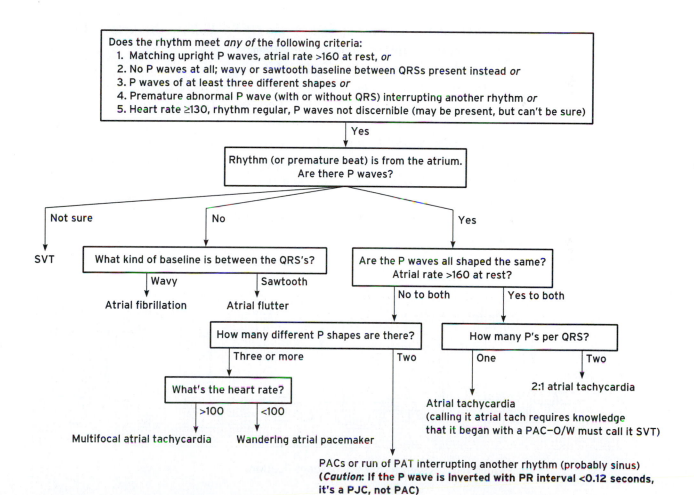

How to Use the Atrial Algorithm

Refer to Figure 11-6. *Does the rhythm meet the criteria?* There are several options for atrial criteria. This rhythm meets criterion 2—no P waves at all; wavy or sawtooth baseline between the QRS complexes present instead. So we follow the arrow to the next question.

Are there P waves? No, none at all. Follow the no arrow to the next question.

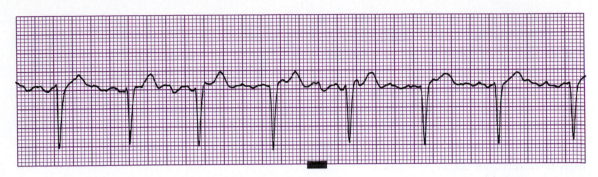

Figure 11-6 Sixth rhythm for identification.

What kind of baseline is between the QRSs? Follow the arrow that says "wavy," and the answer is *atrial fibrillation*.

Let's do another one. See Figure 11-7.

Does the rhythm meet the criteria? Yes. Here we have three different-shaped P waves, meeting the third criterion. Let's go to the next question.

Are there P waves? Yes. Follow the arrow.

Are all Ps shaped the same? Atrial rate greater than 160 at rest? No to both questions. There are three different P wave shapes, and the atrial rate is anywhere from 48 to 60. Follow the no arrow.

How many different P wave shapes are there? Three. Follow the arrow.

What's the heart rate? The heart rate is <100. The rhythm is *wandering atrial pacemaker*.

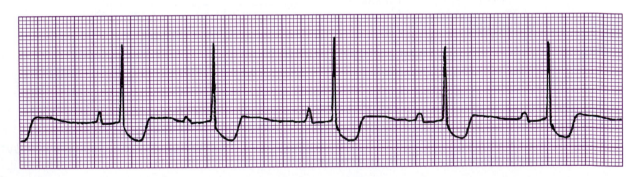

Figure 11-7 Seventh rhythm for identification.

Junctional Algorithm

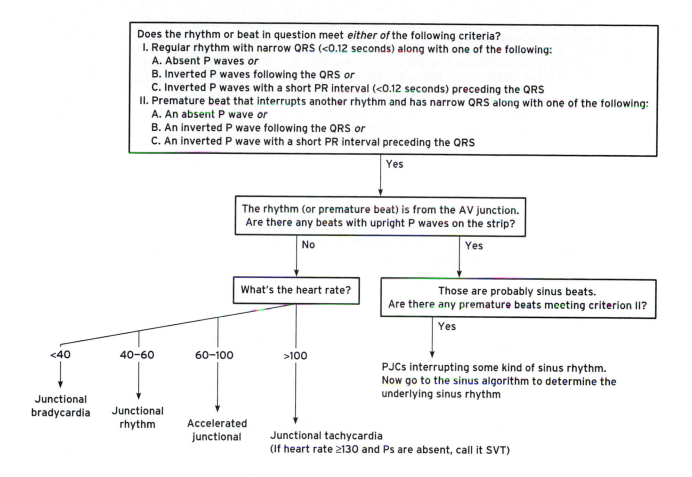

Does the rhythm or beat in question meet *either of* the following criteria?
  I. Regular rhythm with narrow QRS (<0.12 seconds) along with one of the following:
    A. Absent P waves *or*
    B. Inverted P waves following the QRS *or*
    C. Inverted P waves with a short PR interval (<0.12 seconds) preceding the QRS
  II. Premature beat that interrupts another rhythm and has narrow QRS along with one of the following:
    A. An absent P wave *or*
    B. An inverted P wave following the QRS *or*
    C. An inverted P wave with a short PR interval preceding the QRS

Yes

The rhythm (or premature beat) is from the AV junction.
Are there any beats with upright P waves on the strip?

No — What's the heart rate?

Yes — Those are probably sinus beats.
Are there any premature beats meeting criterion II?

Yes

PJCs interrupting some kind of sinus rhythm.
Now go to the sinus algorithm to determine the underlying sinus rhythm

<40 → Junctional bradycardia
40–60 → Junctional rhythm
60–100 → Accelerated junctional
>100 → Junctional tachycardia
(If heart rate ≥130 and Ps are absent, call it SVT)

How to Use the Junctional Algorithm

Refer to Figure 11-8. *Does the rhythm meet the criteria?* Yes. It meets criterion number I(A). The QRS is narrow, the rhythm is regular, and there are no P waves. Follow the arrow to the next question.

Are there any beats with upright P waves on the strip? No. There are no Ps at all. Follow the no arrow to the next question.

What's the heart rate? The heart rate is around 37, so the rhythm is *junctional bradycardia*.

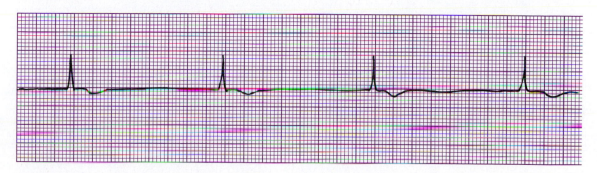

Figure 11-8 Eighth rhythm for identification.

Ventricular Algorithm

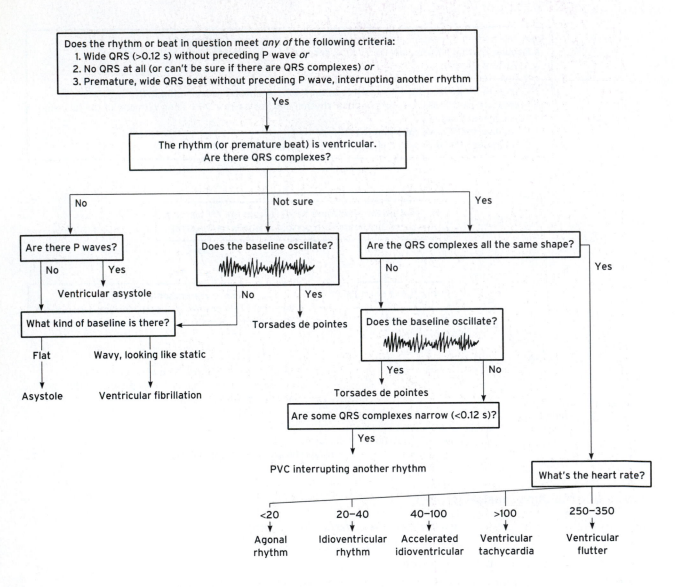

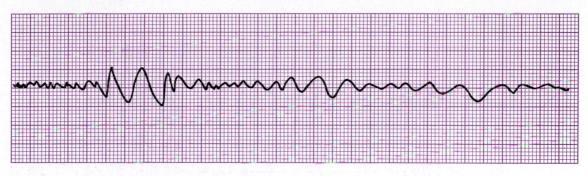

Figure 11-9   Ninth rhythm for identification.

How to Use the Ventricular Algorithm

Refer to Figure 11-9. *Does the rhythm meet the criteria?* Yes. Of the three criteria, this rhythm meets the second one–there are no QRS complexes at all. Go to the next question.

Are there QRS complexes? No, we've already said that. Follow the no arrow to the next question.

Are there P waves? No, there are no P waves at all. Follow the arrow.

What kind of baseline is there? The baseline is wavy, looking like static. The arrow points us to the answer–*ventricular fibrillation*.

Let's do another one. See Figure 11-10.

Does it meet the criteria? Yes, it meets criterion 1. The QRS is wide and there are no preceding P waves. Follow the arrow to the next question.

Are there QRS complexes? Yes. Follow the yes arrow.

Are the QRS complexes all the same shape? Yes. Follow the arrow.

What's the heart rate? The heart rate is about 167, so we follow the arrow labeled ">100" to our answer–*ventricular tachycardia*.

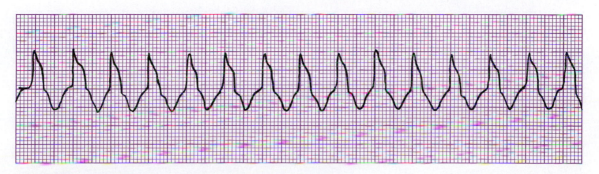

Figure 11-10   Tenth rhythm for identification.

AV Block Algorithm

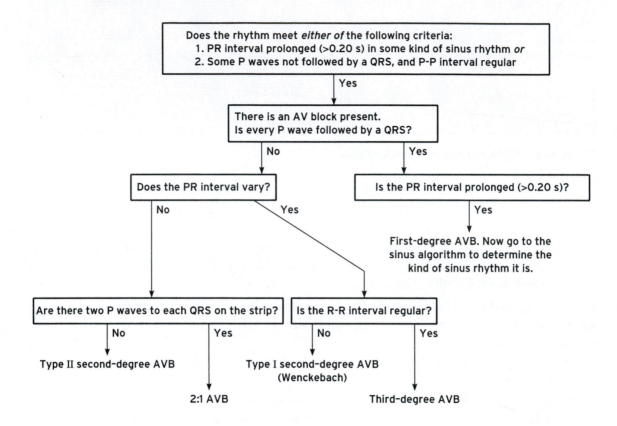

How to Use the AV Block Algorithm

See Figure 11-11. *Does the rhythm meet the criteria?* Yes, it meets the second of the criteria. There are some Ps not followed by a QRS, and the P-P interval is regular.

Is every P followed by a QRS? We've already said no to that, so follow the no arrow.

Does the PR interval vary? Yes. Note that some PRs are very short and others longer. To compare the PR intervals, look only at the P wave directly preceding a QRS. The nonconducted P waves will not have a PR interval.

Is the R-R interval regular? Yes. Follow the arrow to the answer—*third-degree AV block.*

Let's do another one. Refer to Figure 11-12.

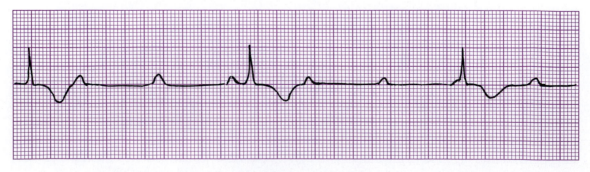

Figure 11-11 Eleventh rhythm for identification.

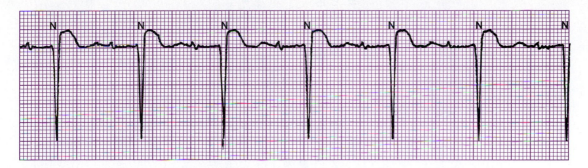

Figure 11-12   Twelfth rhythm for identification.

Does this rhythm meet the criteria? Yes, it meets the first criterion. All the P waves are followed by a QRS, and the PR interval is prolonged (>0.20 s). Go to the next question.

Is every P followed by a QRS? Yes. Go to the next question.

Is the PR interval prolonged (>0.20 s)? Yes. Follow the yes arrow to our answer—*first-degree AV block.* Now go to the sinus algorithm to see what the underlying rhythm is. A first-degree block is not in itself a rhythm—it is an extra feature added onto the rhythm.

Rhythm Summary Sheets

Rhythm Summary: Sinus Rhythms

	RATE	REGULARITY	P WAVE	PR INTERVAL	QRS INTERVAL	CAUSE	ADVERSE EFFECTS	TREATMENT
Sinus rhythm	60-100	Regular	Upright, one per QRS, all shaped the same	0.12-0.20 Constant	<0.12 unless BBB	Normal	None	None
Sinus brady	<60	Regular	Upright, one per QRS, all shaped the same	0.12-0.20 Constant	<0.12 unless BBB	MI, vagal stimulation, hypoxia	None necessarily; maybe decreased cardiac output	Atropine if symptoms Consider O_2
Sinus tachycardia	101-160	Regular	Upright, one per QRS, all shaped the same	0.12-0.20 Constant	<0.12 unless BBB	SNS stimulation, MI, hypoxia, pulmonary embolus, CHF, thyroid storm, fever, vagal inhibition	Maybe none; maybe decreased cardiac output	Treat the cause Consider O_2 and beta blockers
Sinus arrhythmia	Varies ↑ with inspiration, ↓ with expiration	Irregular, R-R varies by ≥0.16 s	Upright, one per QRS, all shaped the same	0.12-0.20 Constant	<0.12 unless BBB	The breathing pattern	Usually none	Atropine if HR slow and symptoms

	RATE	REGULARITY	P WAVE	PR INTERVAL	QRS INTERVAL	CAUSE	ADVERSE EFFECTS	TREATMENT
Sinus arrest	Can occur at any rate	Regular but interrupted	Normal before the pause, different or absent after	Normal before pause, different or absent after	<0.12 unless BBB	Sinus node ischemia, hypoxia, digitoxicity, excessive vagal tone, medication side effects	Maybe none; maybe decreased cardiac output; lower pacemaker takes over after pause	Consider O$_2$; atropine or pacemaker if symptoms
Sinus pause	Can occur at any rate	Regular but interrupted	Normal before and after the pause, all shaped the same	0.12-0.20	<0.12 unless BBB	Sinus node ischemia, hypoxia, digitoxicity, excessive vagal tone	Same as sinus arrest; pause is not a multiple of R-R; sinus resumes after pause	Same as sinus arrest
Sinus exit block	Can occur at any rate	Regular but interrupted	Normal before and after the pause, all shaped the same	0.12-0.20	<0.12 unless BBB	Medication side effects, excessive vagal tone, hypoxia	Same as sinus arrest; pause is a multiple of R-R; Sinus resumes after pause	Same as sinus arrest
Sick sinus syndrome	Varies widely	Irregular	May or may not be present	Varies if present	Varies	Sinus node ischemia, hypoxia, digitoxicity	Decreased cardiac output	Pacemaker, other medications; consider O$_2$

Sinus Rhythms Pictorial Review

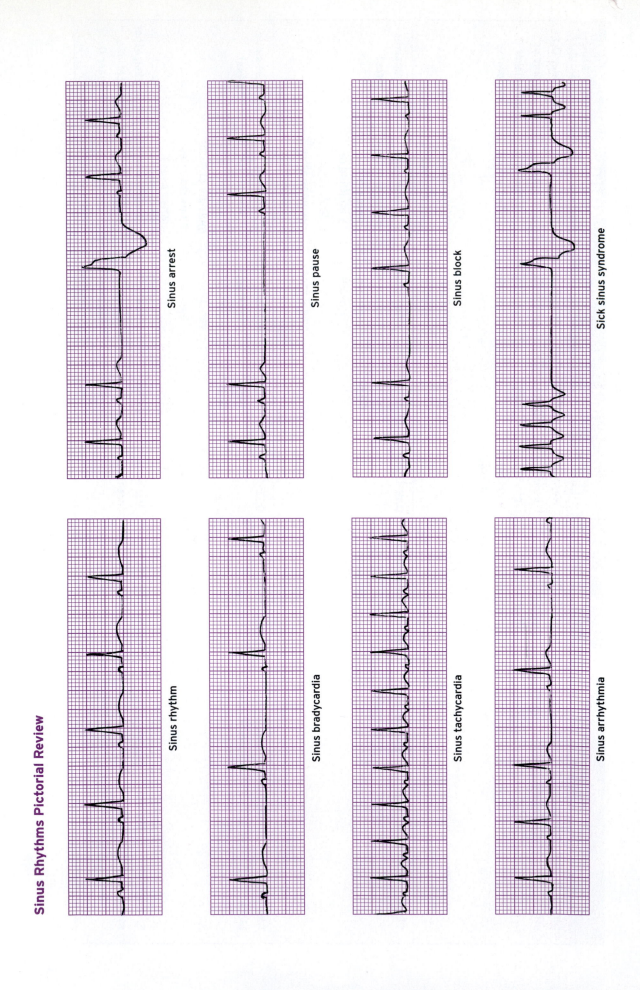

Sinus rhythm

Sinus bradycardia

Sinus tachycardia

Sinus arrhythmia

Sinus arrest

Sinus pause

Sinus block

Sick sinus syndrome

Rhythm Summary: Atrial Rhythms

	RATE	REGULARITY	P WAVE	QRS INTERVAL	CAUSE	ADVERSE EFFECTS	TREATMENT
Wandering atrial pacemaker	<100	Irregular	At least three different shapes, sometimes no P at all on some beats	<0.12 unless BBB	MI, medication side effects, hypoxia, vagal stimulation	Usually no ill effects	Same as sinus brady
PACs	Can occur at any rate	Regular but interrupted	Shaped differently than sinus Ps; often hidden in preceding T wave	<0.12 unless BBB; absent after non-conducted PAC	Stimulants, caffeine, hypoxia, heart disease, or normal	None if occasional; can be a sign of early heart failure	Omit the causes; consider O₂, digitalis, quinidine
Paroxysmal atrial tachycardia (PAT)	161–250 once in atrial tach	Regular but interrupted	Shaped differently than sinus Ps but same as each other	<0.12 unless BBB	Same as PACs	Decreased cardiac output; some people tolerate OK for a while	Digitalis, quinidine, diltiazem, sedation, O₂, adenosine, verapamil, convert, cardioversion
2:1 atrial tachycardia	Atria: 161–250 Ventricle: 80–125	Regular	Two to each QRS; shaped differently than sinus Ps but same as each other	<0.12 unless BBB	Classic digitalis toxicity; can also be caused by MI	Usually no ill effects	Hold digitalis if toxic; give digitalis if not; consider O₂

Rhythm Summary: Atrial Rhythms (continued)

	RATE	REGULARITY	P WAVE	QRS INTERVAL	CAUSE	ADVERSE EFFECTS	TREATMENT
Multifocal atrial tachycardia	Mean rate >100	Irregular	At least three different shapes; some beats may have no P wave	<0.12 unless BBB	Chronic lung disease	Decreased cardiac output with faster rates	Same as atrial tachycardia
Atrial flutter	Atria: 251–350 Ventricle: varies	Regular or irregular	None; flutter waves present (zigzag or sawtooth waves)	<0.12 unless BBB	Heart disease, hypoxia, pulmonary embolus, lung disease, valve disease, thyroid storm	Tolerated OK at normal rate; decreased cardiac output at faster rates	Digitalis, quinidine, calcium channel blockers; consider O₂, carotid massage, cardioversion
Atrial fib	Atria: 350–700 Ventricle: varies	Irregularly irregular	None; fibrillatory waves present (waviness of the baseline)	<0.12 unless BBB	MI, lung disease, valve disease, thyrotoxicosis	Decreased cardiac output; can cause blood clots in atria	Digitalis, quinidine, corvert, adenosine; consider O₂; start Coumadin to prevent clots
SVT	≥130	Regular	May be present but hard to see	<0.12 unless BBB	Same as PAT	Same as PAT	Same as PAT

Atrial Rhythms Pictorial Review

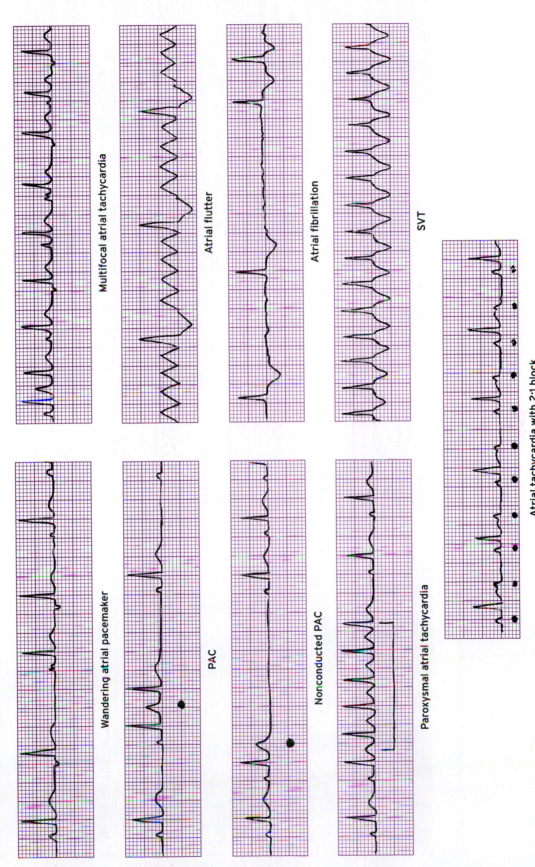

Multifocal atrial tachycardia

Atrial flutter

Atrial fibrillation

SVT

Wandering atrial pacemaker

PAC

Nonconducted PAC

Paroxysmal atrial tachycardia

Atrial tachycardia with 2:1 block

Rhythm Summary: Junctional Rhythms

	RATE	REGULARITY	P WAVE	QRS	CAUSE	ADVERSE EFFECTS	TREATMENT
PJCs	Can occur at any rate	Regular but interrupted	Inverted before or after QRS or hidden inside QRS	<0.12 unless BBB	Same as PACs	Usually no ill effects	Usually none required
Junctional bradycardia	<40	Regular	Inverted before or after QRS or hidden inside QRS	<0.12 unless BBB	Vagal stimulation, hypoxia, sinus node ischemia, MI	Decreased cardiac output	Atropine if symptoms; hold medications that can slow the HR; start O_2
Junctional rhythm	40–60	Regular	Inverted before or after QRS or hidden inside QRS	<0.12 unless BBB	Same as junctional brady	Well tolerated if HR closer to 50–60; decreased cardiac output possible	Same as junctional brady
Accelerated junctional	60–100	Regular	Inverted before or after QRS or hidden inside QRS	<0.12 unless BBB	Heart disease, stimulant drugs, caffeine	Usually no ill effects	Usually none needed
Junctional tach	>100	Regular	Inverted before or after QRS or hidden inside QRS	<0.12 unless BBB	Digitoxicity, heart disease, stimulants, SNS stimulation	Decreased cardiac output if HR too fast	β-blockers, Cardizem, adenosine; consider O_2

Junctional Rhythms Pictorial Review

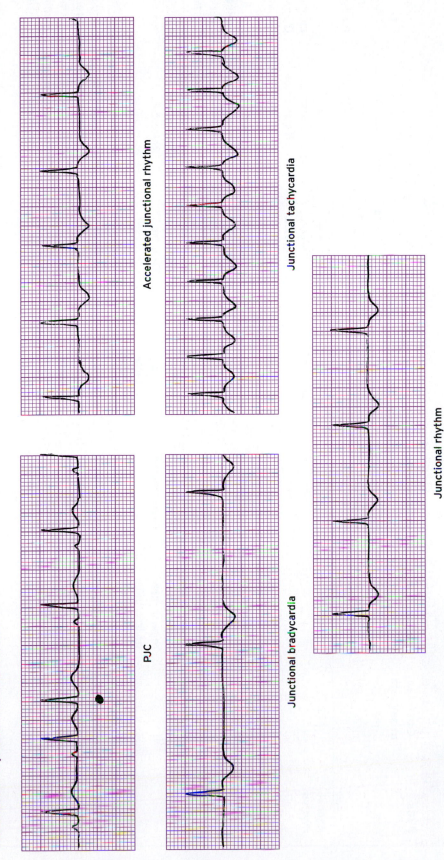

PJC

Accelerated junctional rhythm

Junctional tachycardia

Junctional bradycardia

Junctional rhythm

Rhythm Summary: Ventricular Rhythms

	RATE	REGULARITY	P WAVE	QRS	CAUSE	ADVERSE EFFECTS	TREATMENT
PVCs	Can occur at any rate	Regular but interrupted	Usually none	>0.12, wide and bizarre in shape	Hypoxia, MI, hypokalemia; low magnesium, caffeine, stimulants, stress	Occasional are no problem; can lead to lethal arrhythmias if frequent or after an MI	Lidocaine, O₂, procainamide, amiodarone; atropine for bradycardic PVCs
Agonal rhythm	<20	Irregular	None	>0.12, wide and bizarre in shape	Profound cardiac or other damage, profound hypoxia	Shock, unconsciousness, death if untreated	Atropine, epinephrine, CPR, O₂, pacemaker; *no lidocaine!*
IVR	20–40	Regular	None	>0.12, wide and bizarre in shape	Massive cardiac or other damage, hypoxia	↓CO	Atropine, epinephrine, O₂, pacemaker; *no lidocaine!*
AIVR	40–100	Usually regular—can be irregular at times	Dissociated if even present	>0.12, wide and bizarre in shape	Reperfusion after TPA, MI	Usually well tolerated	Atropine if HR low and symptoms; *no lidocaine!*
V-tach	100–250	Usually regular—can be irregular at times	Dissociated if even present	>0.12, wide and bizarre in shape	Same as PVCs	Tolerated OK for short bursts; can cause shock, unconsciousness, and death if untreated	Lidocaine, O₂, procainamide, amiodarone, cardioversion, or defib; CPR if no pulse

	RATE	REGULARITY	P WAVE	QRS	CAUSE	ADVERSE EFFECTS	TREATMENT
Torsades de pointes	>200	Regular or Irregular	None seen	>0.12, QRS oscillates around an axis	Medications such as quinidine or procainamide; also same as v-tach	Circulatory collapse if sustained; tolerated OK for short bursts	IV magnesium, overdrive pacing, Isuprel, O_2
V-flutter	250–350	Regular	None seen	Zigzag QRS	Same as v-tach	Same as v-tach	Defib usually done
V-fib	Cannot be counted	None detectable	None	None; just a wavy baseline that looks like static	Same as v-tach	Cardiovascular collapse; no pulse, breathing, zero cardiac output	Defibrillation, lidocaine, epinephrine, O_2, CPR, amiodarone
Asystole	Zero	None	None	None	Profound cardiac or other damage, hypoxia	Death if untreated	Atropine, epinephrine, CPR, pacemaker, O_2
Ventricular asystole	Zero	Ps regular	Sinus Ps	None	Same as asystole	Same as asystole	Same as asystole

Ventricular Rhythms Pictorial Review

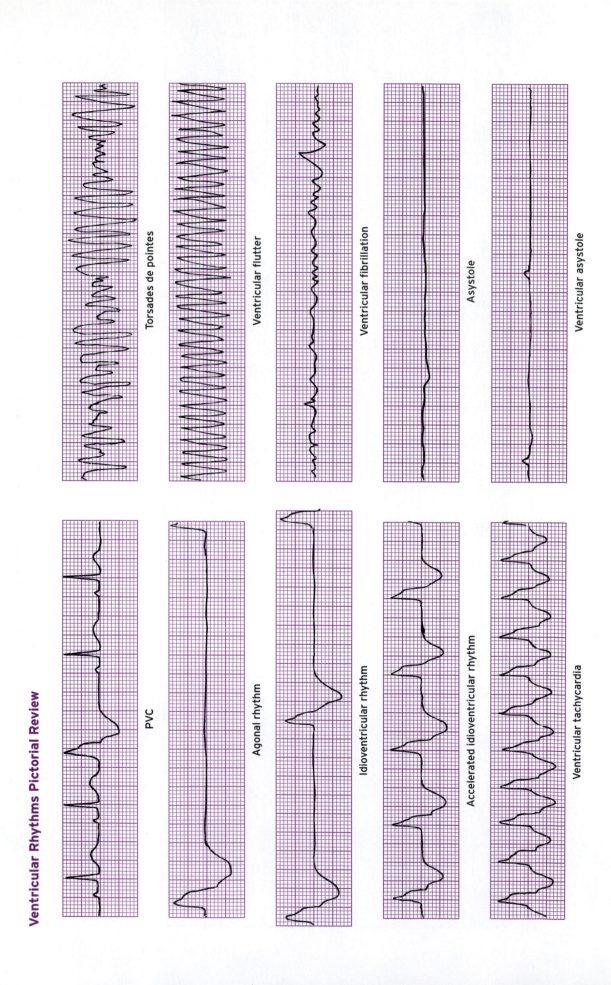

Torsades de pointes

Ventricular flutter

Ventricular fibrillation

Asystole

Ventricular asystole

PVC

Agonal rhythm

Idioventricular rhythm

Accelerated idioventricular rhythm

Ventricular tachycardia

Rhythm Summary: AV Blocks

	RATE	REGULARITY	P WAVE	PR INTERVAL	QRS INTERVAL	CAUSE	ADVERSE EFFECTS	TREATMENT
First-degree AVB	Can occur at any rate	Depends on underlying rhythm	Normal; one per QRS; all shaped the same	>0.20; constant	<0.12 unless BBB	AV node ischemia, prolonged bundle branch depolarization time, digitalis toxicity, other medication side effects	Usually no ill effects	Remove the cause
Type I second-degree AVB	Atria: 60–100 Ventricle: less than atrial rate	Regular but interrupted or irregular; groups of beats, then a pause	Normal; one not followed by a QRS; all shaped the same	Gradually prolongs till a QRS is dropped	<0.12 unless BBB	MI, digitoxicity, medication side effects	Usually well tolerated, but watch for worsening AV block	Atropine if symptoms from low HR
Type II second-degree AVB	Atria: 50–100 Ventricle: less than atrial rate	Regular, regular but interrupted, or irregular	Normal; some not followed by a QRS	Constant on the conducted beats	<0.12 if block at AV node, ≥0.12 if block at bundle branches	MI, conduction system lesion, hypoxia, medication side effects	Decreased cardiac output if HR slow	Atropine, pacemaker, O₂

Rhythm Summary: AV Blocks (continued)

	RATE	REGULARITY	P WAVE	PR INTERVAL	QRS INTERVAL	CAUSE	ADVERSE EFFECTS	TREATMENT
2:1 AVB	Atria: 60–100 Ventricle: half the atrial rate	Regular	Normal; two Ps to each QRS	Constant on the conducted beats	<0.12 unless BBB	Same as Wenckebach and type II	Decreased cardiac output if HR slow	Atropine, pacemaker; consider O₂
Third-degree AVB	Atria: 60–100 Ventricle: 20–60	Regular	Normal; dissociated from QRS	Varies	<0.12 if AV node is the pacemaker, >0.12 if ventricle is the pacemaker	MI, conduction system lesion, hypoxia, medication side effect	Decreased cardiac output if HR slow	Atropine, pacemaker, O₂

AV Blocks Pictorial Review

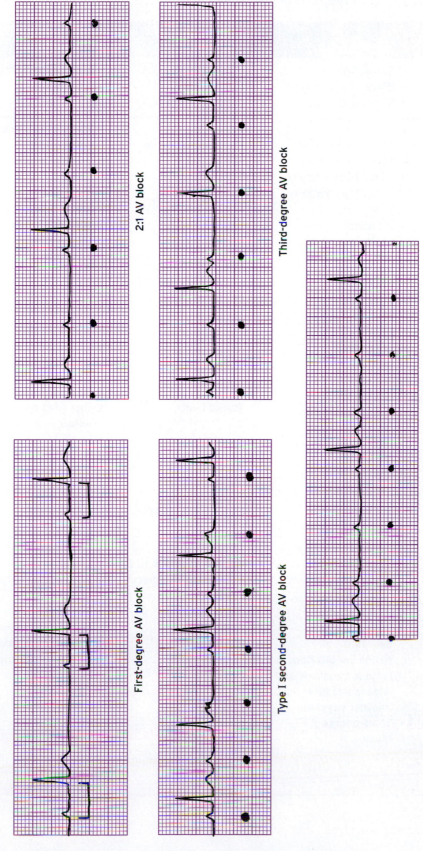

First-degree AV block

Type I second-degree AV block

2:1 AV block

Third-degree AV block

Type II second-degree AV block

127

Rhythm Regularity Summary

The following table points out the type of regularity of each rhythm. *Only rhythms with QRS complexes are shown here.*

ORIGIN OF RHYTHM	REGULAR	REGULAR BUT INTERRUPTED	IRREGULAR
Sinus	• Sinus rhythm • Sinus bradycardia • Sinus tachycardia	• Sinus arrest • Sinus pause • Sinus exit block	• Sinus arrhythmia
Atrial	• SVT • Atrial tachycardia (nonparoxysmal) • Atrial flutter (if the conduction ratio is constant) • 2:1 atrial tachycardia	• PACs • Paroxysmal atrial tachycardia	• Wandering atrial pacemaker • Multifocal atrial tachycardia • Atrial fibrillation • Atrial flutter (if the conduction ratio varies)
Junctional	• Junctional bradycardia • Junctional rhythm • Accelerated junctional rhythm • Junctional tachycardia	• PJCs	• None
Ventricular	• Idioventricular rhythm • Accelerated idioventricular rhythm • Ventricular tachycardia • Ventricular flutter • Paced rhythm	• PVCs • Paced beats	• Agonal rhythm • Torsades de pointes
AV blocks	• First-degree AV block (if the underlying rhythm is regular) • 2:1 AV block • Type II second-degree AV block (if the conduction ratio is constant and it does not interrupt another rhythm) • Third-degree AV block	• Type II second-degree AV block (if it interrupts another rhythm) • Type I second-degree AV block	• First-degree AV block (if the underlying rhythm is irregular) • Wenckebach • Type II second-degree AV block (if the conduction ratio varies)

Rhythms Originating in the Sinus Node

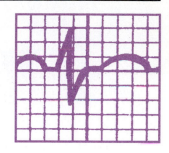

Chapter 12 Objectives

Upon completion of this chapter, the student will be able to:

- State the criteria for each of the sinus rhythms.
- Using the criteria and the algorithms and other rhythm analysis tools, correctly interpret a variety of sinus rhythms.
- State the adverse effects for each of the sinus rhythms.
- State the possible treatment for the sinus rhythms.

Chapter 12 Outline

I.   Introduction
II.   The skinny on sinus rhythms
III. Sinus rhythm
IV.   Sinus bradycardia
V.   Sinus tachycardia
VI.   Sinus arrhythmia
VII. Sinus arrest
VIII. Sinus exit block
IX.   Sinus pause
X.   Sick sinus syndrome
XI.   Practice strips–sinus rhythms
XII. Answers to sinus rhythms practice strips
XIII. Practice quiz
XIV. Practice quiz answers

Chapter 12 Glossary

Bradycardia: Slow heart rate, usually less than 60 beats per minute.

Bundle branch block: An interruption in the transmission of impulses down one of the bundle branches. This results in an abnormally widened QRS complex.

Congestive heart failure: Fluid buildup in the lungs as a result of the heart's inability to pump adequately.

Diaphoresis: Sweating.

Hypoxia: Low blood oxygen level.

Multiple: In referring to the length of pauses, a multiple is an R-R cycle that is exactly two or more times another R-R cycle. For example, a pause of 30 little blocks would be a multiple of a normal R-R cycle of 10 little blocks. Three of the normal R-R cycles would fit exactly into the pause. In order to be a multiple, the fit must be exact.

Pulmonary embolus: Blood clot in the lung. *Pulmonary* refers to lung; *embolus* is a blood clot that has traveled away from its original location.

Supraventricular: Originating in a pacemaker above the ventricle.

Tachycardia: Fast heart rate, greater than 100.

Thyrotoxicosis: Also called *thyroid storm.* A condition in which the thyroid gland so overproduces thyroid hormones that the body's metabolic rate is accelerated to a catastrophic level. Body temperature, heart rate, and blood pressure rise to extreme levels.

Vagal: Pertaining to the vagus nerve.

Introduction

Sinus rhythms originate in the sinus node, travel through the atria to depolarize them, then head down the normal conduction pathway to depolarize the ventricles. Most rhythms from the sinus node are regular rhythms, but as you will see, this is not always the case. You'll recall the sinus node is the normal pacemaker of the heart. See Figure 12-1.

The Skinny on Sinus Rhythms

The sinus node is the acknowledged king of the conduction system's pacemaker cells. And there are only two ways for the sinus node king to relinquish its throne:

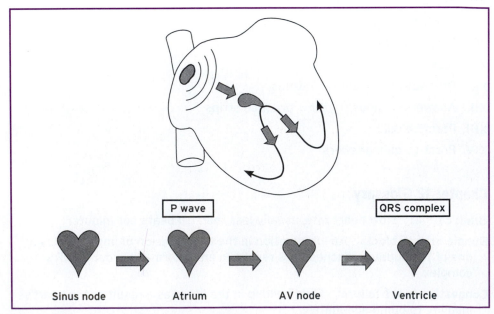

Figure 12-1 Conduction in sinus rhythms.

1. By illness or death, requiring someone to step in for it (escape)
2. By being overthrown by a subordinate (usurpation)

Though they can be irregular at times, sinus rhythms are, for the most part, notoriously regular. They're like the ticking of a clock—predictable and expected. You'll recall the inherent rate of the sinus node is 60 to 100. But also remember that this rate can go higher or lower if the sinus node is acted on by the sympathetic or parasympathetic nervous system. The individual's tolerance of these rhythms will depend in large part on the heart rate. Heart rates that are too fast or too slow can cause symptoms of decreased cardiac output.

Treatment is not needed unless symptoms develop. At that time, the goal is to return the heart rate to normal levels.

Sinus rhythms are the standard against which all other rhythms are compared. Since most of the rhythms you will see in real life will be sinus rhythms, you'll need a thorough understanding of them. Let's look at the criteria for sinus rhythms. *All these criteria must be met for the rhythm to be sinus in origin.*

- Upright matching P waves followed by a QRS *and*
- PR intervals constant *and*
- Heart rate less than or equal to 160 at rest

All matching upright P waves are considered sinus P waves until proven otherwise. The width and deflection of the QRS complex is irrelevant in determining whether a rhythm is sinus. The QRS may be narrow (<0.12 second) or wide (≥0.12 second), depending on the state of conduction through the bundle branches. The deflection of the QRS will depend on the lead in which the patient is being monitored.

The following sinus rhythms that will be covered in this section:

- Sinus rhythm
- Sinus bradycardia
- Sinus tachycardia
- Sinus arrhythmia
- Sinus arrest
- Sinus exit block
- Sinus pause
- Sick sinus syndrome

Now let's look at each of these rhythms in detail.

Sinus Rhythm

What is it? Sinus rhythm is the only normal rhythm. The impulse is born in the sinus node and heads down the conduction pathway to the ventricle. Every P wave is married to a QRS complex, and the heart rate is the normal 60 to 100.

Rate	60 to 100
Regularity	Regular

P waves	Upright in most leads, though may be normally inverted in V_1; one P to each QRS; all P waves have the same shape; *all matching, upright P waves are sinus P waves until proven otherwise* (this is the most crucial criterion to identifying rhythms originating in the sinus node); P-P interval is regular
PR	0.12 to 0.20 second; PR interval is constant from beat to beat
QRS	<0.12 second (can be ≥0.12 s if conduction through the ventricle is abnormal, as in a bundle branch block [BBB]).
Cause	Normal
Adverse effects	None
Treatment	None

In Figure 12-2, there are QRS complexes and they are all shaped the same. The rhythm is regular. Heart rate is 88. P waves are present, one before each QRS complex, and they are all matching and upright. *Remember—all matching upright P waves are sinus P waves until proven otherwise.* P-P interval is regular. PR interval is 0.20, QRS interval is 0.10, both normal. Interpretation: sinus rhythm.

Sinus Bradycardia

What is it? In sinus bradycardia, the sinus node fires at a heart rate slower than normal. The impulse originates in the sinus node and travels the conduction system normally.

Rate	Less than 60
Regularity	Regular
P waves	Upright in most leads, though may be inverted in V_1; one P to each QRS; P waves shaped the same; P-P interval regular
PR	0.12 to 0.20 second, constant from beat to beat
QRS	<0.12 second (will be ≥0.12 s if BBB present)

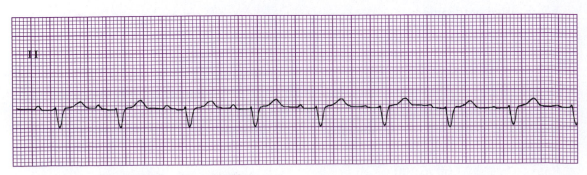

Figure 12-2 Sinus rhythm.

Cause   Vagal stimulation such as vomiting or straining to have a bowel movement, myocardial infarction (MI), **hypoxia** (low blood oxygen level), digitalis toxicity (an overabundance of the medication digitalis in the bloodstream), and other medication side effects. Sinus bradycardia is common in athletes.

Adverse effects   Too slow a heart rate can cause dizziness, weakness, syncope, **diaphoresis** (cold sweat), pallor, and hypotension, all of which are signs of decreased cardiac output. Many individuals, however, tolerate a slow heart rate and do not require treatment.

Treatment   None unless the patient is symptomatic. A medication called *atropine* can be used if needed to speed up the heart rate. Atropine speeds up the rate at which the sinus node propagates (creates) its impulses and also speeds up impulse conduction through the AV node. Thus it causes an increase in heart rate. If atropine is unsuccessful, an electronic pacemaker can be utilized, although that is not usually necessary for sinus bradycardia unless the individual is in shock. Other medications such as epinephrine, dopamine, and Isuprel can also be used to increase the heart rate, but, as with the pacemaker, are usually not necessary for sinus bradycardia. Consider starting oxygen. If the heart does not receive adequate oxygen, conduction system cells become ischemic and may respond by firing at rates above or below their norm. Providing supplemental oxygen can help these stricken cells return to more normal functioning and a more normal heart rate.

In Figure 12-3, there are QRS complexes and they are all shaped the same. The rhythm is regular. Heart rate is 54. P waves are present, one before each QRS complex, and they are upright and matching. P-P interval is regular. PR interval is 0.16, QRS interval is 0.09, both normal. Interpretation: sinus bradycardia. *The only difference between sinus rhythm and sinus bradycardia is the heart rate—the other interpretation criteria are the same.*

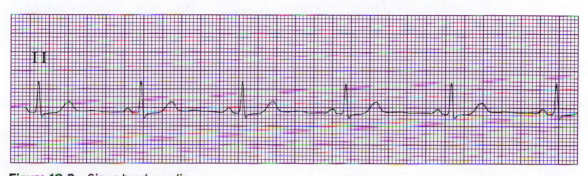

Figure 12-3 Sinus bradycardia.

Sinus Tachycardia

What is it? Sinus tachycardia is a rhythm in which the sinus node fires at a heart rate faster than normal. The impulse originates in the sinus node and travels down the conduction pathway normally.

Rate	101 to 160. According to most experts, the sinus node does not fire at a rate above 160 in supine resting adults. Though this is somewhat controversial, we will adopt this as the upper limit of the sinus node. *All strips in this text are from supine resting adults unless otherwise specified.*
Regularity	Regular
P waves	Upright in most leads, though may be inverted in V_1; one P to each QRS; P waves shaped the same; P-P interval regular
PR	0.12 to 0.20 second, constant from beat to beat
QRS	<0.12 second (≥0.12 s if BBB present)
Cause	Emotional upset, **pulmonary embolus** (blood clot in the lung), MI, congestive heart failure (**CHF**), fever, inhibition of the vagus nerve, hypoxia, and **thyrotoxicosis** (thyroid storm—an emergent medical condition in which the thyroid gland so overproduces thyroid hormones that the heart rate, blood pressure, and temperature all rise to dangerously high levels)
Adverse effects	Increased heart rate causes increased cardiac workload. The faster a muscle works, the more blood and oxygen it requires. This can stress an already weakened heart. Cardiac output can drop. This is especially true in the patient with an acute MI, as the increased blood and oxygen demand cannot easily be met by the damaged heart muscle.
Treatment	Treat the cause. For example, if it's from fever, give medication to decrease the fever. If it's from anxiety, consider sedation. For cardiac patients with persistent sinus tachycardia, a class of medications called **beta-blockers** may be used to slow the heart rate. Consider starting oxygen.

In Figure 12-4, there are QRS complexes, all shaped the same. The rhythm is regular. Heart rate is about 125. P waves are present, one before each QRS, and they are all upright and matching. P-P interval is regular. PR interval is 0.14, QRS interval is 0.06, both within normal limits. Interpretation: sinus tachycardia. *Just as in sinus rhythm and sinus bradycardia, all the criteria for interpretation are the same for sinus tachycardia—the only difference is the heart rate.*

Sinus Arrhythmia

What is it? Sinus arrhythmia is the only **irregular** rhythm from the sinus node, and it has a pattern that is cyclic and usually corresponds with the breathing pattern.

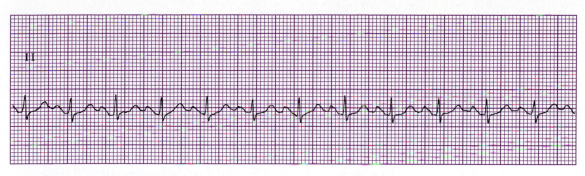

Figure 12-4 Sinus tachycardia.

Rate	Varies with respiratory pattern—faster with inspiration, slower with expiration. The negative pressure in the chest during inspiration sucks up blood from the lower extremities, causing an increase in blood returning to the right atrium. The heart rate speeds up to circulate this extra blood.
Regularity	Irregular in a repetitive pattern; longest R-R cycle exceeds the shortest by ≥0.16 second (four or more little blocks).
P waves	Upright in most leads, though may be inverted in V_1; P waves shaped the same; one P to each QRS; P-P interval is irregular
PR	0.12 to 0.20 second, constant from beat to beat
QRS	<0.12 second (≥0.12 s if BBB present)
Cause	Usually caused by the breathing pattern, but can also be caused by heart disease
Adverse effects	Usually no ill effects
Treatment	Usually none required

In Figure 12-5, there are QRS complexes, all shaped the same. The rhythm is irregular. Heart rate is 62 to 88, with a mean rate of 80. The longest R-R interval (24 little blocks) exceeds the shortest (17 blocks) by four little blocks or more. P waves are present, one before each QRS, and all are

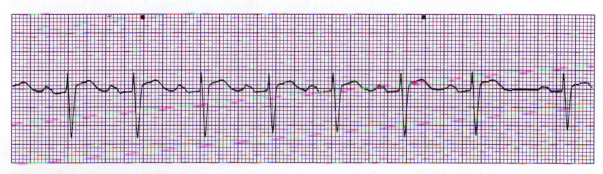

Figure 12-5 Sinus arrhythmia.

upright and shaped the same. P-P interval varies. PR interval is 0.24 seconds (abnormally long), QRS interval is 0.10 (normal). Interpretation: sinus arrhythmia. We'll discuss prolonged PR intervals in Chapter 16.

Sinus Arrest

What is it? A sinus arrest is a pause that occurs when the regularly firing sinus node suddenly stops firing for a brief period. One or more P-QRS-T sequences will be missing. An escape beat from a lower pacemaker then takes over for one or more beats. The sinus node may resume functioning after missing one or more beats, or the lower pacemaker may continue as the pacemaker, creating a new rhythm.

Rate	Can occur at any heart rate
Regularity	Regular but interrupted (by a pause). In any rhythm with a pause, always measure the length of the pause in seconds.
P waves	Normal sinus P waves before the pause, different-shaped Ps (if even present) on the beat ending the pause. P-P interval is usually regular before the pause and may vary after the pause, depending on whether the sinus node regains pacemaking control.
PR	0.12 to 0.20 second before the pause, shorter or absent after the pause
QRS	On the sinus beats, the QRS interval will be <0.12 second (≥0.12 s if BBB present). On the escape beat(s), the QRS will be narrow (<0.12 s) if the AV node escapes as the pacemaker (called a **junctional escape beat**), and wide (>0.12 s) if the ventricle escapes as the pacemaker (called a **ventricular escape beat**). Atrial escape beats are very uncommon and will therefore not be discussed in this text.
Cause	Sinus node ischemia, hypoxia, **digitalis toxicity,** excessive vagal tone, other medication side effects
Adverse effects	Frequent or very long sinus arrests can cause decreased cardiac output.
Treatment	Occasional sinus arrests may not cause a problem—the patient has no ill effects. Frequent sinus arrests may require that the medication causing it be stopped and can require atropine and/or a pacemaker to speed up the heart rate. Consider starting oxygen.

In Figure 12-6, the first three beats are sinus beats firing along regularly. Suddenly there is a long pause, at the end of which is a beat from a lower pacemaker. How do we know the beat that ends the pause (the escape beat) is not a sinus beat? Sinus beats all have matching upright P waves. This beat has no P wave at all, plus its QRS complex is huge, completely unlike the other QRS complexes. Going through our steps now: There are QRS com-

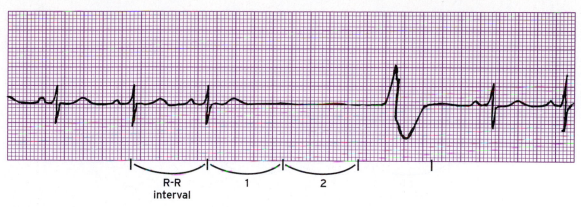

Figure 12-6 Sinus arrest.

plexes, all but one having the same shape. Regularity is regular but interrupted. Heart rate is 30 to 75, with a mean rate of 60. P waves are upright, matching, one before all QRS complexes except the escape beat. PR interval is 0.16, QRS interval is 0.08 on the sinus beats and 0.14 on the escape beat. Interpretation: sinus rhythm interrupted by a 2-second sinus arrest (review Chapter 5 for the number of blocks per second, etc.) and a ventricular escape beat. Note the sinus node resumes functioning after one ventricular escape beat.

Sinus Block (Also Called Sinus Exit Block)

What is it? A sinus block is a pause that occurs when the sinus node fires its impulse on time, but the impulse's exit from the sinus node to the atrial tissue is blocked. *In other words, the beat that the sinus node propagated is not conducted anywhere.* This results in one or more P-QRS-T sequences being missing, creating a pause, the length of which will depend on how many sinus beats are blocked. When conduction of the regularly firing sinus impulses resumes, the sinus beats return on time at the end of the pause. The pause will be a multiple of the previous R-R intervals—that is, exactly two or more R-R cycles will fit into the pause.

Rate	Can occur at any heart rate
Regularity	Regular but interrupted (by a pause)
P waves	Normal sinus Ps both before and after the pause; P waves shaped the same
PR	0.12 to 0.20 second
QRS	<0.12 second (≥0.12 s if BBB present)
Cause	Medication side effects, hypoxia, or strong vagal stimulation
Adverse effects	Same as sinus arrest
Treatment	Same as sinus arrest

In Figure 12-7, there is a pause that lasts exactly eight big blocks. This is exactly twice the R-R interval of the sinus beats that precede and follow the pause. The pause is therefore a multiple of the R-R intervals. The pause ends

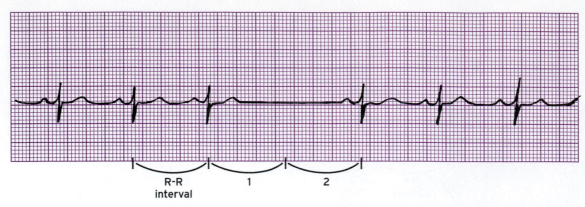

R-R
interval

1

2

Figure 12-7 Sinus block.

with a sinus beat. Going through our steps: There are QRS complexes, all shaped the same. Regularity is regular but interrupted. Heart rate is 37 to 75, with a mean rate of 60. P waves are upright, matching, one before each QRS complex. PR interval is 0.16, QRS interval is 0.08. Interpretation: sinus rhythm with a 1.6-second sinus block.

Sinus Pause

What is it? A sinus pause is a pause that occurs when the sinus node stops firing for a brief period, resulting in a missing P-QRS-T sequence. The sinus then resumes whenever it is able to. The pause ends with a sinus beat, but that sinus beat is not on time. The pause is not a multiple of the R-R cycle lengths.

Rate	Can occur at any heart rate
Regularity	Regular but interrupted (by a pause)
P waves	Normal sinus Ps before and after the pause; P waves shaped the same
PR	0.12 to 0.20 second
QRS	<0.12 second (≥0.12 s if BBB present)
Cause	Sinus node ischemia, hypoxia, digitoxicity, excessive vagal tone
Adverse effects	Same as sinus arrest
Treatment	Same as sinus arrest

In Figure 12-8, there are three sinus beats with an R-R interval of four big blocks, then a pause that lasts seven big blocks. The length of the pause is therefore not a multiple of the previous R-R cycles. The sinus resumes at the end of the pause. Going through our steps: QRS complexes are present and all shaped the same. Regularity is regular but interrupted. Heart rate is 43 to 75, with a mean rate of 70. P waves are upright, matching, one before each QRS complex. PR interval is 0.16, QRS interval is 0.08. Interpretation: sinus rhythm with a 1.4-second sinus pause.

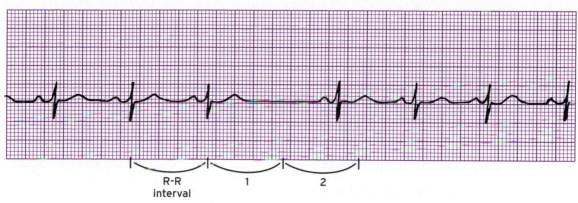

R-R
interval   1   2

Figure 12-8   Sinus pause.

Sick Sinus Syndrome (Also Called Tachy-Brady Syndrome)

What is it? Sick sinus syndrome is not a rhythm per se, but rather a term given to describe a pathology in the sinus node that results in rhythms with wild swings in heart rate. Such rhythms include extremely rapid tachycardias interrupted by profound bradycardias, with sinus arrests, pauses, and blocks. Escape beats are common after prolonged pauses. It's easy to see why this condition is also called *tachy-brady syndrome*.

Rate	Varies wildly
Regularity	Irregular
P waves	May or may not be present; shape may vary
PR interval	Varies if even present
QRS	Varies; will be <0.12 second if the rhythm is **supraventricular** in origin (originating in a pacemaker above the ventricle—i.e., the sinus node, atrium, or AV node); QRS will be >0.12 second if an escape pacemaker in the ventricle has to fire.
Cause	Sinus node ischemia, usually accompanied by some degree of ischemia of the AV node as well; can also be caused by digitalis toxicity
Adverse effects	Signs of decreased cardiac output can occur.
Treatment	This is a complicated problem. The treatment for the tachycardia part of the syndrome would make the bradycardia part too slow, and treating the bradycardia would make the tachycardia even faster. Usually, these individuals receive a permanent pacemaker to prevent the heart rate from going too slow while the tachycardia is treated with medications such as digitalis, calcium channel blockers, beta-blockers, and adenosine. Consider starting oxygen.

In Figure 12-9, this rhythm is all over the place. There are QRS complexes, all the same shape. Regularity is irregular. Heart rate is 30 to 214,

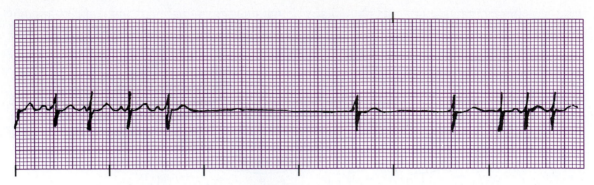

Figure 12-9 Sick sinus syndrome.

with a mean rate of 100. P waves are present before the first four QRS complexes, but not on the next two. There's a small P on the eighth QRS (*do count the blip of a QRS at the beginning of the strip*), and questionable P waves on the last two beats. PR interval is 0.08. QRS interval is 0.08. Interpretation: sinus tachycardia with a 2-second sinus arrest and two junctional escape beats, then SVT. (You'll learn all this soon. . . .) *Remember—sick sinus syndrome is not a rhythm*. It's what *causes* a rhythm to look like this.

Practice Strips: Sinus Rhythms

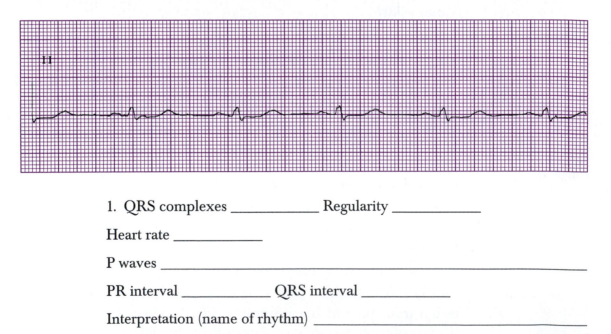

1. QRS complexes _____ Regularity _____

Heart rate _____

P waves _____

PR interval _____ QRS interval _____

Interpretation (name of rhythm) _____

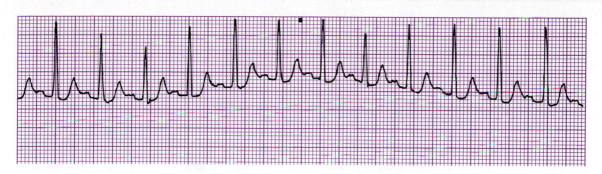

2. QRS complexes _____ Regularity _____

Heart rate _____

P waves _____

PR interval _____ QRS interval _____

Interpretation _____

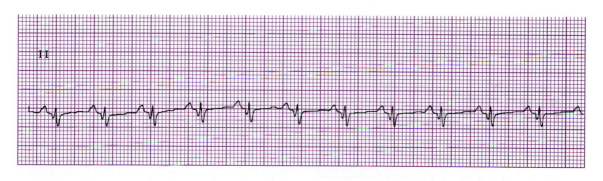

3. QRS complexes _____ Regularity _____

Heart rate _____

P waves _____

PR interval _____ QRS interval _____

Interpretation _____

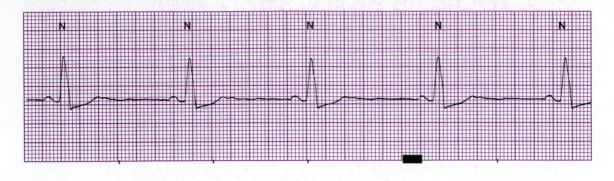

4. QRS complexes _____ Regularity _____

Heart rate _____

P waves _____

PR interval _____ QRS interval _____

Interpretation _____

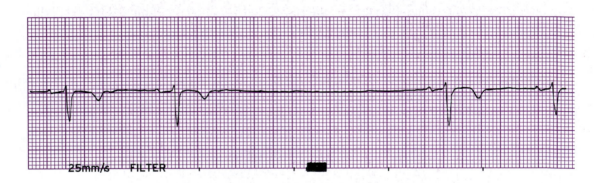

5. QRS complexes _____ Regularity _____

Heart rate _____

P waves _____

PR interval _____ QRS interval _____

Interpretation _____

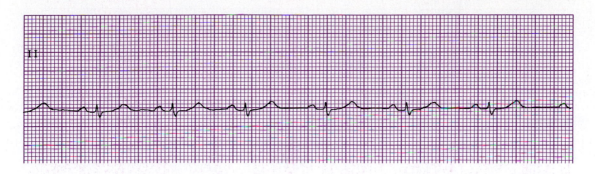

6. QRS complexes _____ Regularity _____

Heart rate _____

P waves _____

PR interval _____ QRS interval _____

Interpretation _____

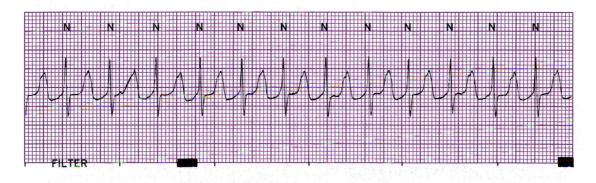

7. QRS complexes _____ Regularity _____

Heart rate _____

P waves _____

PR interval _____ QRS interval _____

Interpretation _____

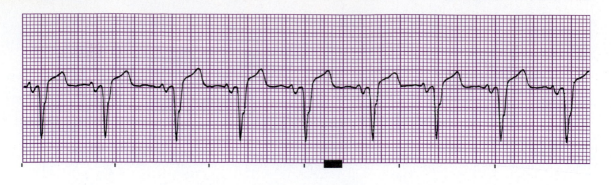

8. QRS complexes _____ Regularity _____

Heart rate _____

P waves _____

PR interval _____ QRS interval _____

Interpretation _____

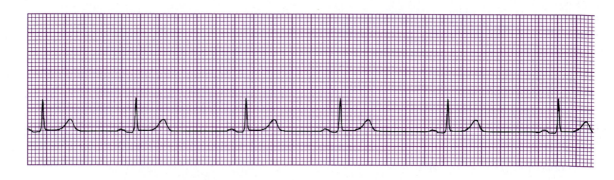

9. QRS complexes _____ Regularity _____

Heart rate _____

P waves _____

PR interval _____ QRS interval _____

Interpretation _____

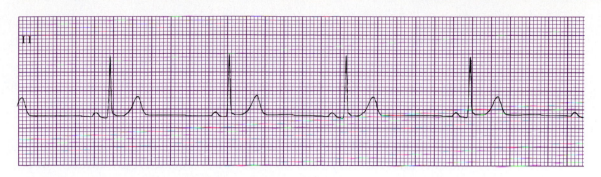

10. QRS complexes _____ Regularity _____

Heart rate _____

P waves _____

PR interval _____ QRS interval _____

Interpretation _____

Answers to Sinus Rhythms Practice Strips

1. **QRS complexes:** present, all shaped the same. **Regularity:** regular. **Heart rate:** 56. **P waves:** upright, matching, one per QRS; P-P interval regular. **PR:** 0.18. **QRS:** 0.12. **Interpretation:** sinus bradycardia with BBB.

2. **QRS complexes:** present, all shaped the same. **Regularity:** regular. **Heart rate:** 125. **P waves:** upright, matching, one per QRS; P-P interval regular. **PR:** 0.14. **QRS:** 0.08. **Interpretation:** sinus tachycardia.

3. **QRS complexes:** present, all shaped the same. **Regularity:** regular. **Heart rate:** 115. **P waves:** upright, matching, one per QRS; P-P interval regular. **PR:** 0.12. **QRS:** 0.10. **Interpretation:** sinus tachycardia.

4. **QRS complexes:** present, all shaped the same. **Regularity:** regular. **Heart rate:** 45. **P waves:** upright, matching, one per QRS; P-P interval regular. **PR:** 0.16. **QRS:** 0.14 (wider than normal). **Interpretation:** sinus bradycardia with bundle branch block.

5. **QRS complexes:** present, all shaped the same. **Regularity:** regular but interrupted (by a pause). **Heart rate:** 21 to 54, with a mean rate of 40. **P waves:** upright, matching, one per QRS; P-P interval irregular due to the pause. **PR:** 0.18. **QRS:** 0.10. **Interpretation:** sinus bradycardia with a 3.08-second sinus pause.

6. **QRS complexes:** present, all shaped the same. **Regularity:** regular (R-R intervals vary by only two small blocks). **Heart rate:** about 68. **P waves:** upright, matching, one per QRS; P-P interval regular. **PR:** 0.16. **QRS:** 0.08. **Interpretation:** sinus rhythm.

7. **QRS complexes:** present, all shaped the same. **Regularity:** regular. **Heart rate:** about 130. **P waves:** upright and matching, one per QRS. The heart rate is so fast that the T waves and P waves merge together. Do you see the notch at the top of the T wave? That's the P wave pop-

ping out. P-P interval regular. **PR:** cannot measure. **QRS:** 0.08. **Interpretation:** sinus tachycardia.

8. **QRS complexes:** present, all shaped the same. **Regularity:** regular. **Heart rate:** 88. **P waves:** biphasic (counts as upright), matching, one per QRS; P-P interval regular. **PR:** 0.12. **QRS:** 0.10. **Interpretation:** sinus rhythm.

9. **QRS complexes:** present, all shaped the same. **Regularity:** irregular; the R-R intervals vary from 25 to 29 small blocks. **Heart rate:** 52 to 60, with a mean rate of 60. **P waves:** upright, matching, one per QRS; P-P interval irregular. **PR:** 0.16. **QRS:** 0.06. **Interpretation:** sinus arrhythmia.

10. **QRS complexes:** present, all shaped the same. **Regularity:** regular. **Heart rate:** about 47. **P waves:** upright, matching, one preceding each QRS; P-P interval regular. **PR:** 0.16. **QRS:** 0.08. **Interpretation:** sinus bradycardia.

Practice Quiz

1. True or false: All rhythms from the sinus node are irregular.

2. The only difference between sinus rhythm, sinus bradycardia, and sinus tachycardia is _____

   _____

3. Sinus arrhythmia is typically caused by _____

4. In what way does a sinus pause differ from a sinus arrest?_____

   _____

5. True or false: Atropine is a medication that is useful in treating sinus tachycardia.

6. What rhythm would be expected in an individual with a fever of 103°F?

   _____

7. A regular rhythm from the sinus node that has a heart rate of 155 is called _____

   _____

8. True or false: All rhythms originating in the sinus node have matching P waves that are upright in most leads.

9. What effect does atropine have on the heart rate? _____

10. Sick sinus syndrome is also called _____

Practice Quiz Answers

1. **False.** Most rhythms from the sinus node are regular rhythms.

2. The only difference between sinus rhythm, sinus bradycardia, and sinus tachycardia is the **heart rate.**

3. Sinus arrhythmia is typically caused by the **breathing pattern.**

4. A sinus pause differs from a sinus arrest in that **a sinus arrest ends with an escape beat from a lower pacemaker, whereas a sinus pause ends with a sinus beat.**

5. **False.** Atropine is inappropriate for sinus tachycardia.

6. An individual with a fever of 103°F would be expected to be in **sinus tachycardia.**

7. A regular rhythm from the sinus node with heart rate of 155 is called **sinus tachycardia.**

8. **True.** That is the most basic criterion for sinus rhythms.

9. **Atropine causes the heart rate to increase.**

10. Sick sinus syndrome is also called **tachy-brady syndrome.**

Rhythms Originating in the Atria

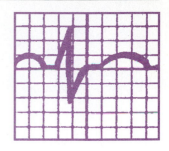

Chapter 13 Objectives

Upon completion of this chapter, the student will be able to:

- State the criteria for each of the atrial rhythms.
- Using the criteria, the algorithms, and other rhythm analysis tools, correctly interpret a variety of atrial rhythms.
- State the adverse effects for each rhythm.
- State the possible treatment for each rhythm.

Chapter 13 Outline

Chapter 13 Glossary

Cardioversion: Converting an abnormal heart rhythm to a normal one by using a small electrical shock to the heart.

Ectopic: Originating in a pacemaker other than the sinus node.

Fibrillation: Wiggling instead of contracting. Can occur in the atria or the ventricles.

Focus: Location. Plural is *foci.*

Paroxysmal: Occurring suddenly and stopping just as suddenly.

Introduction

Atrial rhythms originate in one or more irritable **foci** (locations) in the atria, then depolarize the atria and head down the conduction pathway to the ventricles. Atrial rhythms, and indeed all rhythms that originate in a pacemaker other than the sinus node, are called **ectopic rhythms.** See Figures 13-1 and 13-2.

The Skinny on Atrial Rhythms

The atrium is the pacemaker next in line below the sinus node. Though theoretically this positions it to escape if the sinus node fails (you'll remember the inherent rate of the atrium is 60 to 80), the atrium does not often function in an escape role. In fact, atrial escape beats are very uncommon. The atria like to fire rapidly and are much more likely to become hyper and usurp control from the sinus node than to escape and fire slowly when the sinus node fails. Since atrial rhythms often result in very rapid heart rates, patients are often symptomatic.

Treatment is aimed at converting the rhythm back to sinus rhythm, or, if that is not possible, returning the heart rate to more normal levels.

Atrial rhythms are extremely variable in their presentation. Some rhythms have obvious P waves. Others have no Ps at all–instead, they have fibrillatory or flutter waves between the QRS complexes. Some atrial rhythms are regular and others are completely irregular, even chaotic. Though most atrial rhythms are rapid, a few are slower.

Unlike sinus rhythms, which have a common set of criteria, atrial rhythms have multiple and variable possible criteria. If the rhythm or beat in

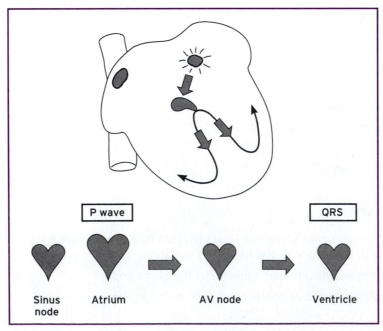

Figure 13-1 Conduction of a single atrial focus.

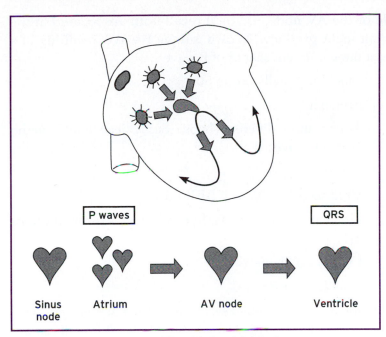

Figure 13-2   Conduction of multiple atrial foci.

question meets *any* of these criteria, it is atrial in origin. Let's look at these criteria now.

- Matching upright Ps, atrial rate >160 at rest *or*
- No Ps at all; wavy or sawtooth baseline between QRSs present instead *or*
- P waves of ≥ three different shapes *or*
- Premature abnormal P wave (with or without QRS) interrupting another rhythm, *or*
- Heart rate ≥130, rhythm regular, P waves not discernible (may be present, but can't be sure)

The atrial rhythms that will be covered in this section are the following:

- Wandering atrial pacemaker
- Premature atrial complexes (PACs)
- Paroxysmal atrial tachycardia
- Atrial tachycardia with 2:1 block
- Multifocal atrial tachycardia (MAT)
- Atrial flutter
- Atrial fibrillation
- Supraventricular tachycardia (SVT)

Let's look at each of these rhythms in detail.

Wandering Atrial Pacemaker

What is it? Wandering atrial pacemaker occurs when the pacemaking impulses originate from varying foci in the atria. One of these atrial foci may be the sinus node or the AV node, as you'll recall both are located in the atria. Each different focus produces its own unique P wave, resulting in a rhythm with at least three different shapes of P waves.

Rate	<100, but usually 50s to 60s
Regularity	Irregular
P waves	At least three different shapes. Some beats may have no visible P waves at all.
PR	Varies
QRS	<0.12 second (≥0.12 s if BBB present)
Cause	Medication side effects, hypoxia, vagal stimulation, or MI
Adverse effects	Usually no ill effects
Treatment	Usually none needed

In Figure 13-3, there are QRS complexes, all shaped the same. Regularity is irregular. Heart rate is 50 to 60, with a mean rate of 50. At least three different shapes of P waves precede the QRS complexes. P-P interval varies. PR interval varies from 0.24 to 0.32. QRS interval is 0.08. Interpretation: wandering atrial pacemaker.

Premature Atrial Complexes (PACs)

What are they? PACs are premature beats that are fired out by irritable atrial tissue before the next sinus beat is due. The premature P wave may or may not be followed by a QRS, depending on how premature the PAC is. If the PAC is very premature, it will not be conducted to the ventricle because it will arrive during the ventricle's refractory period.

Rate	Can occur at any rate
Regularity	Regular but interrupted (by the PACs)
P waves	Shaped differently from sinus P waves. The premature P waves of PACs may be hidden in the T wave of the preceding beat, and if so, will deform the shape of that T wave. Always be suspicious when a T wave suddenly changes shape. If the QRS complexes look the same, then the T waves that belong to them should also look

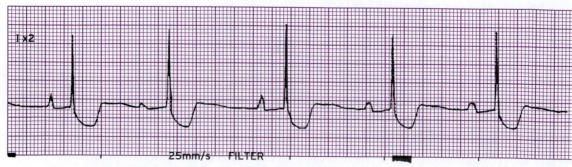

Figure 13-3 Wandering atrial pacemaker.

the same. If one T wave is different, there's probably a P wave hiding in it. If the PAC's P wave is inverted, the PR interval should be 0.12 to 0.20 s.

PR	0.12 to 0.20 second
QRS	<0.12 second (≥0.12 s if BBB present). QRS will be absent after a nonconducted PAC. The most common cause of an unexplained pause is a nonconducted PAC. If you see a pause and you're tempted to call it a sinus pause, sinus arrest, or sinus block, make sure there's no P hiding in the T wave inside the pause. It might just be a nonconducted PAC.
Cause	The atria get hyper and fire early, before the next sinus beat is due. This can be caused by medications (stimulants, caffeine), tobacco, hypoxia, or heart disease. Occasional PACs are normal.
Adverse effects	Frequent PACs can be an early sign of impending heart failure or impending atrial tachycardia or atrial fibrillation. Patients usually have no ill effects from occasional PACs.
Treatment	Omit caffeine, tobacco, and other stimulants. Give digitalis or quinidine to treat PACs. Treat heart failure if present. Consider starting oxygen.

In Figure 13-4, the fourth beat is premature, as evidenced by the shorter R-R interval there. Recall premature beats are followed by a short pause immediately afterward. The QRS complexes are all the same shape. Regularity is regular but interrupted (by a premature beat). Heart rate is 54. P waves precede each QRS complex, and all but the fourth P wave are the same shape. Thus the matching upright P waves are sinus Ps, and the premature P wave is *not* a sinus P since it has a different shape. P-P interval is irregular because of the premature P wave. PR interval is 0.16. QRS interval is 0.08. Interpretation: sinus bradycardia with a PAC.

In Figure 13-5, there are QRS complexes, all the same shape. Regularity is regular but interrupted (by a pause). Heart rate is 43 to 75, with a mean rate of 70. P waves are biphasic and matching, except for the P wave that's at the end of the third beat's T wave. See the little hump there under the dot?

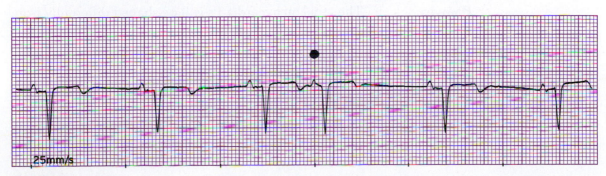

Figure 13-4 PAC.

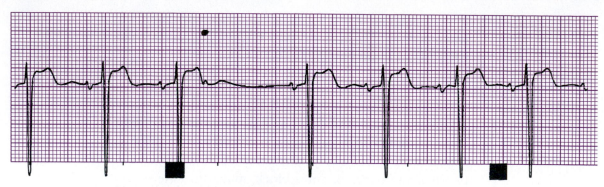

Figure 13-5 Nonconducted PAC.

That's a P wave. That P wave is shaped differently from the sinus P waves, and it is premature. How do we know it's premature? Look at the P-P intervals, the distance between consecutive P waves. All the sinus P waves are about four big blocks apart. This abnormal P wave is only 2½ blocks from the P wave that precedes it. Thus it is premature. A premature P wave that is not followed by a QRS complex is a nonconducted PAC. Note the long pause that this nonconducted PAC causes. Nonconducted PACs are the most common cause of otherwise unexplained pauses. It is important to note that many nonconducted PACs do not have such easily noticeable P waves. Much of the time the premature P wave is hidden inside the T wave of the preceding beat, deforming that T wave's shape. PR interval here is 0.16; QRS interval is 0.10. Interpretation: sinus rhythm with a nonconducted PAC.

Paroxysmal Atrial Tachycardia (PAT)

What is it? The term *paroxysmal* refers to a rhythm that starts and stops suddenly. PAT is simply a sudden burst of three or more PACs in a row that usurps the underlying rhythm and then becomes its *own* rhythm for a period of time. PAT resembles sinus tach, but with a faster heart rate. In order to diagnose PAT, the PAC that initiates it must be seen.

Rate	160 to 250 on the atrial tachycardia itself. The rhythm it interrupts will have a different rate.
Regularity	The atrial tachycardia itself is regular, but since it interrupts another rhythm, the rhythm strip as a whole will be regular but interrupted.
P waves	The atrial tachycardia Ps will be shaped differently from sinus P waves, but all are the same as each other.
PR	0.12 to 0.20 second, constant
QRS	<0.12 second (>0.12 s if BBB present)
Cause	Same as PACs or sinus tach
Adverse effects	Prolonged runs of PAT can cause decreased cardiac output. Healthy people can tolerate this rhythm for a while without symptoms, but those with heart disease may develop symptoms rapidly.

Treatment   Digitalis, quinidine, Cardizem, sedation, adenosine, verapamil, oxygen. Synchronized electrical **cardioversion,** electric shock to the heart, can be used in cases in which the medications are unsuccessful or in which the patient's condition deteriorates. Cardioversion is not usually a first choice in treating a rhythm unless it is an emergency.

In Figure 13-6, there are four sinus beats and then a run of five PACs. This run of PACs is called PAT. There are QRS complexes, all the same shape. Regularity is regular but interrupted (by a run of premature beats). Heart rate is 75 for the sinus rhythm, and 187 for the atrial tachycardia. P waves precede each QRS complex but are not all the same shape. The sinus beats have one shape of P wave, and the atrial tachycardia has a different shape P that is deforming the T waves. Note the dots over the premature P waves. P-P interval is regular during the sinus rhythm, and regular, though different, during the atrial tachycardia, but irregular when the strip as a whole is looked at. PR interval is 0.16; QRS 0.08. The PR interval was measured on the sinus beats. The atrial tachycardia PR interval cannot be determined since the P waves are inside the T waves. Interpretation: sinus rhythm with a five-beat run of PAT.

Atrial Tachycardia with 2:1 Block

What is it? Atrial tachycardia with 2:1 block is an atrial tachycardia in which only every second P wave results in a QRS complex. This is because the AV node, as a protective mechanism, allows only every other atrial impulse to get through to the ventricle.

Rate   Atrial rate (from P-P) 160 to 250. Ventricular rate is half the atrial rate.

Regularity   Regular

P waves   Shaped differently from sinus P waves, but the same as each other; two P waves to each QRS. Some P waves may be difficult to see because they may be hidden in the T wave of the preceding beat.

PR   0.12 to 0.20 second, constant

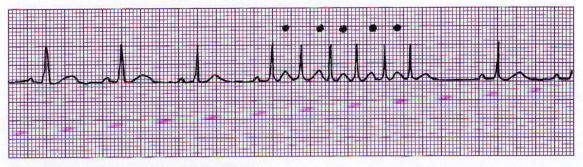

Figure 13-6 Paroxysmal atrial tachycardia.

QRS	<0.12 second (≥0.12 s if BBB present)
Cause	Classically caused by digitalis toxicity, but can also be caused by heart disease
Adverse effects	Usually tolerated well because the heart rate (the ventricular rate) is not too high
Treatment	Hold digitalis if the digitalis level is elevated. Treat with digitalis if it's not the cause. Consider starting oxygen.

In Figure 13-7, there are QRS complexes, all shaped the same. Regularity is regular. Heart rate is 94, atrial rate 187. The atria are tachycardic, as evidenced by the atrial rate. P waves are present, two preceding each QRS complex. P-P interval is regular. The P waves are the same shape, but the P wave closest to the QRS is deformed by the proximity of the QRS. PR interval is approximately 0.12. It's difficult to measure, since the P wave is essentially on top of the QRS. QRS interval is approximately 0.06. Interpretation: atrial tachycardia with 2:1 block.

Multifocal Atrial Tachycardia (MAT)

What is it? Multifocal atrial tachycardia is the same rhythm as wandering atrial pacemaker, but with a mean heart rate greater than 100.

Rate	>100 mean rate
Regularity	Irregular
P waves	At least three different shapes. MAT is simply a run of six or more PACs in a row from different locations. It's the same as WAP but with a faster rate.
PR	Varies
QRS	<0.12 second (≥0.12 s if BBB present)
Cause	Almost always associated with chronic lung disease
Adverse effects	Decreased cardiac output with faster rates
Treatment	Same as atrial tachycardia

In Figure 13-8, there are QRS complexes, all the same shape. Rhythm is irregular. Heart rate is 107 to 187, with a mean rate of 120. P waves vary in shape from beat to beat. P-P interval is irregular. PR interval varies; QRS interval is 0.06. Interpretation: multifocal atrial tachycardia.

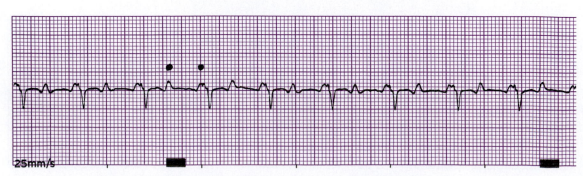

25mm/s

Figure 13-7 Atrial tachycardia with 2:1 block.

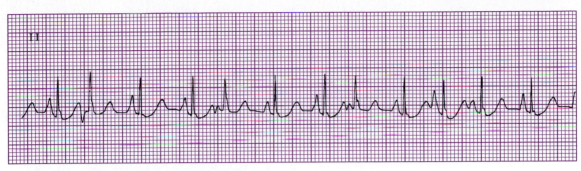

Figure 13-8 Multifocal atrial tachycardia.

Atrial Flutter

What is it? Atrial flutter results when one irritable atrial focus fires out regular impulses at a rate so rapid that a fluttery pattern is produced instead of P waves. The atrial rate is so rapid that the AV node cannot depolarize fast enough to keep up, so many of the impulses never get through to the ventricle.

Rate	Atrial rate 250 to 350. Ventricular rate depends on the conduction ratio.
Regularity	Regular if the conduction ratio is constant; irregular if the conduction ratio varies; can look regular but interrupted at times
P waves	No P waves present. Flutter waves are present instead. These are zigzag or sawtooth-shaped waves between the QRS complexes. Flutter waves are also described as picket-fence-shaped, V-shaped, or upside-down-V shaped. There will be two or more flutter waves to each QRS. All flutter waves march out—they're all the same distance apart. Flutter waves are always regular. They do not interrupt themselves to allow a QRS complex to pop in. Some flutter waves will therefore be hidden inside QRS complexes or T waves. The easiest way to find all the flutter waves is to find two flutter waves back-to-back and note the distance between the two (measure from either the top or bottom of the flutter waves; go from top to top of the flutter waves or bottom to bottom). Then march out where the rest of the flutter waves should be using this interval. Though most flutter waves will be easily visible using this method, some flutter waves will not be as obvious, as they are hidden inside the QRS or the T wave. Even though you can't see these flutter waves, they are there and they still count. The downstroke of the flutter waves indicates atrial depolarization, and the upstroke denotes atrial repolarization.
PR	Not measured, since there are no real P waves
QRS	<0.12 second (≥0.12 s if BBB present)

Cause	Almost always implies heart disease. Other causes include pulmonary embolus, valvular heart disease, thyrotoxicosis, or lung disease.
Adverse effects	Can be very well tolerated at normal ventricular rates. At higher rates, signs of decreased cardiac output can occur. Cardiac output is influenced not by the atrial rate, but by the heart rate.
Treatment	Digitalis, quinidine, ibutilide, adenosine, carotid sinus massage to slow the ventricular rate. Electrical cardioversion can be done if medications are ineffective or the patient's condition deteriorates.

In Figure 13-9, there are QRS complexes, all shaped the same. Regularity is regular. Atrial rate is 300; heart rate is 100. P waves are not present; flutter waves are present instead, as evidenced by the zigzag pattern of waves between the QRS complexes. Flutter waves are all regular. PR interval is not measured in atrial flutter. QRS interval is approximately 0.10, though it's difficult to measure as the flutter waves distort the QRS complex. Interpretation: atrial flutter with 3:1 conduction (three flutter waves to each QRS). See the dots under the flutter waves? There are three dots for each QRS. What if we measured from the top of the flutter waves instead of the bottom? Same thing. See the asterisks above the flutter waves? There are three of them (the third flutter wave is *inside* the QRS, but it still counts) to each QRS complex.

Atrial Fibrillation

What is it? In atrial fibrillation there are hundreds of atrial impulses from different locations all firing off at the same time. As a result, the atria depolarize not as a unit as they usually do, but rather in small sections. This causes the atria to wiggle instead of contract. The AV node is bombarded with all these impulses and simply cannot depolarize fast enough to let them all through. Every now and then one of these impulses does get through to the ventricle and provides a QRS.

Rate	Atrial rate is 350 to 700; ventricular rate varies. Atrial fibrillation with a ventricular rate >150 is called uncontrolled atrial fib; a ventricular rate of >100 is called rapid

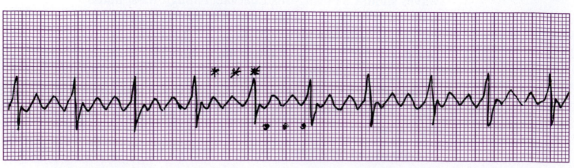

Figure 13-9 Atrial flutter.

atrial fib; a ventricular rate of <60 is slow atrial fib. Remember ventricular rate is the same as heart rate.

Regularity	Irregularly irregular, completely unpredictable
P waves	No P waves are present. Fibrillatory waves are present instead. These are undulations or waviness of the baseline between QRSs. If there are P waves, the rhythm is not atrial fibrillation.
PR	Since there are no P waves, there is no PR interval.
QRS	<0.12 second (>0.12 s if BBB present)
Cause	MI, lung disease, valvular heart disease, hyperthyroidism
Adverse effects	Atrial fibrillation can cause a drop in cardiac output because of the loss of the atrial kick, which accounts for 15 to 30% of the cardiac output. One possible complication of atrial fibrillation is blood clots, which can collect in the sluggish atria. This can result in MI, strokes, or blood clots in the lung.
Treatment	Digitalis, quinidine, ibutilide, Cardizem. An anticoagulant called Coumadin can be given to prevent blood clots from forming. Electrical cardioversion can be done if the medications don't work or the patient's condition deteriorates. Consider starting oxygen.

In Figure 13-10, there are QRS complexes, all the same shape. Regularity is irregular. Heart rate is 65 to 100, with a mean rate of 90. P waves are absent; fibrillatory waves are present instead. PR interval is not applicable; QRS interval is 0.10. Interpretation: atrial fibrillation.

Supraventricular Tachycardia (SVT)

What is it? SVT is a term given to tachycardias that originate above the ventricles (hence the term supraventricular) in either the sinus node, the atrium, or the AV node, but whose exact origin cannot be identified because P waves are not discernible. SVT can include rhythms such as atrial tachycardia, sinus tachycardia, junctional tachycardia, and atrial flutter with 2:1 conduction.

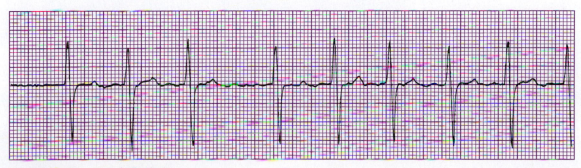

Figure 13-10 Atrial fibrillation.

Rate	About 130 or higher
Regularity	Regular
P waves	Not discernible
PR	Cannot be measured since P waves cannot be positively identified
QRS	<0.12 second (≥0.12 s if BBB present)
Cause	Same as PAT
Adverse effects	Decreased cardiac output secondary to the rapid heart rate
Treatment	Digitalis, ibutilide, calcium channel blockers, beta-blockers. Consider starting oxygen.

In Figure 13-11, there are QRS complexes, all shaped the same. Rhythm is regular. Heart rate is 150. P waves are not identifiable. PR interval is not measurable. QRS interval is 0.08. Interpretation: SVT. Could it be atrial flutter? Sure. Could it be sinus tachycardia with the P inside the T wave? Possibly. The point is the origin of this rhythm is not clear, but we know that it originated in a pacemaker above the ventricle, since the QRS complex is narrow, less than 0.12 second. (Rhythms that originate in the ventricle have a wide QRS complex, greater than 0.12 second.) Bottom line: If the QRS is <0.12 second, the heart rate is around 130 or higher, the rhythm is regular, and you can't pick out the P waves, call the rhythm SVT.

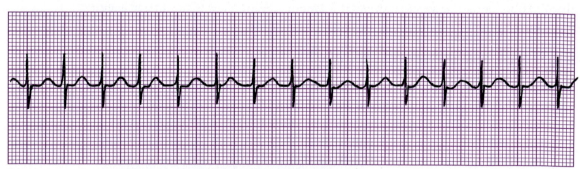

Figure 13-11 Supraventricular tachycardia.

Practice Strips: Atrial Rhythms

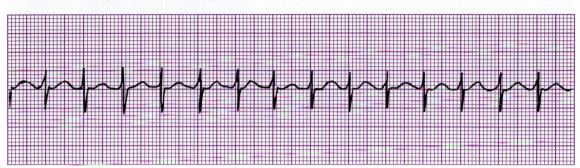

1. QRS complexes _____ Regularity _____

Heart rate _____

P waves _____

PR interval _____ QRS interval _____

Interpretation (name of rhythm) _____

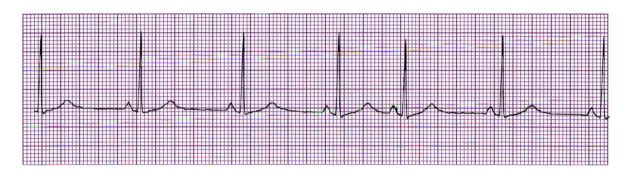

2. QRS complexes _____ Regularity _____

Heart rate _____

P waves _____

PR interval _____ QRS interval _____

Interpretation _____

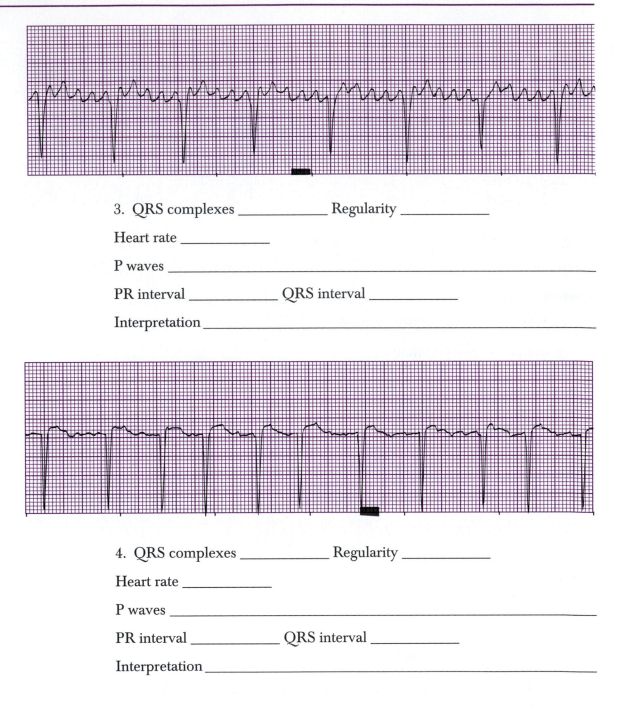

3. QRS complexes _____ Regularity _____

Heart rate _____

P waves _____

PR interval _____ QRS interval _____

Interpretation _____

4. QRS complexes _____ Regularity _____

Heart rate _____

P waves _____

PR interval _____ QRS interval _____

Interpretation _____

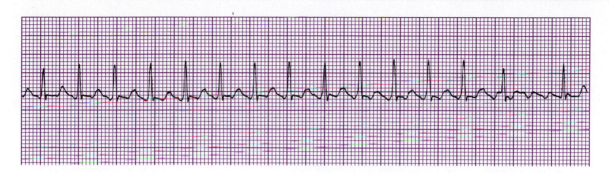

5. QRS complexes _____ Regularity _____

Heart rate _____

P waves _____

PR interval _____ QRS interval _____

Interpretation _____

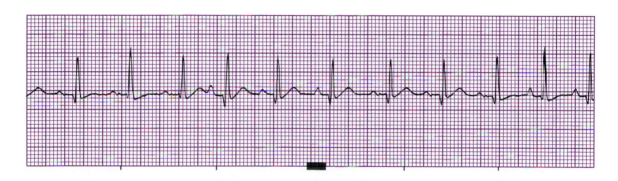

6. QRS complexes _____ Regularity _____

Heart rate _____

P waves _____

PR interval _____ QRS interval _____

Interpretation _____

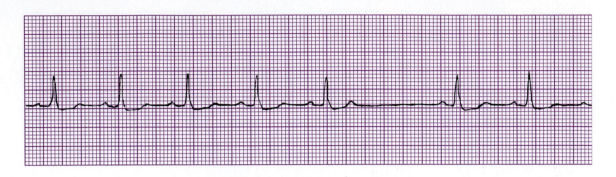

7. QRS complexes _____ Regularity _____

Heart rate _____

P waves _____

PR interval _____ QRS interval _____

Interpretation _____

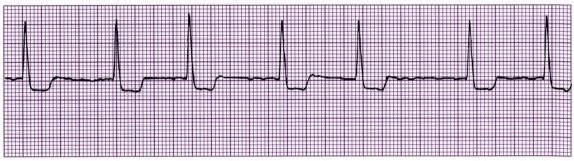

8. QRS complexes _____ Regularity _____

Heart rate _____

P waves _____

PR interval _____ QRS interval _____

Interpretation _____

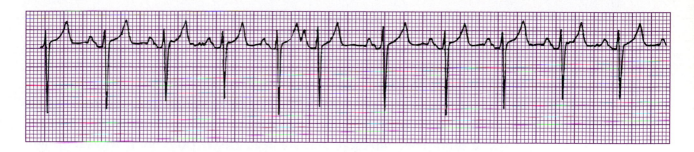

9. QRS complexes _____ Regularity _____

Heart rate _____

P waves _____

PR interval _____ QRS interval _____

Interpretation _____

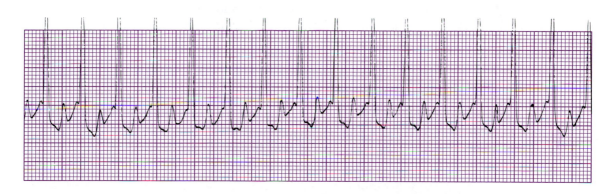

10. QRS complexes _____ Regularity _____

Heart rate _____

P waves _____

PR interval _____ QRS interval _____

Interpretation _____

Answers to Atrial Rhythms Practice Strips

1. **QRS complexes:** present, all shaped the same. **Regularity:** regular. **Heart rate:** 150. **P waves:** none visible. **PR:** not applicable. **QRS:** 0.08. **Interpretation:** SVT.

2. **QRS complexes:** present, all shaped the same. **Regularity:** regular but interrupted (by a premature beat). Remember it's normal to have a short pause after a premature beat. **Heart rate:** 56. **P waves:** upright and matching, except for the fourth P wave, which is premature and shaped differently. (There is a tiny notch on the downstroke of the premature P wave.) P-P interval irregular because of the premature beat. **PR:** 0.12. **QRS:** 0.08. **Interpretation:** sinus bradycardia with a PAC.

3. **QRS complexes:** present, all shaped the same. **Regularity:** regular. **Heart rate:** atrial rate 375; ventricular rate 79. **P waves:** none present; flutter waves present instead. **PR:** not applicable. **QRS:** 0.10. **Interpretation:** atrial flutter with 5:1 and 6:1 conduction.

4. **QRS complexes:** present, all shaped the same. **Regularity:** irregular. **Heart rate:** 88 to 137, with a mean rate of 110. **P waves:** none present; wavy baseline present instead. **PR:** not applicable. **QRS:** 0.08. **Interpretation:** atrial fibrillation.

5. **QRS complexes:** present, all shaped the same. **Regularity:** regular but interrupted (by a pause). **Heart rate:** atrial rate 300; ventricular rate 98 to 158, with a mean rate of 150. **P waves:** none present; flutter waves present instead. **PR:** not applicable. **QRS:** 0.08. **Interpretation:** atrial flutter with 2:1 and 4:1 conduction.

6. **QRS complexes:** present, all shaped the same. **Regularity:** irregular. **Heart rate:** 100 to 125, with a mean rate of 110. **P waves:** at least three different shapes. P-P interval irregular. **PR:** varies. **QRS:** 0.08. **Interpretation:** multifocal atrial tachycardia.

7. **QRS complexes:** present, all shaped the same. **Regularity:** regular but interrupted (by a pause). **Heart rate:** 43 to 83. **P waves:** upright and matching, one before each beat. See the T wave of the last beat before the pause? It's a bit taller than the other Ts. There is a P hiding inside it, distorting its normal shape. That P in the T is premature, so that makes it a PAC. **PR:** 0.16. **QRS:** 0.10. **Interpretation:** sinus rhythm with a nonconducted PAC.

8. **QRS complexes:** present, all shaped the same. **Regularity:** irregular. **Heart rate:** 52 to 75, with a mean rate of 70. **P waves:** none present; wavy baseline present instead. **PR:** not applicable. **QRS:** 0.10. **Interpretation:** atrial fibrillation.

9. **QRS complexes:** present, all shaped the same. **Regularity:** regular but interrupted (by a premature beat). **Heart rate:** 100. **P waves:** upright, all matching except for the premature P wave preceding the sixth QRS complex. There is one P wave preceding each QRS complex. P-P interval irregular. **PR:** 0.16. **QRS:** 0.08. **Interpretation:** sinus rhythm with a PAC.

10. **QRS complexes:** present, all shaped the same. **Regularity:** regular. **Heart rate:** about 150. **P waves:** Is that a tall pointy P wave distorting the T waves? Maybe. But it's also a possibility that those are flutter waves between the QRS complexes. We just can't be sure. **PR:** not applicable. **QRS:** 0.08. **Interpretation:** SVT.

Practice Quiz

1. What common complication of atrial fibrillation is treated with anticoagulant medications?_____

   _____

2. The rhythm that is the same as wandering atrial pacemaker except for the heart rate is _____

   _____

3. The rhythm that produces a zigzag pattern between QRS complexes is

   _____

4. Atrial rhythms take what path to the ventricles? _____

5. All rhythms that originate in a pacemaker other than the sinus node are called _____

   _____

6. Synchronized electrical cardioversion can be used to treat which atrial arrhythmias? _____

   _____

7. True or false: All PACs conduct through to the ventricles.

8. The classic cause of multifocal atrial tachycardia is_____

9. The classic cause of atrial tachycardia with 2:1 block is _____

10. If the rhythm is regular, heart rate is 130 or greater, and P waves cannot be identified, the rhythm is called_____

Practice Quiz Answers

1. The complication of atrial fibrillation that is treated with anticoagulants is **blood clots.**

2. The rhythm that is the same as wandering atrial pacemaker except for the heart rate is **multifocal atrial tachycardia.**

3. The rhythm that produces a zigzag pattern between QRS complexes is **atrial flutter.**

4. Atrial rhythms take **the normal conduction pathway to the ventricles after depolarizing the atria.**

5. All rhythms that originate in a pacemaker other than the sinus node are called **ectopic rhythms.**

6. Synchronized electrical cardioversion can be used to treat **PAT, atrial flutter, atrial fibrillation,** and **SVT.**

7. **False.** Some PACs are nonconducted.

8. The classic cause of multifocal atrial tachycardia is **chronic lung disease.**

9. The classic cause of atrial tachycardia with 2:1 block is **digitalis toxicity.**

10. If the rhythm is regular, heart rate is 130 or greater, and P waves cannot be identified, the rhythm is called **SVT.**

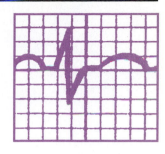

Rhythms Originating in the AV Node

Chapter 14 Objectives

Upon completion of this chapter, the student will be able to:

- State the criteria for each junctional rhythm.
- Differentiate between *high, low,* and *midjunctional.*
- Correctly identify the junctional rhythms using the criteria and the rhythm strip analysis tools.
- State the adverse effects of each junctional rhythm.
- State the possible treatment for the junctional rhythms.
- State which junctional rhythms occur mostly because of escape and which imply usurpation.

Chapter 14 Outline

I.   Introduction
II.   The skinny on junctional rhythms
III.   PJCs
IV.   Junctional bradycardia
V.   Junctional rhythm
VI.   Accelerated junctional rhythm
VII.   Junctional tachycardia
VIII.   Practice strips: junctional rhythms
IX.   Answers to junctional rhythms practice strips
X.   Practice quiz
XI.   Practice quiz answers

Chapter 14 Glossary

Antegrade: In a forward direction.
Inverted: Upside down.
Retrograde: In a backward direction.

Introduction

Though it was once thought that these rhythms originated only in the AV node itself, it is now recognized that they also arise from the **AV junction,** the tissue immediately surrounding the AV node. All these rhythms are blanketed under the term **junctional rhythms.**

With junctional rhythms, the impulse travels **antegrade,** or forward, toward the ventricle, and **retrograde,** or backward, toward the atria. Thus the impulse travels in two directions. The AV junctional area can be divided into regions—high, mid, and low—and whichever of these regions initiates the impulse will determine the location of the P wave.

If the impulse originates high in the AV junction, close to the atria, it will arrive at the atria first and write an **inverted** (upside down) P wave. The P wave is inverted because the impulse is going in a backward direction to reach the atria. Then the forward impulses reach the ventricle and write the QRS complex. The PR interval is short, less than 0.12 second. Because the impulse starts out in the AV junction, halfway to the ventricle, it simply doesn't have as far to go as sinus impulses would. Bottom line: If the impulse originates high in the AV junction, the resultant rhythm or beat will have an inverted P wave preceding the QRS, and the PR interval should be less than 0.12 second.

If the impulse originates midway in the AV junction, the impulses will reach the atria and ventricles simultaneously. Therefore, the P wave will be swallowed up by the QRS complex. Bottom line: Midjunctional impulses have no visible P waves.

If the impulse originates low in the AV junction, the impulses will reach the ventricle first, writing a QRS complex, and then reaching the atria and writing the P wave. Thus the P wave will follow the QRS and, since the impulses must travel backward to reach the atria, the P wave will be inverted. Bottom line: Impulses originating from low in the AV junction have inverted P waves following the QRS complex. See Figure 14-1.

The Skinny on Junctional Rhythms

Junctional rhythms are seen less often than sinus or atrial rhythms. Though the inherent rate of the AV node is 40 to 60, the heart rate may actually go much faster or slower, which can result in symptoms. More normal heart rates are less likely to cause symptoms.

Treatment is aimed at alleviating the cause of the junctional rhythm. More active treatment is not usually necessary unless symptoms develop, at which time the goal is to return the sinus node to control or to return the heart rate to more normal levels.

Junctional rhythms are very easy to identify. Let's look at the criteria.

- Regular rhythm or premature beat with narrow QRS and one of the following:
  Absent P waves
  Inverted P waves following the QRS
  Inverted P waves with short PR interval preceding the QRS

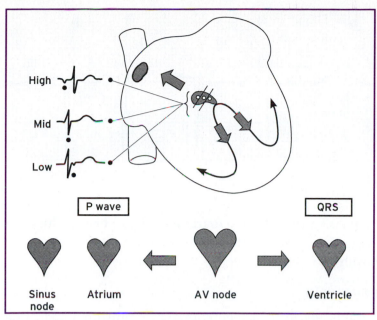

Figure 14-1   Conduction and P wave location in junctional rhythms.

The following junctional rhythms will be covered in this section:

- Premature junctional complexes (PJCs)
- Junctional bradycardia
- Junctional rhythm
- Accelerated junctional rhythm
- Junctional tachycardia

Let's look at each of these rhythms in detail.

Premature Junctional Complexes (PJCs)

What are they? PJCs are premature beats that originate in the AV junction before the next sinus beat is due. This is caused by irritable tissue in the AV node region firing off and usurping the sinus node for that beat.

Rate	Can occur at any rate
Regularity	Regular but interrupted
P waves	Inverted before or after the QRS, or hidden inside the QRS
PR	<0.12 second if the P wave precedes the QRS
QRS	<0.12 second (≥0.12 s if BBB present)
Cause	Stimulants (such as caffeine or drugs), nicotine, hypoxia, heart disease
Adverse effects	Usually no ill effects
Treatment	Usually none required aside from removal of the cause

In Figure 14-2, there are QRS complexes, all shaped the same. Regularity is regular but interrupted (by two premature beats). Heart rate is 71. P waves

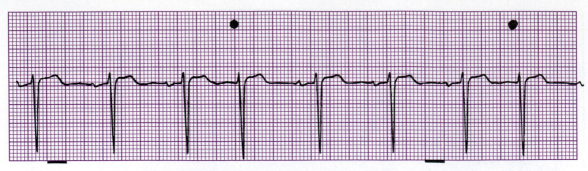

Figure 14-2 PJC.

are matching and biphasic except for the fourth and eighth beats, which are premature and have no P waves. PR interval is 0.16; QRS is 0.10. Interpretation: sinus rhythm with two PJCs.

Junctional Bradycardia

What is it? Junctional bradycardia is a junctional rhythm with a heart rate slower than usual. A higher pacemaker has failed, and the AV node has to escape to save the patient's life.

Rate	<40
Regularity	Regular
P waves	Inverted before or after the QRS, or hidden inside the QRS
PR	<0.12 second if the P precedes the QRS
QRS	<0.12 second (≥0.12 s if BBB present)
Cause	Vagal stimulation, hypoxia, ischemia of the sinus node, heart disease
Adverse effects	The slow heart rate can cause decreased cardiac output.
Treatment	Atropine if the patient is symptomatic. Hold or withdraw any medications that can slow the heart rate. A pacemaker can be utilized if atropine is unsuccessful and the patient is symptomatic. Start oxygen.

In Figure 14-3, there are QRS complexes, all shaped the same. Regularity is regular. Heart rate is 23. P waves are absent, or at least not visible. There is

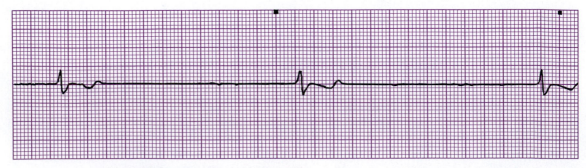

Figure 14-3 Junctional bradycardia.

some somatic tremor artifact causing the baseline to look a bit jittery. PR interval is not applicable. QRS interval is 0.12. Interpretation: junctional bradycardia.

Junctional Rhythm

What is it? Junctional rhythm is a rhythm that originates in the AV junction at its inherent rate of 40 to 60. It is usually an escape rhythm.

Rate	40 to 60
Regularity	Regular
P waves	Inverted before or after the QRS, or hidden inside the QRS
PR	<0.12 second if the P precedes the QRS
QRS	<0.12 second (≥0.12 s if BBB present)
Cause	Vagal stimulation, hypoxia, sinus node ischemia, heart disease
Adverse effects	Very often there are no ill effects if the heart rate is closer to the 50s to 60s range. Signs of decreased cardiac output are possible at slower heart rates.
Treatment	Atropine if symptomatic from the slow heart rate. Withdraw or decrease any medications that can slow the heart rate. Consider starting oxygen.

In Figure 14-4, there are QRS complexes, all the same shape. Regularity is regular. Heart rate is 58. P waves are absent. (Those are not P waves after the QRS; those are S waves, a part of the QRS.) PR interval is not applicable. QRS interval is 0.12. Interpretation: junctional rhythm. Though this example of junctional rhythm has no visible P waves, it could just as easily have had an inverted P wave with a short PR interval preceding the QRS, or an inverted P wave following the QRS. Remember, the location of the P wave is dependent upon the region of the AV junction in which the impulse originates.

Accelerated Junctional Rhythm

What is it? Accelerated junctional rhythm can occur because of escape or usurpation. If the sinus node slows down, the AV junction can become stimulated to escape and take over as the pacemaker. Or an irritable spot in the

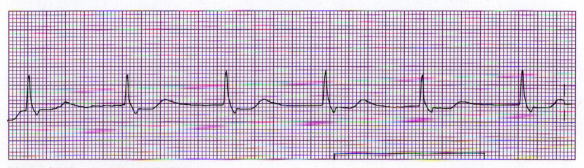

Figure 14-4 Junctional rhythm.

AV junction can usurp control from the slower sinus node and become the heart's pacemaker at a heart rate faster than the AV junction normally fires.

Rate	60 to 100
Regularity	Regular
P waves	Inverted before or after the QRS, or hidden inside the QRS
PR	<0.12 second if the P precedes the QRS
QRS	<0.12 second (≥0.12 s if BBB present)
Cause	Heart disease, stimulant drugs, and caffeine
Adverse effects	Usually no ill effects because the heart rate is within normal limits
Treatment	Usually none required aside from removal of the cause

In Figure 14-5, there are QRS complexes, all the same shape. Regularity is regular. Heart rate is 75. P waves are absent. PR interval is not applicable. QRS interval is 0.08. Interpretation: accelerated junctional rhythm.

Junctional Tachycardia

What is it? An irritable spot in the AV junction has taken over as the pacemaker, and the heart rate is very rapid. This is usually a result of usurpation. Junctional tachycardia is best called SVT if there are no visible P waves, as the origin of the rhythm could not be identified.

Rate	>100
Regularity	Regular
P waves	Inverted before or after the QRS, or hidden inside the QRS
PR	<0.12 second if the P precedes the QRS
QRS	<0.12 second (≥0.12 s if BBB present)
Cause	Most often caused by digitalis toxicity, but can be caused by heart disease, stimulants, or anything else that stimulates the sympathetic nervous system to speed up the heart rate

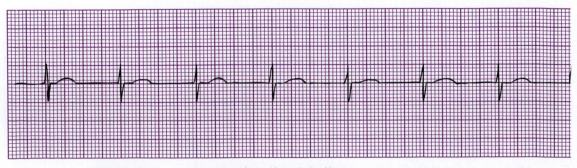

Figure 14-5 Accelerated junctional rhythm.

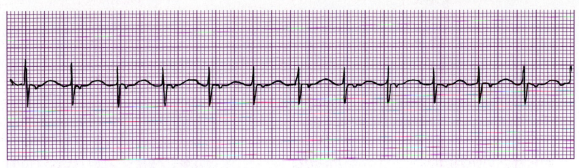

Figure 14-6 Junctional tachycardia.

Adverse effects   Decreased cardiac output possible if the heart rate is fast enough

Treatment   Beta-blockers, calcium channel blockers, adenosine. Consider starting oxygen.

In Figure 14-6, there are QRS complexes, all the same shape. Regularity is regular. Heart rate is 125. P waves are present, inverted, following the QRS complex. PR interval is not applicable. QRS interval is 0.08. Interpretation: junctional tachycardia.

Practice Strips: Junctional Rhythms

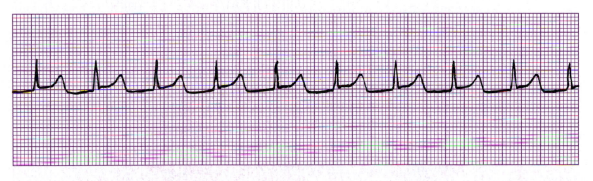

1. QRS complexes _____ Regularity _____

Heart rate _____

P waves _____

PR interval _____ QRS interval _____

Interpretation (name of rhythm) _____

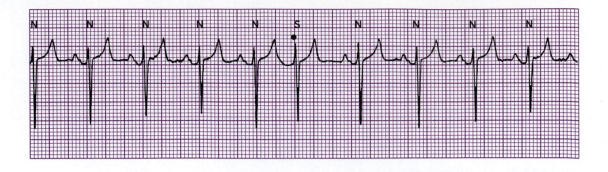

2. QRS complexes _____ Regularity _____

Heart rate _____

P waves _____

PR interval _____ QRS interval _____

Interpretation _____

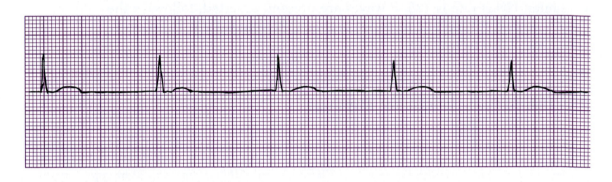

3. QRS complexes _____ Regularity _____

Heart rate _____

P waves _____

PR interval _____ QRS interval _____

Interpretation _____

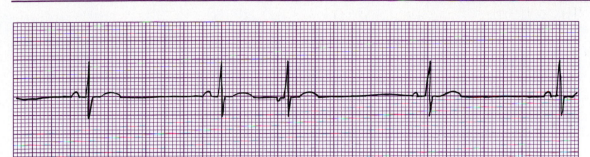

4. QRS complexes _____ Regularity _____

Heart rate _____

P waves _____

PR interval _____ QRS interval _____

Interpretation _____

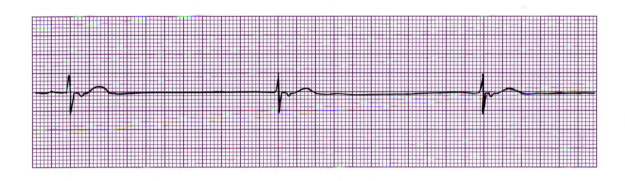

5. QRS complexes _____ Regularity _____

Heart rate _____

P waves _____

PR interval _____ QRS interval _____

Interpretation _____

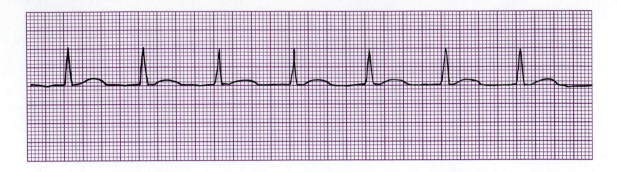

6. QRS complexes _____ Regularity _____

Heart rate _____

P waves _____

PR interval _____ QRS interval _____

Interpretation _____

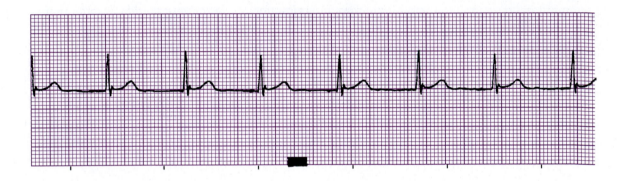

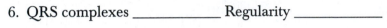

7. QRS complexes _____ Regularity _____

Heart rate _____

P waves _____

PR interval _____ QRS interval _____

Interpretation _____

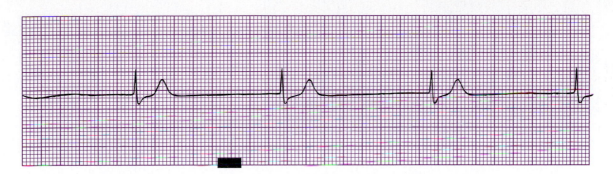

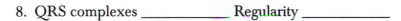

8. QRS complexes _____ Regularity _____

Heart rate _____

P waves _____

PR interval _____ QRS interval _____

Interpretation _____

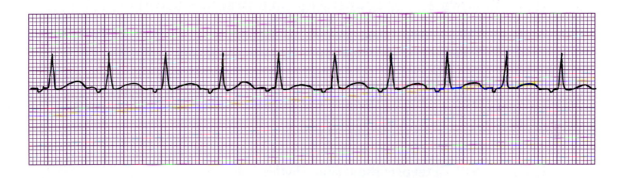

9. QRS complexes _____ Regularity _____

Heart rate _____

P waves _____

PR interval _____ QRS interval _____

Interpretation _____

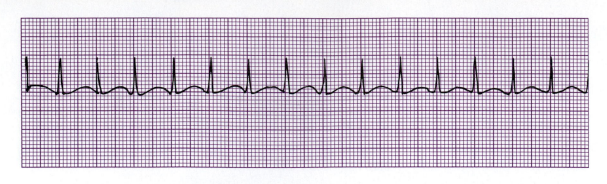

10. QRS complexes _____ Regularity _____

Heart rate _____

P waves _____

PR interval _____ QRS interval _____

Interpretation _____

Answers to Junctional Rhythms Practice Strips

1. **QRS complexes:** present, all shaped the same. **Regularity:** regular. **Heart rate:** 94. **P waves:** none visible. **PR:** not applicable. **QRS:** 0.08. **Interpretation:** accelerated junctional rhythm.

2. **QRS complexes:** present, all shaped the same. **Regularity:** regular but interrupted. **Heart rate:** 100. **P waves:** matching and upright on all except the sixth beat. That beat has no visible P wave at all. P-P interval is regular except for that sixth beat, which is premature. **PR:** 0.14. **QRS:** 0.08. **Interpretation:** sinus rhythm with a PJC.

3. **QRS complexes:** present, all shaped the same. **Regularity:** regular. **Heart rate:** 48. **P waves:** none visible. **PR:** not applicable. **QRS:** 0.08. **Interpretation:** junctional rhythm.

4. **QRS complexes:** present, all shaped the same. **Regularity:** regular but interrupted. **Heart rate:** 47. **P waves:** matching upright Ps present except on the third beat, which has an inverted P wave preceding the QRS. **PR:** 0.16 on the beats with upright Ps; 0.06 on the third beat. **QRS:** 0.08. **Interpretation:** sinus bradycardia with a PJC. Remember it is normal for the R-R cycle immediately following a premature beat to be a little longer than usual. Consider this when determining the regularity.

5. **QRS complexes:** present, all shaped the same. **Regularity:** regular. **Heart rate:** 28. **P waves:** inverted following the QRS complexes. **PR:** not applicable. **QRS:** 0.08. **Interpretation:** junctional bradycardia.

6. **QRS complexes:** present, all shaped the same. **Regularity:** regular. **Heart rate:** 75. **P waves:** none visible. **PR:** not applicable. **QRS:** 0.08. **Interpretation:** accelerated junctional rhythm.

7. **QRS complexes:** present, all shaped the same. **Regularity:** regular. **Heart rate:** 72. **P waves:** none visible. **PR:** not applicable. **QRS:** 0.10. **Interpretation:** accelerated junctional rhythm.

8. **QRS complexes:** present, all shaped the same. **Regularity:** regular. **Heart rate:** 38. **P waves:** none visible. **PR:** not applicable. **QRS:** 0.10. **Interpretation:** junctional bradycardia.

9. **QRS complexes:** present, all shaped the same. **Regularity:** regular. **Heart rate:** 100. **P waves:** inverted preceding each QRS. **PR:** 0.10 to 0.12. **QRS:** 0.08. **Interpretation:** accelerated junctional rhythm.

10. **QRS complexes:** present, all shaped the same. **Regularity:** regular. **Heart rate:** 150. **P waves:** none visible. **PR:** not applicable. **QRS:** 0.08. **Interpretation:** SVT. Though this could indeed be a junctional tachycardia, it is best to call this SVT since P waves cannot be seen. Had there been an inverted P wave present, we'd have known for sure the rhythm was junctional in origin. Without those P waves, we can't be sure the rhythm is junctional. It could be atrial or even sinus in origin (with the P waves hidden inside the T waves).

Practice Quiz

1. What are the three possible locations for the P waves in junctional rhythms?_____

   _____

   _____

2. Why is the P wave inverted in junctional rhythms? _____

   _____

3. A junctional rhythm with a heart rate greater than 100 is _____

4. True or false: PJCs are a sign that the heart is going to develop a lethal arrhythmia.

5. A junctional rhythm with a heart rate less than 40 is _____

6. Treatment for junctional bradycardia would consist of_____

   _____

   _____

7. PJCs cause the regularity to be _____

8. Is junctional bradycardia usually a result of escape or usurpation?_____

   _____

9. Junctional tachycardia is best called SVT if the P waves are located where? _____

   _____

10. Is junctional tachycardia a result of escape or usurpation?_____

Practice Quiz Answers

1. The three possible locations for the P waves in junctional rhythms are **before the QRS complex, after the QRS complex,** and **hidden inside the QRS complex.**

2. The P wave is inverted in junctional rhythms because **the impulse travels in a backward direction to reach the atria.**

3. A junctional rhythm with a heart rate greater than 100 is **junctional tachycardia.**

4. **False.** PJCs do not imply that a lethal arrhythmia is imminent.

5. A junctional rhythm with a heart rate less than 40 is **junctional bradycardia.**

6. Treatment for junctional bradycardia would consist of **atropine if the patient is symptomatic, consideration of starting oxygen, discontinuing or decreasing the dosage of any medications that could slow the heart rate down, and consideration of a pacemaker.**

7. PJCs cause the regularity to be **regular but interrupted.**

8. Junctional bradycardia is usually the result of **escape.**

9. Junctional tachycardia is best called SVT if the P waves are **hidden inside the QRS.**

10. Junctional tachycardia is the result of **usurpation.**

Rhythms Originating in the Ventricles

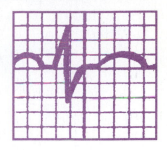

Chapter 15 Objectives

Upon completion of this chapter, the student will be able to:

- State the criteria for each of the ventricular rhythms.
- Using the criteria and the other rhythm analysis tools, correctly identify ventricular rhythms on a variety of strips.
- State the adverse effects for each ventricular rhythm.
- State the possible treatment for the ventricular rhythms.

Chapter 15 Outline

I.   Introduction
II.   The skinny on ventricular rhythms
III. PVCs
IV.   Agonal rhythm
V.   Idioventricular rhythm
VI.   Accelerated idioventricular rhythm
VII. Ventricular tachycardia
VIII. Torsades de pointes
IX.   Ventricular flutter
X.   Ventricular fibrillation
XI.   Asystole
XII. Pacemaker rhythms
XIII. Practice strips: ventricular rhythms
XIV. Answers to ventricular rhythms practice strips
XV.   Practice quiz
XVI. Practice quiz answers

Chapter 15 Glossary

Bigeminy: Every other beat is an abnormal beat.

Couplet: A pair of beats.

Defibrillation: Asynchronous electrical shock to the heart, used to treat ventricular fibrillation and pulseless ventricular tachycardia.

Hypokalemia: Low blood potassium level.

Multifocal: Coming from more than one location.

Quadrigeminy: Every fourth beat is an abnormal beat.

Trigeminy: Every third beat is an abnormal beat.

Unifocal: Coming from one location.

Introduction

Ventricular rhythms originate in one or more irritable foci in the ventricular tissue and do not have the benefit of the conduction system to speed the depolarization there. The result is that the impulses trudge very slowly, cell by cell, through the ventricle, producing a very wide QRS complex that measures >0.12 seconds. The impulse does sometimes travel backward to depolarize the atria, but the resultant P wave is usually lost in the mammoth QRS complex. Slow ventricular rhythms are the heart's last gasp as a pacemaker, kicking in when the higher pacemakers can't. Rapid ventricular arrhythmias can result in drastically decreased cardiac output, cardiovascular collapse, and death. See Figures 15-1 and 15-2.

The Skinny on Ventricular Rhythms

Ventricular rhythms are by far the most potentially lethal of all the rhythms. They therefore command great respect from healthcare personnel. Ventricular rhythms can result from escape (you'll recall the inherent rate of the ventricle is 20 to 40) or usurpation, and can have a heart rate varying from 0 to over 250 beats per minute. Though some ventricular rhythms can be well tolerated, most will cause symptoms of decreased cardiac output, if not frank cardiac standstill.

Most ventricular rhythms respond well to medications. Oddly enough, however, some of the very medications used to treat ventricular rhythms can

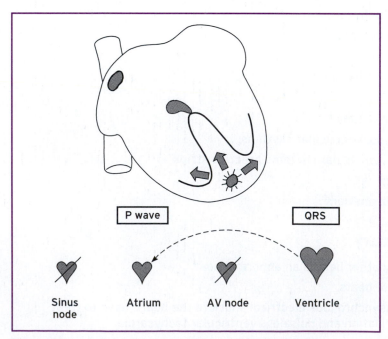

Figure 15-1   Conduction of a single ventricular focus.

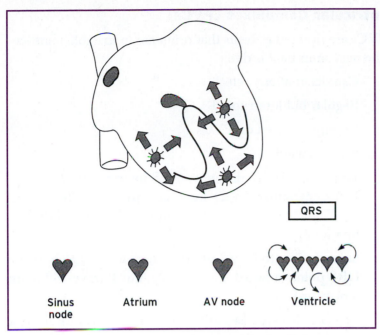

Figure 15-2   Conduction of multiple ventricular foci.

cause them in some circumstances. Some ventricular rhythms can only be treated by electric shock to the heart. And others, despite aggressive treatment, are usually lethal.

Ventricular beats have wide, bizarre QRS complexes. Some ventricular rhythms, however, have no QRS complexes at all. If the rhythm or beat in question meets *any* of the criteria below, it is ventricular in origin. Let's look at the criteria.

- Wide QRS (>0.12 second) without preceding P wave *or*
- No QRS at all (*or* can't be sure if there are QRS complexes), *or*
- Premature, wide QRS beat without preceding P wave, interrupting another rhythm

The ventricular rhythms that will be covered in this section are the following:

- Premature ventricular complexes (PVCs)
- Agonal rhythm
- Idioventricular rhythm
- Accelerated idioventricular rhythm
- Ventricular tachycardia
- Torsades de pointes
- Ventricular flutter
- Ventricular fibrillation
- Asystole
- Ventricular asystole
- Pacemaker rhythms

Let's look at each of these rhythms in detail.

Premature Ventricular Complexes (PVCs)

What are they? PVCs are premature beats that originate in irritable ventricular tissue before the next sinus beat is due.

Rate	Can occur at any rate
Regularity	Regular but interrupted
P waves	Usually not seen on PVCs
PR	Not applicable
QRS	Wide and bizarre in shape. QRS interval >0.12 second. Left-ventricular PVCs have an upward deflection in V_1. Right-ventricular PVCs have a downward deflection in V_1.
T wave	Slopes off in the opposite direction to the QRS. If the QRS points upward, for example, the T wave will point downward.
Cause	The big three causes are heart disease, **hypokalemia** (low blood potassium level), and hypoxia. Other causes include low blood magnesium level, stimulants, caffeine, stress, or anxiety. All these things can cause the ventricle to become irritable and fire off early beats.
Adverse effects	Occasional PVCs are of no concern. Frequent PVCs (six or more per minute) or PVCs that are very close to the preceding T wave can progress to lethal arrhythmias like ventricular tachycardia or ventricular fibrillation. Multifocal PVCs are also cause for concern, since it means that there are multiple irritable areas.
Treatment	Occasional PVCs don't require treatment. They can occur in normal healthy individuals. If PVCs are more frequent, treat the cause. If the potassium level is low, give supplemental potassium. Start oxygen. Lidocaine is the medication most commonly used to treat PVCs that are frequent or close to the T wave. Procainamide can also be used, as can amiodarone or a number of other medications to decrease ventricular irritability and prevent lethal arrhythmias. Frequent PVCs in the presence of a slow bradycardia are not treated with lidocaine, however. They are treated with atropine. Bradycardic rhythm PVCs are the heart's attempt to increase the heart rate by providing another beat from *somewhere* . . . anywhere. Giving lidocaine would knock out the PVCs, leaving a slower heart rate. Atropine would speed up the underlying rhythm and the PVCs would go away on their own. See Figure 15-3.

In Figure 15-3, there are QRS complexes, all except the fourth beat having the same shape. The fourth beat has a very wide QRS complex. Regular-

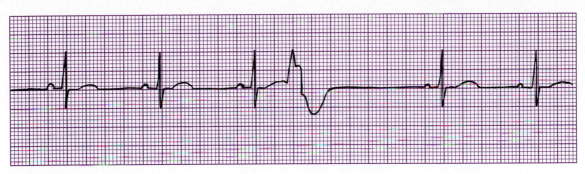

Figure 15-3   PVC.

ity is regular but interrupted. Heart rate is 60. There are matching upright P waves on all beats except the fourth beat, which has no P wave at all. PR interval is 0.16 on the sinus beats, no PR on the PVC. QRS interval is 0.08 on the sinus beats, 0.14 on the PVC. Interpretation: sinus rhythm with one PVC.

PVCs that come from a single focus all look alike. They're called **unifocal** PVCs. PVCs from different foci look different. They're called **multifocal** PVCs. See Figure 15-4.

Note in Figure 15-4 that A's PVCs are shaped the same–they're unifocal. B's PVCs are shaped differently–they're multifocal.

Two consecutive PVCs are called a **couplet.** Couplets can be either unifocal or multifocal. See Figure 15-5.

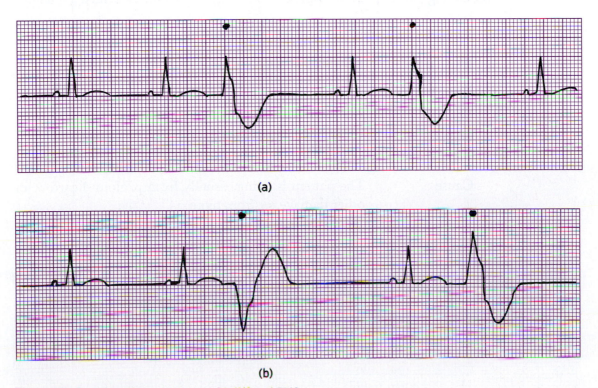

(a)

(b)

Figure 15-4   (a) Unifocal PVCs. (b) Multifocal PVCs.

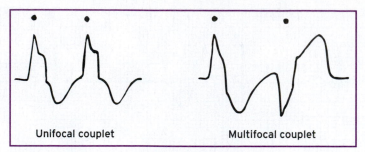

Figure 15-5   Unifocal and multifocal couplets.

PVCs can be very regular at times. If every other beat is a PVC, it's called ventricular **bigeminy.** If every third beat is a PVC, it's called ventricular **trigeminy.** If every fourth beat is a PVC, it's ventricular **quadrigeminy.** See Figure 15-6.

In Figure 15-6, note every third beat is a PVC. This is ventricular trigeminy.

PVCs usually have a pause, called a **complete compensatory pause,** after them. This allows the regular rhythm to resume right on time as if the PVC had never happened. A complete compensatory pause measures two R-R cycles from the beat preceding the PVC to the beat following the PVC. See Figure 15-7.

Agonal Rhythm (Dying Heart)

What is it? Agonal rhythm is a very irregular rhythm in which the severely impaired heart is only able to "cough out" an occasional beat from its only remaining pacemaker, the ventricle. The higher pacemakers have all failed.

Rate	<20, though an occasional beat might come in at a slightly higher rate
Regularity	Irregular
P waves	None
PR	Not applicable
QRS	Wide and bizarre, QRS interval >0.12 second
T wave	Slopes off in the opposite direction to the QRS
Cause	The patient is dying, usually from profound cardiac or other damage, or from hypoxia.

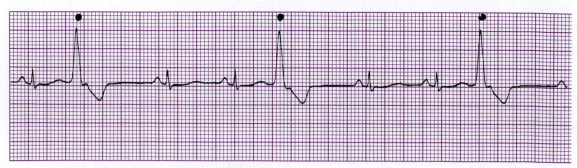

Figure 15-6   Ventricular trigeminy.

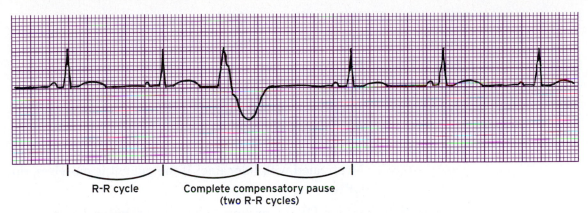

R-R cycle   Complete compensatory pause
(two R-R cycles)

Figure 15-7   Complete compensatory pause.

Adverse effects	Profound shock, unconsciousness; death if untreated. Agonal rhythm usually does not provide a pulse.
Treatment	Atropine to speed up the heart rate, CPR, epinephrine, dopamine, pacemaker, oxygen. Not treated with lidocaine! Lidocaine would knock out the only functioning pacemaker left–the ventricle–and would leave no heart rate at all.

In Figure 15-8, there are two QRS complexes, both the same shape, wide and bizarre. Regularity is indeterminate on this strip because there are only two QRS complexes. (Three are needed to determine regularity.) Heart rate is about 12. There are no P waves, therefore no PR interval. QRS interval is 0.28, extremely wide. Interpretation: agonal rhythm.

Idioventricular Rhythm (IVR)

What is it? IVR is a rhythm originating in the ventricle at its inherent rate. Higher pacemakers have failed, so the ventricle escapes to save the patient's life.

Rate	20 to 40
Regularity	Regular
P waves	None
PR	Not applicable

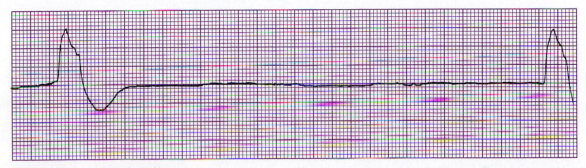

Figure 15-8   Agonal rhythm.

QRS	Wide and bizarre, QRS interval >0.12 second
T wave	Slopes off in the opposite direction to the QRS
Cause	Usually implies massive cardiac or other damage, hypoxia
Adverse effects	Decreased cardiac output, cardiovascular collapse. IVR may or may not result in a pulse.
Treatment	Atropine, epinephrine, pacemaker, oxygen, dopamine. Not treated with lidocaine! If the patient is pulseless, do CPR.

In Figure 15-9, there are QRS complexes, all wide and bizarre. Regularity is regular. Heart rate is 37. There are no P waves, therefore no PR interval. QRS interval is 0.20, extremely wide. Interpretation: idioventricular rhythm.

Accelerated Idioventricular Rhythm (AIVR)

What is it? This is a rhythm originating in the ventricle, with a heart rate faster than the ventricle's normal. It can result from escape or usurpation.

Rate	40 to 100
Regularity	Usually regular, but can be a little irregular at times
P waves	Usually not seen
QRS	Wide and bizarre, QRS interval >0.12 second
T wave	Slopes off in the opposite direction to the QRS
Cause	Very common after an MI. Can be caused by the same things that cause PVCs. AIVR is also very common after administration of thrombolytic medications, and in that context it is considered a **reperfusion arrhythmia,** meaning it implies the heart muscle is once again getting blood flow.
	Imagine it this way: Suppose you hadn't eaten anything in several days, and then when you did eat, it was a huge meal. You'd probably feel pretty sick. It's the same with the heart. It's been without blood flow for a period of time because of the blood clot in the coronary artery. Then here comes a tidal wave of blood and oxy-

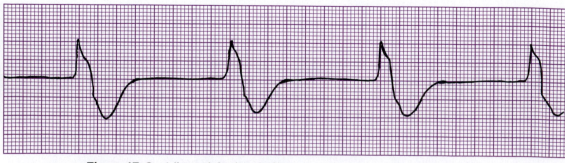

Figure 15-9 Idioventricular rhythm.

gen after the thrombolytic medication dissolves the clot. The ventricular tissue doesn't feel so good for a while after that, so it gets a little irritable and goes into AIVR. But just like your stomach, it'll get back to normal soon.

Adverse effects   Usually no ill effects because the heart rate is close to normal

Treatment   Not treated with lidocaine! Could be treated with atropine if the heart rate is around 40 and the patient is symptomatic. Consider starting oxygen. Usually no treatment is necessary as AIVR tends to be a self-limiting rhythm.

In Figure 15-10, there are QRS complexes, all wide and bizarre. Regularity is regular. Heart rate is 60. There are no P waves and thus no PR interval. QRS interval is about 0.18, very wide. Interpretation: accelerated idioventricular rhythm.

Ventricular Tachycardia (V-Tach)

What is it? An irritable focus in the ventricle has usurped the sinus node to become the pacemaker and is firing very rapidly.

Rate   100 to 250

Regularity   Usually regular, but can be a little irregular at times

P waves   Usually none, but dissociated from the QRS if present

PR   Will vary if even present

QRS   Wide and bizarre, QRS >0.12 second

T wave   Slopes off in the opposite direction to the QRS

Cause   Same as PVCs

Adverse effects   This rhythm may be tolerated for short bursts, but prolonged runs of v-tach can cause profound shock, unconsciousness, and death if untreated.

Treatment   Lidocaine, procainamide, amiodarone. Electric shock to the heart (cardioversion or defibrillation) may be necessary. Also treat the cause (low potassium or oxygen levels, etc.). CPR is indicated if the patient is pulseless.

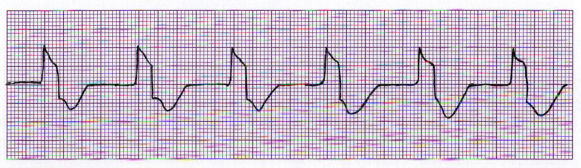

Figure 15-10   AIVR.

In Figure 15-11, there are QRS complexes, all wide and bizarre. Regularity is regular. Heart rate is 107. P waves are absent. PR interval is not applicable. QRS interval is 0.16. Interpretation: ventricular tachycardia.

Torsades de Pointes

What is it? *Torsades de pointes* is a French term meaning "twisting of the points." It's a form of ventricular tachycardia that is recognized primarily by its classic shape—it oscillates around an axis, with the QRS complexes pointing up, then becoming smaller, then rotating around until they point down. Torsades is not usually well tolerated in longer bursts, and often deteriorates into ventricular fibrillation.

Rate	>200
Regularity	May be regular or irregular
P waves	None seen
PR	Not applicable
QRS	Wide and bizarre, >0.12 second; often hard to measure the QRS interval
T wave	Opposite the QRS, but may not be seen due to the rapidity of the rhythm
Cause	Can be caused by antiarrhythmic medications such as quinidine or procainamide, which cause an increased QT interval. Otherwise it is caused by the same things that cause v-tach and v-fib.
Adverse effects	May be tolerated for short runs, but usually results in cardiac arrest if sustained
Treatment	Intravenous magnesium is the usual treatment. Electrical cardioversion may be needed. Isoproterenol is an option if other measures fail. Start oxygen.

In Figure 15-12, there are QRS complexes, not all the same shape. Some point downward, some point upward, and others are very small. Regularity is regular. Heart rate is about 375. P waves are absent, therefore there is no PR interval. QRS interval is 0.16. Interpretation: torsades de pointes. The big clue here is the oscillating character of the QRS complexes—bigger, then smaller, then bigger again, and so on. That's classic for torsades.

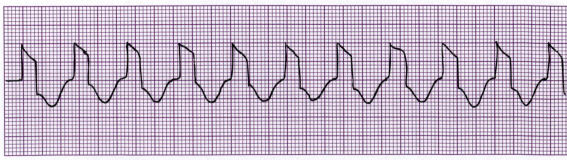

Figure 15-11   Ventricular tachycardia.

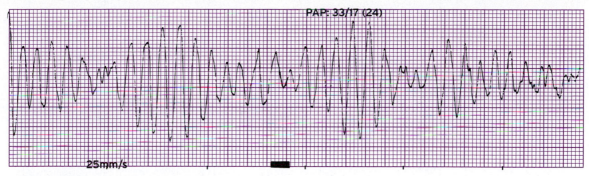

Figure 15-12   Torsades de pointes.

Ventricular Flutter (V-Flutter)

What is it? An irritable ventricular focus has become the pacemaker, and the rate is so fast that a zigzag or sawtooth pattern is created, rather than clearly defined QRS complexes. This is usually an intermediate pattern between v-tach and v-fib.

Rate	250 to 350
Regularity	Regular
P waves	None seen
PR	Not applicable
QRS	Usually hard to pick out QRS complexes; just a zigzag pattern seen
T wave	Usually not seen as it blends in with the QRS
Cause	Same as v-tach
Adverse effects	Same as v-tach
Treatment	Same as v-tach, but usually electric shock required

In Figure 15-13, there is a zigzag pattern of QRS complexes. Regularity is regular. Heart rate is 300. There are no P waves, therefore no PR interval. QRS interval is 0.12 (guesstimate–it's hard to tell where QRS ends and T wave begins). Interpretation: ventricular flutter. If you're thinking this looks a lot like ventricular tachycardia, you're right–but here the heart rate is faster than v-tach normally fires.

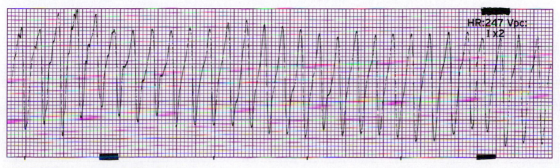

Figure 15-13   Ventricular flutter.

Ventricular Fibrillation (V-Fib)

What is it? Hundreds of impulses in the ventricle are firing off, each depolarizing its own little piece of territory. As a result, the ventricles wiggle instead of contract. The heart's electrical system is in chaos, and the resultant rhythm looks like static.

Rate	Cannot be counted
Regularity	None detectable
P waves	None
QRS	None detectable; just a wavy or spiked baseline
T wave	None
Cause	Same as v-tach; also can be caused by drowning, drug overdoses, accidental electric shock
Adverse effects	Profound cardiovascular collapse. There is no cardiac output whatsoever. There is no pulse, no breathing, nothing. The patient is functionally dead. New onset v-fib has coarse fibrillatory waves. These waves get progressively finer the longer it lasts.
Treatment	Immediate defibrillation (electric shock to the heart), epinephrine, lidocaine, CPR, procainamide, amiodarone, oxygen. The rhythm will not be converted with just medications. Defibrillation must be done. The medications make the defibrillation more successful and can prevent recurrences of v-fib.

In Figure 15-14, there are no identifiable QRS complexes—just a wavy, spiked baseline resembling static. Regularity is not determinable. Heart rate is not measurable since there are no QRS complexes. P waves are not present. PR and QRS intervals cannot be measured. Interpretation: ventricular fibrillation.

Asystole

What is it? Asystole is flat-line EKG. Every one of the heart's pacemakers has failed.

Rate	Zero
Regularity	None

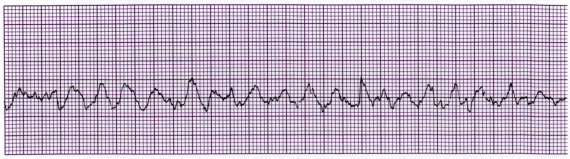

Figure 15-14 Ventricular fibrillation.

P waves	None
PR	None
QRS	None
T wave	None
Cause	Profound cardiac or other body system damage; profound hypoxia. Even with vigorous resuscitative efforts, this is usually a terminal rhythm.
Adverse effects	Death if untreated
Treatment	Atropine to reverse any vagal influence, epinephrine, CPR, pacemaker, dopamine, oxygen

In Figure 15-15, there are no QRS complexes, only a flat line. There is no regularity. Heart rate is zero. There are no P waves, no PR interval, and no QRS interval. Interpretation: asystole.

There is another kind of asystole in which there are no QRS complexes but there are still P waves. This is called **ventricular asystole.** The still-functioning sinus node fires out its impulses, but they do not cause ventricular depolarization as the ventricle is too damaged to respond to the stimulus. Since the atria depolarize but the ventricles don't, there is no QRS after the Ps. Eventually the sinus impulses will slow and stop, since there is no cardiac output to feed blood to the sinus node. Remember—if there is no QRS complex, there is no cardiac output. Treatment is the same as for asystole.

In Figure 15-16, there are no QRS complexes. Regularity is not applica-

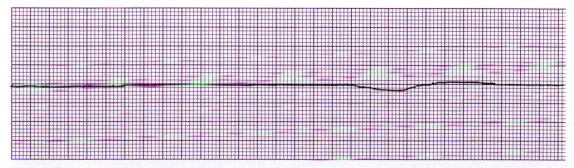

Figure 15-15   Asystole.

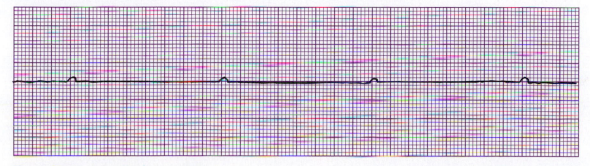

Figure 15-16   Ventricular asystole.

ble. Heart rate is zero. P waves are present, regular, with an atrial rate of 37. There is no PR interval or QRS interval. Interpretation: ventricular asystole.

Pacemakers

Pacemakers are electronic devices that can be implanted into or attached to the patient to send out an electrical impulse to cause the heart to depolarize. Pacemakers are used when the heart is temporarily or permanently unable to generate or transmit its own impulses, or when it does so too slowly to provide a reasonable cardiac output. They can be used to pace the atria, the ventricles, or both.

When the pacemaker sends out its signal, a vertical spike is recorded on the EKG paper. Ventricular pacing provides a spike followed by a wide QRS. Atrial pacing has a spike followed by a P wave. Dual-chamber pacing (both atrium and ventricle) has a spike before the P and a spike before the QRS. See Figure 15-17.

In Figure 15-17(a), there are QRS complexes, all wide, all shaped the same. Each QRS is preceded by a pacemaker spike. Regularity is regular. Heart rate is 50. There are no P waves, therefore no PR interval. QRS interval is 0.24 second. Interpretation: ventricular pacing.

In Figure 15-17(b), there are QRS complexes, all wide, all shaped the same. Regularity is regular. Heart rate is 50. There are matching P waves, each preceded by a pacemaker spike. PR interval is not measured in paced rhythms. The **AV interval** (the interval between atrial and ventricular pacing spikes) is 0.16 second and should be constant as this interval is preset when the pacemaker is implanted. QRS interval is 0.24 second. Interpretation: dual-chamber pacing (also called AV pacing).

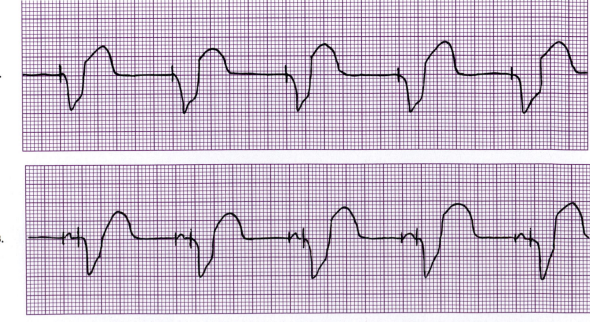

A.

B.

Figure 15-17   Pacemakers: (a) Ventricular pacing; (b) dual chamber pacing.

Practice Strips: Ventricular Rhythms

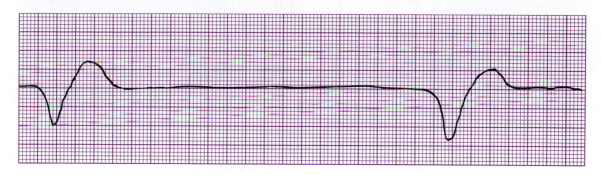

1. QRS complexes _____ Regularity _____

Heart rate _____

P waves _____

PR interval _____ QRS interval _____

Interpretation (name of rhythm) _____

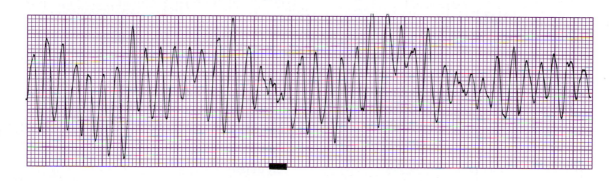

2. QRS complexes _____ Regularity _____

Heart rate _____

P waves _____

PR interval _____ QRS interval _____

Interpretation _____

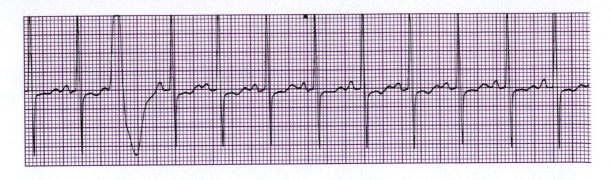

3. QRS complexes _____ Regularity _____

Heart rate _____

P waves _____

PR interval _____ QRS interval _____

Interpretation _____

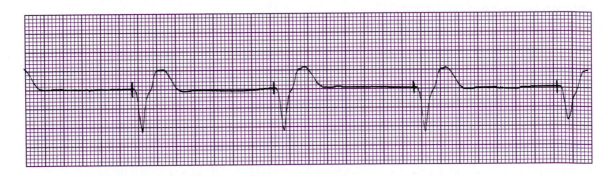

4. QRS complexes _____ Regularity _____

Heart rate _____

P waves _____

PR interval _____ QRS interval _____

Interpretation _____

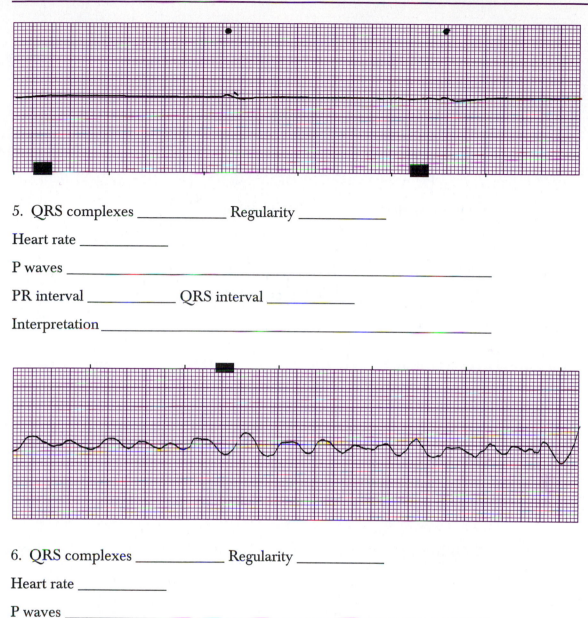

5. QRS complexes _____ Regularity _____

Heart rate _____

P waves _____

PR interval _____ QRS interval _____

Interpretation _____

6. QRS complexes _____ Regularity _____

Heart rate _____

P waves _____

PR interval _____ QRS interval _____

Interpretation _____

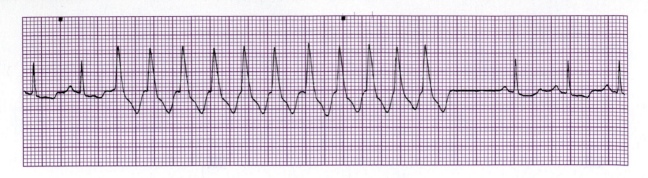

7. QRS complexes _____ Regularity _____

Heart rate _____

P waves _____

PR interval _____ QRS interval _____

Interpretation _____

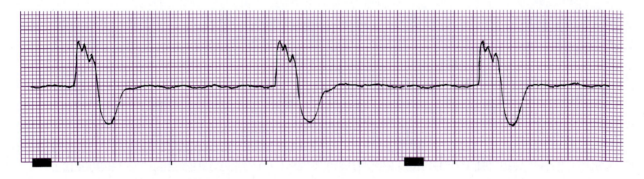

8. QRS complexes _____ Regularity _____

Heart rate _____

P waves _____

PR interval _____ QRS interval _____

Interpretation _____

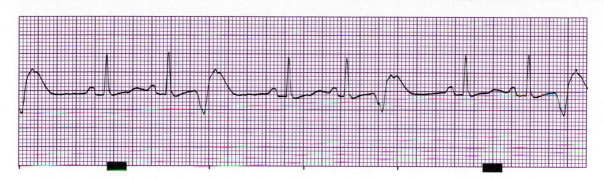

9. QRS complexes _____ Regularity _____

Heart rate _____

P waves _____

PR interval _____ QRS interval _____

Interpretation _____

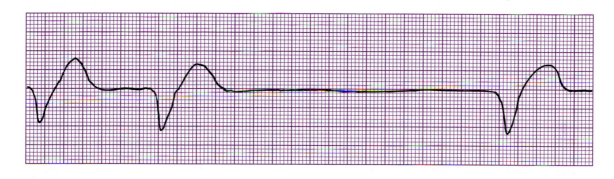

10. QRS complexes _____ Regularity _____

Heart rate _____

P waves _____

PR interval _____ QRS interval _____

Interpretation _____

Answers to Ventricular Rhythms Practice Strips

1. **QRS complexes:** present, both shaped the same—very wide and bizarre. **Regularity:** cannot tell as only two QRS complexes are shown. **Heart rate:** 14. **P waves:** not present. **PR:** not applicable. **QRS:** 0.38. **Interpretation:** agonal rhythm.

2. **QRS complexes:** present, varying in shapes and sizes. **Regularity:** irregular. **Heart rate:** 375 to 500. **P waves:** absent. **PR:** not applicable. **QRS:** varies—some QRS intervals are unmeasurable, others are 0.12. **Interpretation:** torsades de pointes.

3. **QRS complexes:** present, all but the third QRS shaped the same. The third QRS is wider. **Regularity:** regular but interrupted (by a premature beat). **Heart rate:** 115. **P waves:** matching and upright on all beats except the third, which has no P wave. **PR:** 0.12 on the sinus beats. **QRS:** 0.10 on the sinus beats; 0.16 on the premature beat. **Interpretation:** sinus tachycardia with one PVC.

4. **QRS complexes:** present, wide, all shaped the same; spike noted preceding each QRS complex. **Regularity:** regular. **Heart rate:** 40. **P waves:** none noted. **PR:** not applicable. **QRS:** 0.16. **Interpretation:** paced ventricular rhythm.

5. **QRS complexes:** absent. **Regularity:** not applicable. **Heart rate:** zero. **P waves:** upright, matching, atrial rate 26. **PR:** not applicable. **QRS:** not applicable. **Interpretation:** ventricular asystole.

6. **QRS complexes:** absent; wavy baseline present instead. **Regularity:** not applicable. **Heart rate:** unmeasurable. **P waves:** absent. **PR:** not applicable. **QRS:** not applicable. **Interpretation:** ventricular fibrillation.

7. **QRS complexes:** present, two different shapes—some narrow, others wide and bizarre. **Regularity:** regular but interrupted (by a run of premature beats). **Heart rate:** 107 while in sinus; 187 when in ventricular tachycardia. **P waves:** upright and matching on the narrow beats; none noted on the wide beats. **PR:** 0.12 on the narrow beats; no P waves on the wide beats. **QRS:** 0.06 on the narrow beats; 0.12 on the wide beats. **Interpretation:** sinus tachycardia with an 11-beat run of ventricular tachycardia.

8. **QRS complexes:** present, all shaped the same—extremely wide and bizarre. **Regularity:** regular. **Heart rate:** 28. **P waves:** absent. **PR:** not applicable. **QRS:** 0.28. **Interpretation:** idioventricular rhythm.

9. **QRS complexes:** present, every third beat wider than the rest. **Regularity:** regular but interrupted (by premature beats). **Heart rate:** 94. **P waves:** matching and upright on all narrow beats. P waves are noted in the T waves of the wide beats. **PR:** 0.16. **QRS:** 0.06 on the narrow beats; 0.14 on the wide beats. **Interpretation:** sinus rhythm with PVCs in trigeminy.

10. **QRS complexes:** present, all shaped the same—wide QRS complexes. **Regularity:** irregular. **Heart rate:** 16 to 47, with a mean rate of 30. **P**

waves: none noted. **PR:** not applicable. **QRS:** 0.28. **Interpretation:** agonal rhythm. Though in places this rate exceeds 20, the very irregular nature of it points to agonal rhythm rather than idioventricular rhythm.

Practice Quiz

1. The three main causes of PVCs are _____

   _____

   _____

2. The rhythm that has no QRS complexes, but instead has a wavy, static-looking baseline is _____

3. Appropriate treatment for PVCs interrupting a sinus bradycardia with a heart rate of 32 would be _____

4. Torsades de pointes is a French term that means_____

5. How does asystole differ from ventricular asystole? _____

   _____

6. Your patient has a ventricular rhythm with a heart rate of 39, but no pulse. What treatment would be appropriate?_____

   _____

7. True or false: Asystole is treated with electric shock to the heart.

8. The treatment of choice for ventricular fibrillation is _____

   _____

9. True or false: Pacemakers can pace the atrium, the ventricle, or both.

10. True or false: Lidocaine should be given to treat agonal rhythm.

Practice Quiz Answers

1. The three main causes of PVCs are **heart disease, hypokalemia,** and **hypoxia.**

2. The rhythm that has no QRS complexes, but instead has a wavy, static-looking baseline is **ventricular fibrillation.**

3. Appropriate treatment for PVCs interrupting a sinus bradycardia with a heart rate of 32 would be **atropine** or **epinephrine** to increase the heart rate. Do not give lidocaine!

4. Torsades de pointes is a French term meaning **twisting of the points.**

5. Asystole differs from ventricular asystole in that **asystole is flat-line** and **ventricular asystole still has P waves.**

6. For a patient with a ventricular rhythm with a heart rate of 39 and no pulse, the treatment would be **CPR, epinephrine, atropine, oxygen, dopamine.**

7. **False.** Asystole is *not* treated with electric shock to the heart. Electric shock's goal is to recoordinate the heart's electrical activity. In asystole, there is no electrical activity to coordinate.

8. The treatment of choice for ventricular fibrillation is **defibrillation.**

9. **True.** Pacemakers can pace the atrium, the ventricle, or both.

10. **False.** Lidocaine should *not* be used to treat agonal rhythm. The lidocaine would suppress the only pacemaker this person has left—the ventricle—and would likely be fatal. Try atropine or epinephrine instead to speed up the heart rate.

AV Blocks

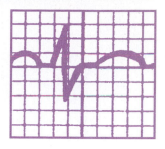

Chapter 16 Objectives

Upon completion of this chapter, the student will be able to:

- State the criteria for each type of AV block.
- State whether the block is at the AV node or the bundle branches.
- Identify each type of AV block using the criteria and the rhythm strip analysis tools.
- State the adverse effects for each type of AV block.
- State the possible treatment for each type of AV block.

Chapter 16 Outline

Chapter 16 Glossary

AV dissociation (atrioventricular dissociation): A condition in which the atria and ventricles depolarize and contract independently of each other.

Introduction

With AV blocks, there is a partial or complete interruption in the transmission of impulses from the sinus node to the ventricles. The site of the block is either at the AV node or at the bundle branches. See Figures 16-1 and 16-2.

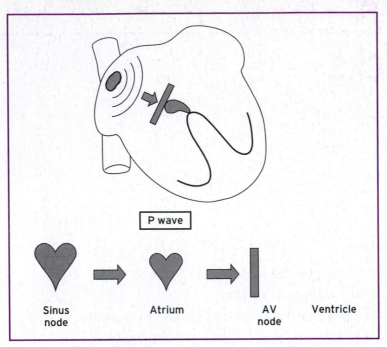

Figure 16-1 Block at the AV node.

Degrees of AV Block

There are three degrees of block, varying in severity from benign to life-threatening.

- **First-degree AV block.** Just as a first-degree burn is the least dangerous type of burn, a first-degree AV block is the least dangerous type of AV block. There is a delay in impulse transmission from the sinus node

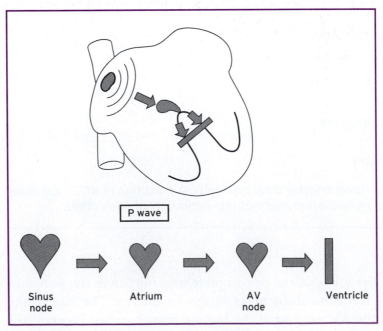

Figure 16-2 Block at the bundle branches.

to the ventricles, but every impulse does get there—it just takes a little longer. The site of block is the AV node.

- **Second-degree AV block.** Some impulses from the sinus node get through to the ventricles; some don't. The site of block is the AV node or the bundle branches. This type of AV block is more serious—like a second-degree burn.

- **Third-degree AV block.** Due to a block at the AV node or the bundle branches, none of the impulses from the sinus node get through to the ventricles. Third-degree AV block, like a third-degree burn, can be life-threatening. A lower pacemaker has to escape to provide stimulus to the ventricle.

The Skinny on AV Blocks

In AV blocks, the underlying rhythm is sinus. The impulse is born in the sinus node and heads down the conduction pathway as usual. Thus the P waves are normal sinus P waves. Further down the conduction pathway, however, there is a roadblock. This can result in either a simple delay in impulse transmission or a complete or partial interruption in the conduction of sinus impulses to the ventricle. Heart rates can be normal or very slow, and symptoms may be present or absent. Treatment is aimed at increasing the heart rate and improving AV conduction.

There are two possible criteria for AV blocks. *If either of these criteria is met, there is an AV block.* Let's look at the criteria:

- PR interval prolonged (>0.20 s) in some kind of sinus rhythm, *or*
- Some Ps not followed by a QRS; P-P interval regular

The following AV blocks will be covered in this section:

- First-degree AV block
- Type I second-degree AV block (Wenckebach)
- Type II second-degree AV block
- 2:1 AV block
- Third-degree AV block

Let's look at each of these rhythms in detail.

First-Degree AV Block

What is it? First-degree AV block is a prolonged PR interval that results from a delay in the AV node's conduction of sinus impulses to the ventricle. All the sinus impulses do get through; they just take longer than normal because the AV node is ischemic or otherwise suppressed.

Rate	Can occur at any rate
Regularity	Depends on the underlying rhythm
P waves	Upright, matching; one P to each QRS
PR interval	Prolonged (>0.20 s), constant
QRS	<0.12 second (≥0.12 s if BBB present)

Cause	AV node ischemia, digitalis toxicity, or a side effect of other medications such as beta-blockers or calcium channel blockers. This is a benign type of block, but be alert for worsening AV block. First-degree block is usually seen only with rhythms originating in the sinus node.
Adverse effects	The first-degree AV block itself causes no symptoms.
Treatment	Remove any medication causing it. Otherwise, treat the cause.

In Figure 16-3, there are QRS complexes, all shaped the same. Regularity is regular. Heart rate is 62. P waves are upright, matching, one to each QRS. PR interval is 0.28. QRS interval is 0.08. Interpretation is sinus rhythm with a first-degree AV block.

Type I Second-Degree AV Block (Wenckebach)

What is it? Usually a transient block, Wenckebach usually lasts only a few days. It occurs when the AV node becomes progressively sicker and less able to conduct the sinus impulses until finally it is unable to send the impulse down to the ventricle at all. As a result, the PR intervals grow progressively longer until there is a P wave that has no QRS behind it.

Rate	Atrial rate usually 60 to 100; ventricular rate less than the atrial rate due to nonconducted beats
Regularity	Usually irregular, but can look regular but interrupted at times. A hallmark of Wenckebach is groups of beats, then a pause.
P waves	Normal sinus P waves. All Ps except the blocked P are followed by a QRS. P-P interval is regular. There may be P waves that are hidden in the QRS complex or the T wave. Find two consecutive P waves and then march out where the rest of the P waves are, keeping in mind they will all have the same P-P interval, so they'll all be the same distance apart.
PR interval	The PR gradually prolongs until a QRS is dropped.
QRS	<0.12 second (≥0.12 s if BBB present)

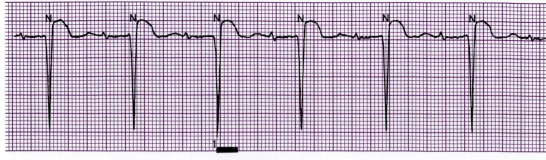

Figure 16-3 First-degree AV block.

Cause	Myocardial infarction (MI), digitalis toxicity, medication side effects
Adverse effects	Usually no ill effects. Watch for worsening block.
Treatment	Atropine if the heart rate is slow and the patient is symptomatic. A pacemaker can be used if atropine is unsuccessful. Most patients with Wenckebach require nothing more than cautious observation.

In Figure 16-4, there are QRS complexes, all shaped the same. Regularity is irregular. Heart rate is 50 to 83, with a mean rate of 70. P waves are matching, upright, some not followed by a QRS. Some Ps are at the end of the T waves. P-P interval is regular. Atrial rate is 83. PR interval varies from 0.04 to 0.28. Note the relatively short PR of the first beat on the strip. Compare this to the third beat. The PR interval prolongs from beat to beat until the fourth P wave does not conduct through to the ventricle at all. The cycle then repeats, with prolonging PR intervals, until the eighth P wave is not conducted. QRS interval is 0.10. Interpretation: sinus rhythm with type I second-degree AV block (Wenckebach). Where did the sinus rhythm part of the interpretation come from? Remember, the underlying rhythm in all AV blocks is a sinus rhythm of some sort. The atrial rate will tell you which sinus rhythm it is. An atrial rate of 60 to 100 would be sinus rhythm; an atrial rate of less than 60 would be sinus bradycardia; and an atrial rate greater than 100 would be sinus tachycardia.

Type II Second-Degree AV Block

What is it? Type II results from an intermittent block at the AV node or the bundle branches, preventing some sinus impulses from getting to the ventricles. With AV node block, the resultant QRS complexes will be narrow. With block at the bundle branches, the QRS will be wide. Usually, type II patients already have a bundle branch block, meaning one of their bundle branches does not let impulses through. They are therefore dependent on the other bundle branch to conduct the impulses through to the ventricles. When that other bundle branch becomes suddenly blocked, none of the sinus impulses can get through. Some sinus P waves conduct through normally to the ventricles when the one bundle branch is open, and others never get through at all when both bundle branches are blocked. The impulses that do get through do so with an unchanging PR interval.

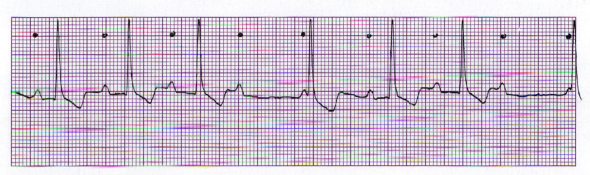

Figure 16-4 Wenckebach.

Rate	Atrial rate usually 60 to 100; ventricular rate less than atrial rate due to dropped beats
Regularity	May be regular, irregular, or regular but interrupted
P waves	Normal sinus P waves. All Ps except the blocked Ps have a QRS behind them. P-P interval is regular. Some P waves may be hidden inside QRS complexes or T waves.
PR interval	Unchanging on the conducted beats
QRS	<0.12 second if the block is at the AV node, ≥0.12 second if the block is at the bundle branches
Cause	MI, conduction system lesion, medication side effect, hypoxia
Adverse effects	Since the heart rate can be very slow, the patient may have signs of decreased cardiac output. Type II can progress to third-degree block if untreated.
Treatment	Atropine first. Depending on where the block is, atropine may or may not work. Atropine speeds up the rate of sinus node firing and improves AV node conduction. If the block is at the AV node, atropine will improve the conduction, and the impulse will travel on down the pathway. If the block is at the bundle branches, however, the impulse will blast through the AV node and head down the pathway only to find that both bundle branches are still blocked. Atropine has no effect on the bundle branches. Patients with type II will usually receive epinephrine to increase their heart rate until a temporary pacemaker can be inserted, because the risk is very high that they will soon be in a worse block. Consider starting oxygen.

In Figure 16-5, there are QRS complexes, all the same shape. Regularity is regular. Heart rate is 44. P waves are upright, matching, some not followed by a QRS. P-P interval is regular. Atrial rate is 137. PR interval is constant at 0.12. QRS interval is 0.12. Interpretation is sinus tachycardia with type II second-degree AV block and a BBB.

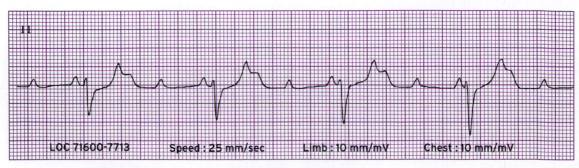

LOC 71600-7713   Speed : 25 mm/sec   Limb : 10 mm/mV   Chest : 10 mm/mV

Figure 16-5 Type II second-degree AV block.

2:1 AV Block

What is it? 2:1 AV block is a type of second-degree block in which there are two P waves to each QRS complex. The first P wave in each pair of P waves is blocked. 2:1 AV block can be caused by either Wenckebach or type II. In order to differentiate the two, it is necessary to have two conducted beats in a row to see if the PR is constant or if it gradually prolongs until a beat is dropped. If the entire strip shows nothing but two Ps to each QRS, the atrial rate is 60 to 100, and the PR is constant, the rhythm is simply called 2:1 AV block. If, however, the 2:1 AV block is preceded or followed by an obvious Wenckebach, then it is probably also Wenckebach. If it's preceded or followed by an obvious type II, then it is probably also type II. Another clue—if the QRS is <0.12 second and the PR is prolonged, it's probably Wenckebach. If the QRS is >0.12 second with a normal PR interval, it's probably type II.

Rate	Atrial rate 60 to 100; ventricular rate half the atrial rate
Regularity	Regular
P waves	Normal sinus P waves; two Ps to each QRS; P-P interval is regular.
QRS	<0.12 second (≥0.12 s if BBB present)
Cause	Same as Wenckebach or type II
Adverse effects	Decreased cardiac output if the heart rate is too slow
Treatment	Atropine first if the patient is symptomatic; epinephrine, dopamine, pacemaker if the block continues and symptoms are present. Consider starting oxygen.

In Figure 16-6, there are QRS complexes, all the same shape. Regularity is regular. Heart rate is 37. Atrial rate is 75. P waves are upright and matching, two to each QRS. P-P interval is regular. PR interval is 0.16. QRS interval is 0.08. Interpretation: 2:1 AV block.

Third-Degree AV Block (Complete Heart Block)

What is it? In third-degree block, the sinus node sends out its impulses as usual, *but not a single one of them ever gets to the ventricles,* because there is a block at the AV node or the bundle branches. Meanwhile, the AV node and

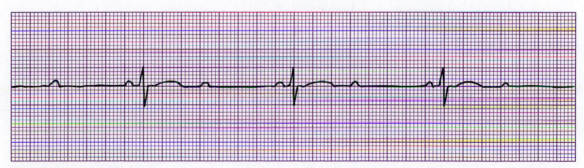

Figure 16-6 2:1 AV block.

the ventricle wait patiently for the sinus impulses to reach them. When it's obvious that the sinus impulse isn't coming, the lower pacemakers assume the sinus node has failed. One of them then escapes and assumes pacemaking control to provide a QRS complex. If the AV node is the location of the block, a lower spot in the AV node takes over as pacemaker and provides a heart rate of 40 to 60. If the block is at the bundle branches, the only pacemaker left below that is the ventricle, with a heart rate of 20 to 40. Even though the lower pacemaker has assumed control of providing the QRS complex, the sinus node is unaware of that, so it continues firing out its impulses as usual.

Rate	Atrial rate usually 60 to 100; ventricular rate usually 20 to 60
Regularity	Regular
P waves	Normal sinus P waves; P-P interval is regular; P waves may be hidden inside QRS complexes or T waves. P waves are not associated with any of the QRS complexes, even though there may at times appear to be a relationship. This is called **AV dissociation,** and it is a hallmark of third-degree block. AV dissociation means the sinus node is firing at its normal rate, and the lower pacemaker is firing at its slower rate, and the two have nothing to do with each other. AV dissociation results in independent beating of the atria and the ventricles. Here's another way to describe AV dissociation as seen in third-degree AV block: Imagine the lower pacemaker that controls the ventricles as an old man jogging around a circular racetrack at 2 miles per hour. The sinus node is an 18-year-old boy sprinting at 4 miles per hour. Since the boy is going faster than the old man, he will periodically catch up with him and then pass him. An onlooker might see the boy at the split second he's side by side with the old man and assume they are together and that there is a relationship between the two. There isn't, of course. Their being side by side was just coincidence, just as it's coincidence that a sinus P wave might land right in front of a QRS and make it seem as though there is a relationship there.
PR interval	Varies
QRS	Normal (<0.12 s) or wide (>0.12 s), depending on the location of the block. If the block is at the AV node, the junction will become the pacemaker and the QRS will be narrow. If the block is at the bundle branches, the ventricle will become the pacemaker, with a wide QRS.
Cause	MI, conduction system lesion, medication side effects, hypoxia

Adverse effects   Signs of low cardiac output may occur. The patient with third-degree block may be very symptomatic or may feel fine, depending on the heart rate.

Treatment   A temporary pacemaker will usually be necessary until the rhythm returns to normal or until a permanent pacemaker can be inserted. Atropine, epinephrine, or dopamine can be given until a pacemaker can be inserted. Start oxygen.

In Figure 16-7, there are QRS complexes, all shaped the same. Regularity is regular. Heart rate is 37. P waves are upright and matching. Atrial rate is 60. P-P interval is regular. One P wave is hidden in the ST segment of the third QRS complex. PR interval varies. QRS interval is 0.20. Interpretation: sinus rhythm with third-degree AV block and an idioventricular rhythm. Idioventricular rhythm? We know the sinus node is controlling the atria and providing the P waves. We also know, since the QRS is wide, that the ventricle is the pacemaker controlling the ventricles. Since the ventricular rate is between 20 and 40, the rhythm is idioventricular rhythm. Put the two together and we come up with our interpretation. If the AV junction had been the pacemaker, the QRS would have been narrow.

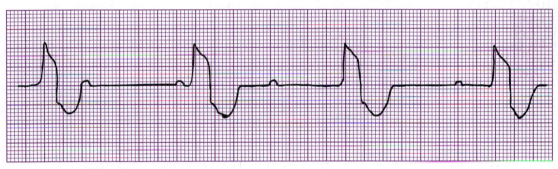

Figure 16-7   Third-degree AV block.

Practice Strips: AV Blocks

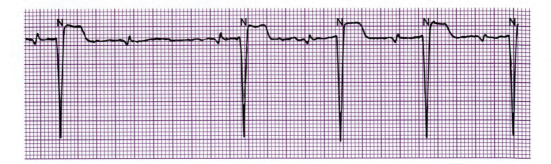

1. QRS complexes _____ Regularity _____

Heart rate _____

P waves _____

PR interval _____ QRS interval _____

Interpretation (name of rhythm) _____

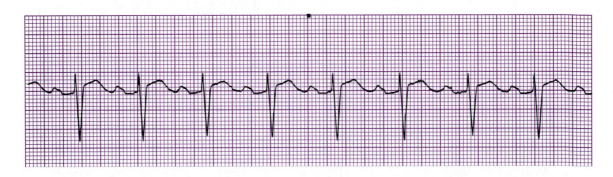

2. QRS complexes _____ Regularity _____

Heart rate _____

P waves _____

PR interval _____ QRS interval _____

Interpretation _____

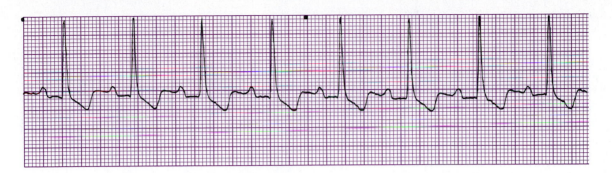

3. QRS complexes _____ Regularity _____

Heart rate _____

P waves _____

PR interval _____ QRS interval _____

Interpretation _____

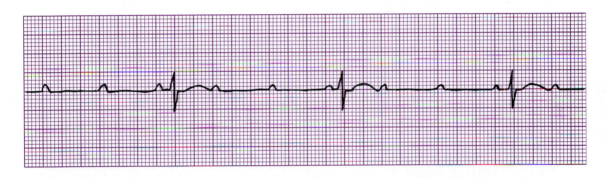

4. QRS complexes _____ Regularity _____

Heart rate _____

P waves _____

PR interval _____ QRS interval _____

Interpretation _____

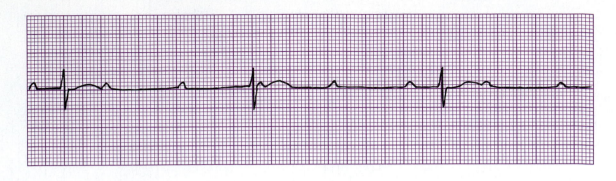

5. QRS complexes _____ Regularity _____

Heart rate _____

P waves _____

PR interval _____ QRS interval _____

Interpretation _____

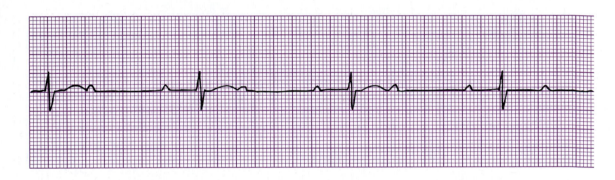

6. QRS complexes _____ Regularity _____

Heart rate _____

P waves _____

PR interval _____ QRS interval _____

Interpretation _____

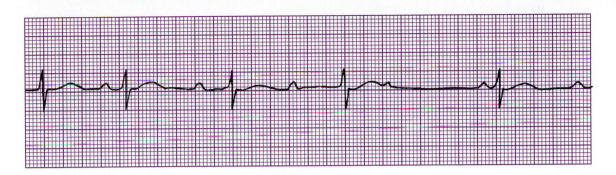

7. QRS complexes _____ Regularity _____

Heart rate _____

P waves _____

PR interval _____ QRS interval _____

Interpretation _____

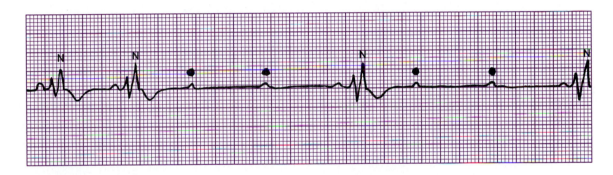

8. QRS complexes _____ Regularity _____

Heart rate _____

P waves _____

PR interval _____ QRS interval _____

Interpretation _____

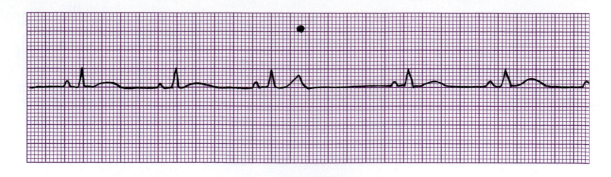

9. QRS complexes _____ Regularity _____

Heart rate _____

P waves _____

PR interval _____ QRS interval _____

Interpretation _____

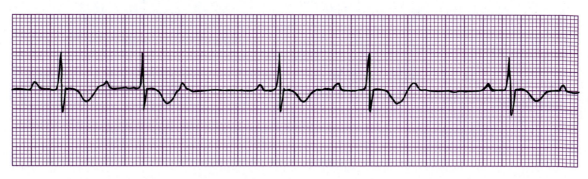

10. QRS complexes _____ Regularity _____

Heart rate _____

P waves _____

PR interval _____ QRS interval _____

Interpretation _____

Answers to AV Blocks Practice Strips

1. **QRS complexes:** present, all shaped the same. **Regularity:** regular but interrupted (by a pause). **Heart rate:** 31 to 68, with a mean rate of 50. **P waves:** biphasic, matching, more than one per QRS at times. P-P interval is regular. Atrial rate is 62. **PR:** varies. **QRS:** 0.08. **Interpretation:** sinus rhythm with type I second-degree AV block (Wenckebach). Look at the P directly preceding the second QRS complex. The PR interval there is 0.24. The PR preceding the last QRS on the strip is 0.28. The PR interval prolongs and there are blocked P waves. The rhythm starts out as 2:1 AV block, then becomes an obvious Wenckebach. The 2:1 AV block here is therefore also Wenckebach.

2. **QRS complexes:** present, all shaped the same. **Regularity:** regular. **Heart rate:** 88. **P waves:** upright, matching, one to each QRS complex; atrial rate is 88; P-P interval is regular. **PR:** 0.24. **QRS:** 0.10. **Interpretation:** sinus rhythm with first-degree AV block.

3. **QRS complexes:** present, all shaped the same. **Regularity:** regular. **Heart rate:** 83. **P waves:** upright, matching, one to each QRS; P-P interval is regular; atrial rate is 83. **PR:** 0.24. **QRS:** 0.10. **Interpretation:** sinus rhythm with first-degree AV block.

4. **QRS complexes:** present, all shaped the same. **Regularity:** regular. **Heart rate:** 33. **P waves:** upright, matching, three to each QRS; P-P interval is regular; atrial rate is 100. **PR:** 0.16. **QRS:** 0.08. **Interpretation:** sinus rhythm with type II second-degree AV block. The block here is probably at the AV node, as evidenced by the narrow QRS. This can also be called a **high-grade AV block,** as more than half the P waves are not conducted.

5. **QRS complexes:** present, all shaped the same. **Regularity:** regular. **Heart rate:** 30. **P waves:** upright, matching, more than one per QRS; P-P interval is regular; atrial rate is 75. **PR:** varies. **QRS:** 0.08. **Interpretation:** Sinus rhythm with third-degree AV block and a junctional bradycardia.

6. **QRS complexes:** present, all shaped the same. **Regularity:** regular. **Heart rate:** 37. **P waves:** upright, matching, two per QRS; P-P interval is regular; atrial rate is 75. **PR:** 0.36. **QRS:** 0.08. **Interpretation:** 2:1 AV block (probably Wenckebach, since the QRS is narrow and there is a prolonged PR interval).

7. **QRS complexes:** present, all shaped the same. **Regularity:** irregular. **Heart rate:** 37 to 68. **P waves:** upright, matching, one to each QRS except for the fifth QRS, which has two P waves preceding it; P-P interval is regular; atrial rate is 60. **PR:** varies—prolongs progressively. **QRS:** 0.08. **Interpretation:** sinus rhythm with type I second-degree AV block (Wenckebach).

8. **QRS complexes:** present, all the same shape. **Regularity:** irregular. **Heart rate:** 25 to 75, with a mean rate of 40. **P waves:** matching, upright, one for the first two QRS complexes, then three per QRS; P-P

interval is regular; atrial rate is 75. **PR:** 0.16. **QRS:** 0.16. **Interpretation:** sinus rhythm with type II second-degree AV block and a bundle branch block. The first two beats are sinus rhythm with BBB, then suddenly the other bundle branch goes down and the sinus impulses can't get through. When they do finally get through, they do so with the same PR interval they started with.

9. **QRS complexes:** present, all shaped the same. **Regularity:** regular but interrupted (by a pause). **Heart rate:** 42 to 60, with a mean rate of 50. **P waves:** matching, upright, one preceding each QRS except the fourth QRS, which has two P waves preceding it (there's a P in the T wave of the third beat); P-P interval is *irregular;* atrial rate is 60 to 125. **PR:** 0.16. **QRS:** 0.108. **Interpretation:** sinus rhythm with a nonconducted PAC. "Wait a minute," you exclaim. "That's not fair! We're doing AV blocks, not atrial rhythms!" Mea culpa. But there's a method to this madness. Do you see how easy it is to mistake a nonconducted PAC for an AV block? How do you tell the difference? Simple. AV blocks have regular P-P intervals. Here the P-P is *not regular,* is it? One P is premature. That makes it a PAC. And since there's no QRS following it, that makes it a nonconducted PAC. Piece of cake. . . .

10. **QRS complexes:** present, all shaped the same. **Regularity:** regular but interrupted (by pauses). **Heart rate:** 42 to 68, with a mean rate of 50. **P waves:** upright, matching, more than one per QRS at times; P-P interval is regular; atrial rate is 75. **PR:** varies. **QRS:** 0.08. **Interpretation:** sinus rhythm with type I second-degree AV block (Wenckebach).

Practice Quiz

1. Name the two typical locations of the block in AV blocks. _____

2. True or false: People with a first-degree AV block need a pacemaker inserted.

3. Wenckebach is another name for which kind of block? _____

4. AV dissociation is a hallmark of which kind of AV block?_____

5. True or false: Atropine is effective in all types of AV blocks, whether the block is at the AV node or the bundle branches.

6. The AV block that merely provides a prolonged PR interval is _____

7. What is atropine's mode of action?_____

8. The most dangerous type of AV block is _____

9. The least dangerous type of AV block is _____

10. True or false: All AV blocks require atropine or epinephrine to increase the heart rate.

Practice Quiz Answers

1. The two typical locations for the block in AV blocks are the **AV node** and the **bundle branches.**

2. **False.** First-degree AV block causes no symptoms and does not require pacemaker insertion.

3. Wenckebach is another name for **type I second-degree AV block.**

4. AV dissociation is a hallmark of **third-degree AV block.**

5. **False.** Atropine has no effect on blocks at the bundle branches.

6. The AV block that provides merely a prolonged PR interval is **first-degree AV block.**

7. Atropine's mode of action is **to speed up the sinus node's rate of firing and to accelerate conduction through the AV node.**

8. The most dangerous type of AV block is **third-degree AV block.**

9. The least dangerous type of AV block is **first-degree AV block.**

10. **False.** First-degree AV blocks do not require atropine or epinephrine.

Artifact Masquerading as Rhythms

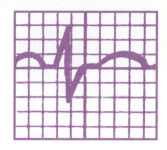

Chapter 17 Objectives

Upon completion of this chapter, the student will be able to:

- Name the rhythms that can be mimicked by artifact.
- Tell how to differentiate between artifact and the real thing.
- Correctly identify artifact versus rhythm.

Chapter 17 Outline

I.   Introduction
II.   Artifact masquerading as asystole
III.   "Toothbrush tachycardia"
IV.   Is it real or is it artifact?
V.   CPR artifact
VI.   Artifact in three leads monitored simultaneously
VII.   Practice strips: artifact masquerading as rhythms
VIII. Answers to artifact practice strips
IX.   Practice quiz
X.   Practice quiz answers

Chapter 17 Glossary

There are no new terms in this chapter.

Introduction

Artifact can mimic rhythms quite convincingly, so much so that emergency teams are sometimes summoned to deal with patients with "life-threatening" rhythms that are later discovered to be nothing but artifact. The scenarios that follow will emphasize the importance of assessing the patient who has a change in rhythm. In other words, *do not always believe what you see on the rhythm strip. Check your patient.*

Artifact Masquerading as Asystole

Figure 17-1 is from an elderly man who'd had an MI two days prior. He was on the telemetry floor wearing a portable heart monitor. The nurse at the monitoring station saw this rhythm on the screen and ran into the patient's room. The patient was awake and feeling fine, but his rhythm indicated that his heart had completely stopped beating. Since this obviously was not the case, the nurse checked the man's monitor patches and wires and discovered several were loose or disconnected. She reconnected them and his rhythm pattern then returned to normal. Thus the rhythm in Figure 17-1 was *not* really a rhythm, but rather was **artifact** masquerading as a rhythm.

Now look at Figure 17-2. This is a strip of a heart that has indeed stopped beating. Notice the similarity between this strip and Figure 17-1.

"Toothbrush Tachycardia"

Mr. Johnson was brushing his teeth when the strip in Figure 17-3 printed out at the nurses's station, along with an auditory alarm that indicated the patient was experiencing a potentially fatal arrhythmia. The nurse, thinking Mr. Johnson was in ventricular flutter, yelled for help and ran into Mr. Johnson's room to find him brushing his teeth and in no distress (though he was shocked at having the nurses come racing into his room as if he were dying). The repetitive arm movements of his toothbrushing jiggled the EKG lead wires and caused a common type of artifact that healthcare workers refer to as "toothbrush tachycardia." When he stopped brushing his teeth, Mr. Johnson's rhythm strip returned to normal.

Now see Figure 17-4, this time of a patient in ventricular flutter, a lethal arrhythmia. Note the similarity.

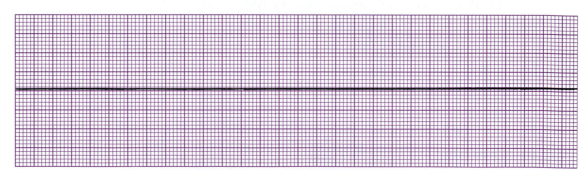

Figure 17-1   Artifact masquerading as asystole.

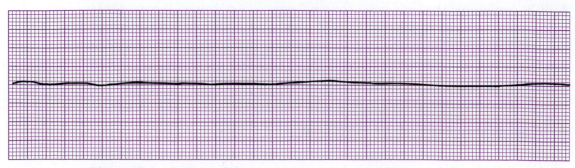

Figure 17-2   True asystole.

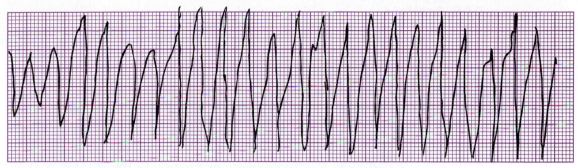

Figure 17-3   "Toothbrush tachycardia" masquerading as a rhythm.

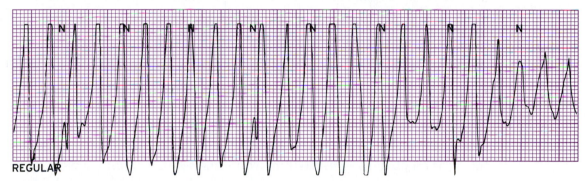

Figure 17-4   Ventricular flutter.

Is It Real or Is It Artifact?

What do you see in Figure 17-5?

If you say sinus tachycardia with a PVC, look again. That's not a PVC. It's a sinus beat obscured by artifact. See the dot on the strip? The normal QRS is right beneath it. One trick to finding artifact that suddenly pops up on a strip is to follow the R-R intervals. Where should the next QRS be? If you can see the normal QRS spike in the midst of what looks like something else, the "something else" is most likely artifact.

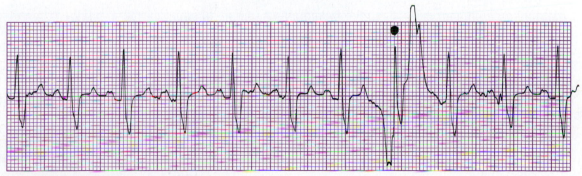

Figure 17-5   Is it real or is it artifact?

CPR Artifact

Artifact is seen frequently during resuscitation efforts. The external chest compressions of CPR produce artifact that resembles rhythms. See Figure 17-6, in which the pattern resembles a ventricular rhythm with very wide QRS complexes. In fact, it looks like a sine wave pattern that implies severe hyperkalemia (we'll get to that in Chapter 20). But look closer. See the dots? Look beneath them. See how the pattern changes a bit there? Those are the patient's own QRS complexes popping out. Now look at Figure 17-7. Here CPR was stopped momentarily to allow evaluation of the rhythm without CPR artifact.

In Figure 17-7, there is one QRS complex and then asystole. This is the patient's true rhythm. The two QRS complexes in the first strip were obviously agonal rhythm (dying heart). The rest of the pattern in the first strip were simply pseudo-QRS complexes produced by CPR.

Artifact in Three Leads Monitored Simultaneously

Figure 17-8 is a beautiful example of artifact masquerading as a rhythm. This patient was being monitored simultaneously in three different leads–V_1, lead II, and lead I. *Since the three are recorded simultaneously, all three are the same rhythm, just seen in different leads.* Note that leads II and I look like atrial flutter, but V_1 is an obvious sinus rhythm, with some somatic tremor artifact. How can that be? The strips all have to be the same rhythm. Think about this for a moment. Consider the location of the electrodes composing each lead.

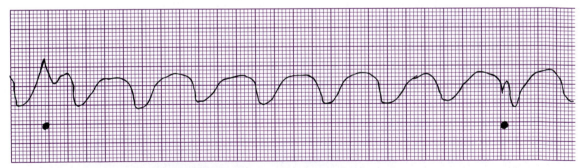

Figure 17-6 CPR artifact.

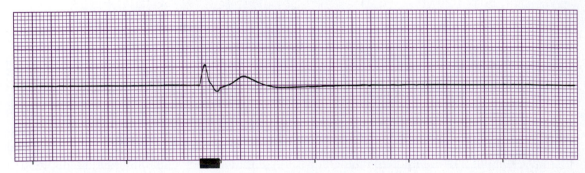

Figure 17-7 Rhythm without CPR artifact.

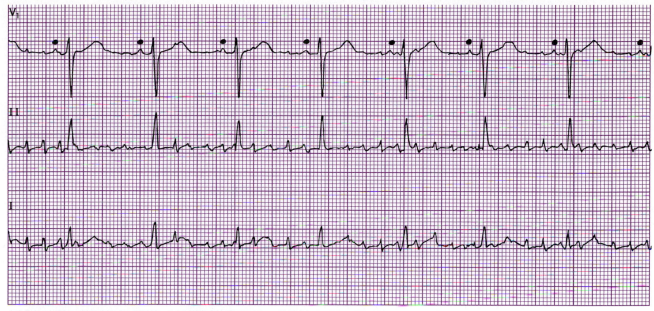

Figure 17-8 Artifact in three leads monitored simultaneously.

The answer is simple. The true rhythm is sinus rhythm. Leads II and I have artifact that obscures the P wave and provides what looks like flutter waves. You'll recall that leads II and I are limb leads and are therefore subject to artifact from muscle movement. Since V_1 is a precordial lead and is located on the chest, it picks up less artifact. Also note that the "flutter waves" here do not march out, as true flutter waves will. That is a clue that this is artifact and not the true rhythm. This patient, it turns out, had tremors from Parkinson's disease.

As you've seen, artifact can be very deceptive. Experts can pore over rhythm strips for quite a while trying to determine the legitimacy of the rhythm. *So how do you know if the rhythm you see is real or artifact?*

- If the rhythm you see is different from the patient's previous rhythm, *go check your patient.* Ask how he or she feels and check vital signs (respiratory rate, heart rate, and blood pressure). This is especially important if the rhythm appears to be life-threatening. Patients with life-threatening arrhythmias will exhibit symptoms of low cardiac output and/or cardiovascular collapse. Artifact will not produce such symptoms.

- Observe the rhythm in another lead, preferably a lead such as V_1 or MCL_1, which has minimal muscle artifact.

- Check to be sure the "rhythm" meets all its normal criteria. If it doesn't, be suspicious and check another lead.

- Check the patient's monitor wires and patches to see if they are loose or detached.

- See if the patient is having any muscle activity that could cause artifact mimicking a rhythm.

- The bottom line is this:

Always check your patient, not just the monitor!

Practice Strips: Artifact Masquerading as Rhythms

On the strips that follow, tell what the rhythm is.

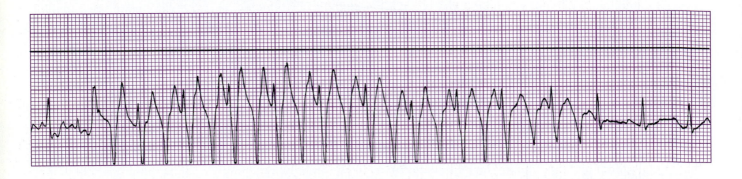

1. _____

_____

_____

_____

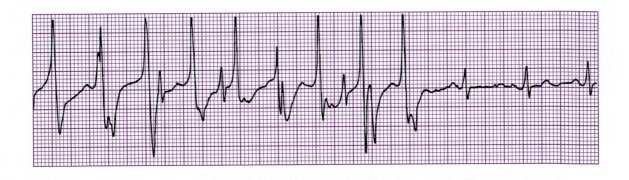

2. _____

_____

_____

_____

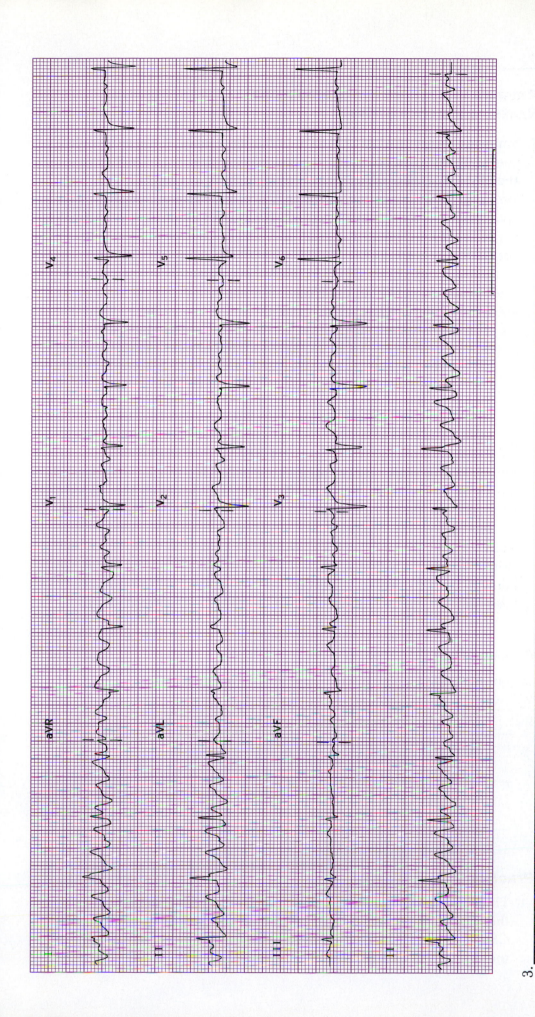

3.

Answers to Artifact Masquerading as Rhythms Practice Strips

1. **Sinus tachycardia with artifact mimicking v-tach.** If this strip fooled you, you're in good company. It also fooled several experienced nurses and physicians, all of whom initially thought this was a run of v-tach. Let's look at it in depth. See the last three QRS complexes on the strip? The middle one has a very obvious upright P wave preceding it, and the heart rate is about 125, making it a sinus beat. There is a P wave preceding the last QRS also, but it is a bit distorted by artifact. Look at the R-R intervals on those last three beats. The R-R interval is constant. Now march the R-R intervals *backward* from these beats and you'll find normal QRS complexes at regular intervals. The rest of the spikes are artifact. This is not v-tach. It's simply sinus tachycardia with artifact. Here's a clue: Always be suspicious of a rhythm that looks like v-tach but has *extra spikes* scattered throughout the rhythm. Those extra spikes may just be the normal QRS complexes visible through the artifact.

2. **Sinus rhythm with artifact.** This strip also fooled some experienced healthcare personnel. Again, note the sinus beats on the strip. March out the R-R intervals to find the other normal QRS complexes.

3. **Sinus rhythm with artifact mimicking atrial flutter.** At first glance, this looks like atrial flutter, doesn't it? In many leads on this 12-lead EKG, it looks like there are flutter waves between the QRS complexes. But look at lead III. See the P waves preceding each QRS? And look at leads V_4 to V_6. You can see the P waves there also. Though the rhythm strip of lead II at the bottom of the EKG page looks like atrial flutter, we know it's merely artifact distorting the sinus rhythm. Had there only been lead II to go by, this patient might have been unnecessarily treated for atrial flutter.

Practice Quiz

1. List three ways to determine if a rhythm is real or artifact. _____
   _____
   _____

2. "Toothbrush tachycardia" is a type of artifact caused by _____
   _____

3. List three rhythms that artifact can mimic._____
   _____
   _____

Practice Quiz Answers

1. Three ways to determine if a rhythm is real or artifact are any three of the following: **Observe the rhythm in another lead such as V_1. Check to see if the rhythm meets the normal criteria. Check the monitor wires and patches. See if the patient is having any mus-**

cle activity that could cause artifact. **Check the patient's vital signs for evidence of decreased cardiac output.**

2. "Toothbrush tachycardia" is caused by **repetitive arm movements from toothbrushing or similar activities.**

3. Artifact can mimic any of these rhythms: **asystole, atrial flutter, atrial fibrillation, ventricular flutter, other ventricular rhythms, PVCs.**

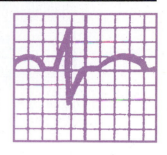

Rhythm Practice Strips

Chapter 18 Objectives

Upon completion of this chapter, the student will be able to:

- Correctly identify the rhythms in this chapter.
- Practice the five steps to rhythm interpretation covered in Chapter 11.
- Correctly determine PR, QRS, and QT intervals on a variety of rhythm strips.
- Identify any weak areas for further study.

Chapter 18 Outline

I.   Rhythm strips for interpretation

II. Answers to rhythms

Chapter 18 Glossary

There are no new terms in this chapter.

Rhythm Strips for Interpretation

This chapter contains practice strips of all rhythm types. Some strips are on solid-line paper, others are on dotted-line paper. *Do not let that distract you!* That does not change anything in terms of intervals, rhythm interpretation, and so forth.

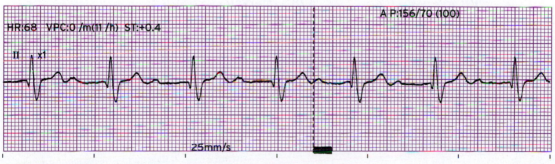

1. QRS complexes _____ Regularity _____

Heart rate _____

P waves _____

PR interval _____ QRS interval _____

Interpretation (name of rhythm) _____

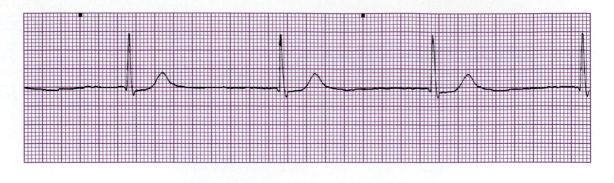

2. QRS complexes _____ Regularity _____

Heart rate _____

P waves _____

PR interval _____ QRS interval _____

Interpretation _____

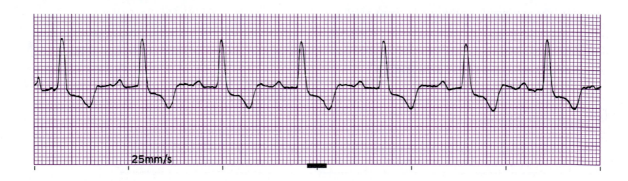

25mm/s

3. QRS complexes _____ Regularity _____

Heart rate _____

P waves _____

PR interval _____ QRS interval _____

Interpretation _____

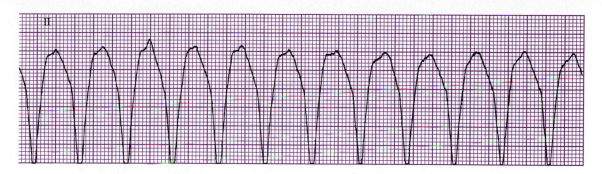

4. QRS complexes _____ Regularity _____

Heart rate _____

P waves _____

PR interval _____ QRS interval _____

Interpretation _____

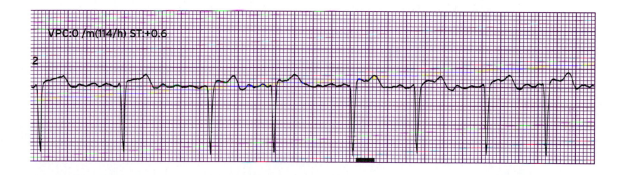

5. QRS complexes _____ Regularity _____

Heart rate _____

P waves _____

PR interval _____ QRS interval _____

Interpretation _____

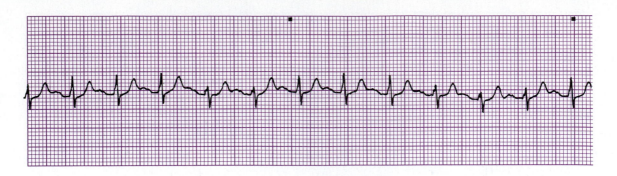

6. QRS complexes _____ Regularity _____

Heart rate _____

P waves _____

PR interval _____ QRS interval _____

Interpretation _____

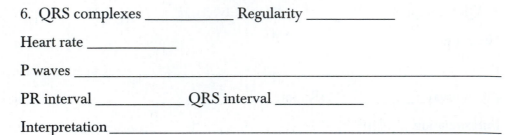

7. QRS complexes _____ Regularity _____

Heart rate _____

P waves _____

PR interval _____ QRS interval _____

Interpretation _____

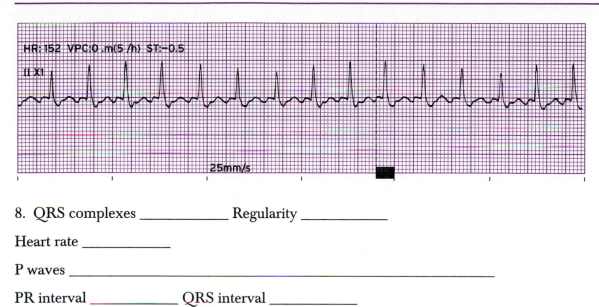

HR: 152 VPC:0 .m(5 /h) ST:-0.5

II X1

25mm/s

8. QRS complexes _____ Regularity _____

Heart rate _____

P waves _____

PR interval _____ QRS interval _____

Interpretation _____

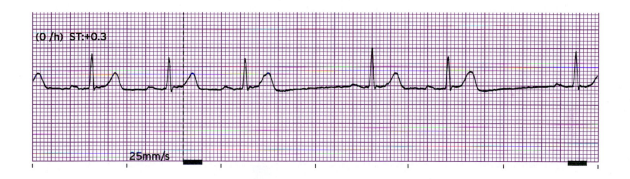

(0 /h) ST:+0.3

25mm/s

9. QRS complexes _____ Regularity _____

Heart rate _____

P waves _____

PR interval _____ QRS interval _____

Interpretation _____

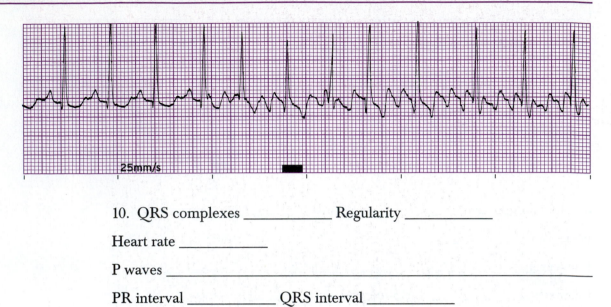

25mm/s

10. QRS complexes _____ Regularity _____

Heart rate _____

P waves _____

PR interval _____ QRS interval _____

Interpretation _____

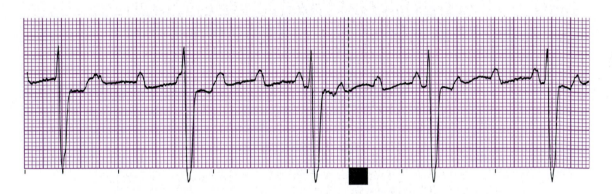

11. QRS complexes _____ Regularity _____

Heart rate _____

P waves _____

PR interval _____ QRS interval _____

Interpretation _____

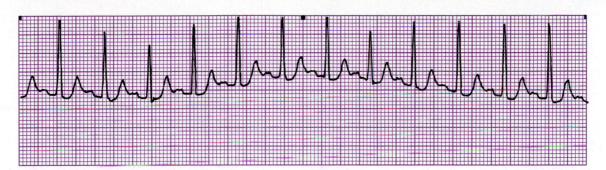

12. QRS complexes _____ Regularity _____

Heart rate _____

P waves _____

PR interval _____ QRS interval _____

Interpretation _____

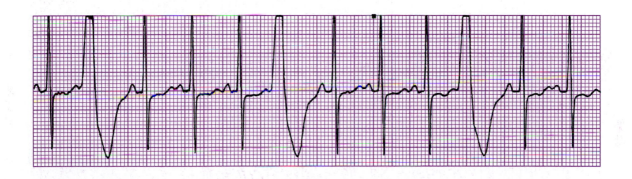

13. QRS complexes _____ Regularity _____

Heart rate _____

P waves _____

PR interval _____ QRS interval _____

Interpretation _____

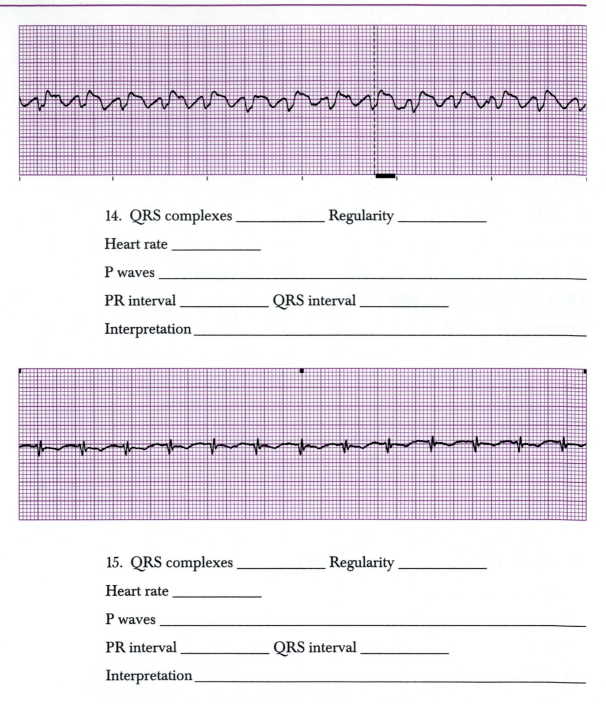

14. QRS complexes _____ Regularity _____

Heart rate _____

P waves _____

PR interval _____ QRS interval _____

Interpretation _____

15. QRS complexes _____ Regularity _____

Heart rate _____

P waves _____

PR interval _____ QRS interval _____

Interpretation _____

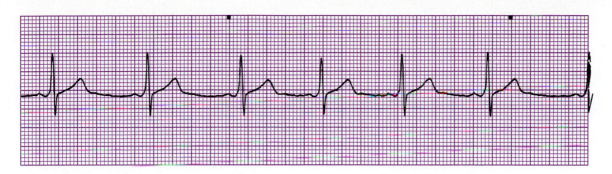

16. QRS complexes _____ Regularity _____

Heart rate _____

P waves _____

PR interval _____ QRS interval _____

Interpretation _____

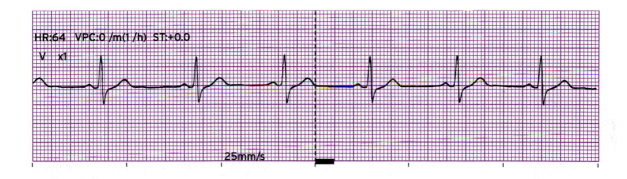

17. QRS complexes _____ Regularity _____

Heart rate _____

P waves _____

PR interval _____ QRS interval _____

Interpretation _____

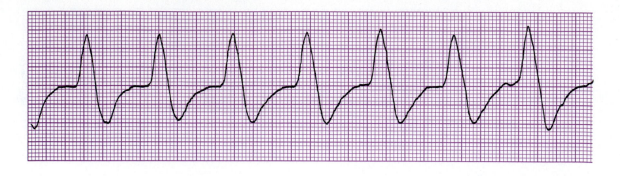

18. QRS complexes _____ Regularity _____

Heart rate _____

P waves _____

PR interval _____ QRS interval _____

Interpretation _____

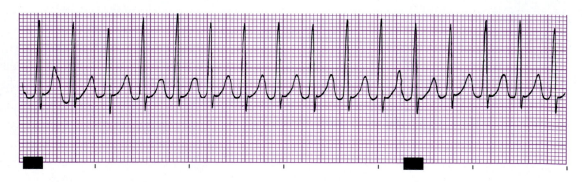

19. QRS complexes _____ Regularity _____

Heart rate _____

P waves _____

PR interval _____ QRS interval _____

Interpretation _____

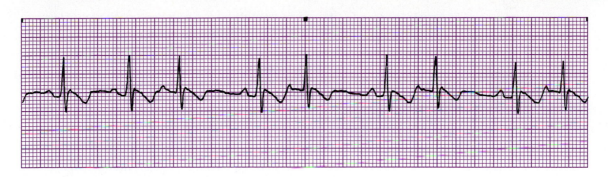

20. QRS complexes _____ Regularity _____

Heart rate _____

P waves _____

PR interval _____ QRS interval _____

Interpretation _____

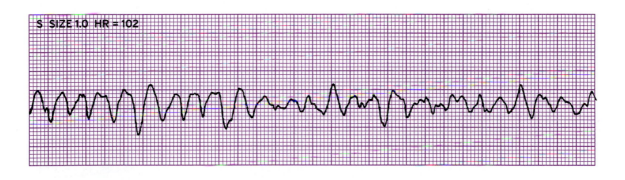

21. QRS complexes _____ Regularity _____

Heart rate _____

P waves _____

PR interval _____ QRS interval _____

Interpretation _____

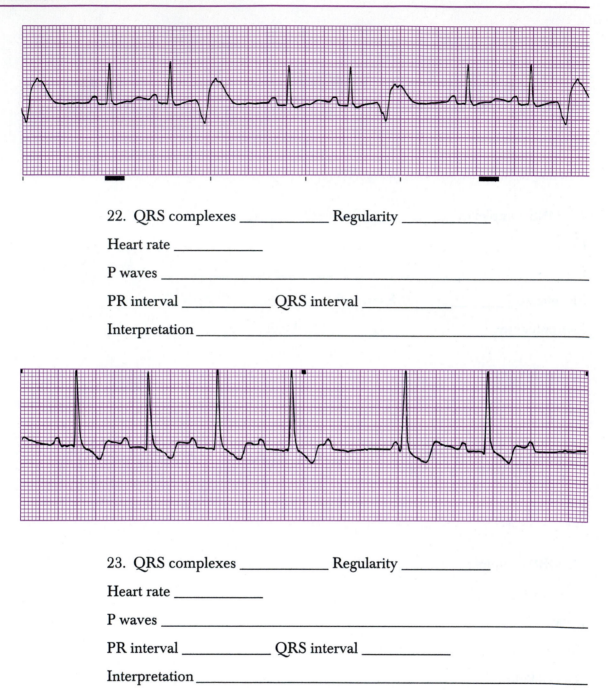

22. QRS complexes _____ Regularity _____

Heart rate _____

P waves _____

PR interval _____ QRS interval _____

Interpretation _____

23. QRS complexes _____ Regularity _____

Heart rate _____

P waves _____

PR interval _____ QRS interval _____

Interpretation _____

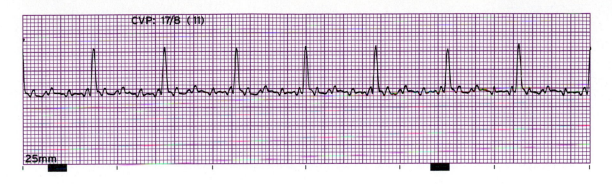

24. QRS complexes _____ Regularity _____

Heart rate _____

P waves _____

PR interval _____ QRS interval _____

Interpretation _____

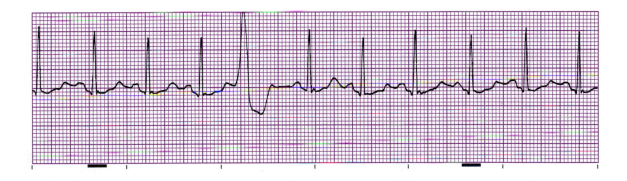

25. QRS complexes _____ Regularity _____

Heart rate _____

P waves _____

PR interval _____ QRS interval _____

Interpretation _____

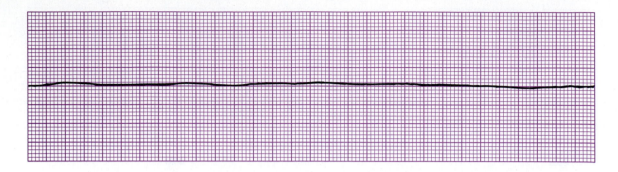

26. QRS complexes _____ Regularity _____

Heart rate _____

P waves _____

PR interval _____ QRS interval _____

Interpretation _____

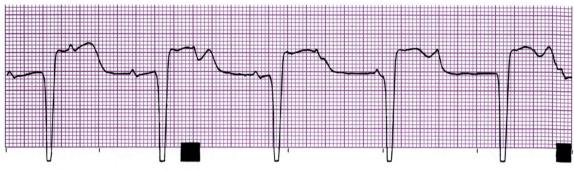

27. QRS complexes _____ Regularity _____

Heart rate _____

P waves _____

PR interval _____ QRS interval _____

Interpretation _____

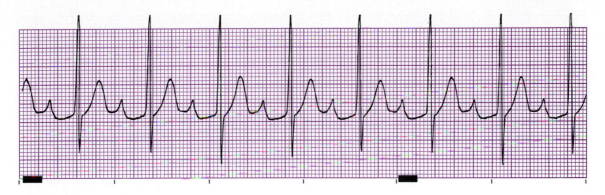

28. QRS complexes _____ Regularity _____

Heart rate _____

P waves _____

PR interval _____ QRS interval _____

Interpretation _____

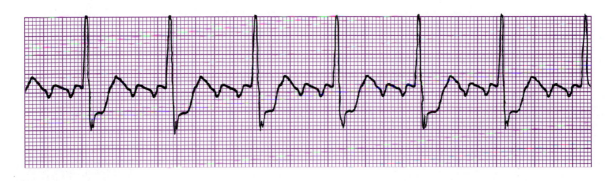

29. QRS complexes _____ Regularity _____

Heart rate _____

P waves _____

PR interval _____ QRS interval _____

Interpretation _____

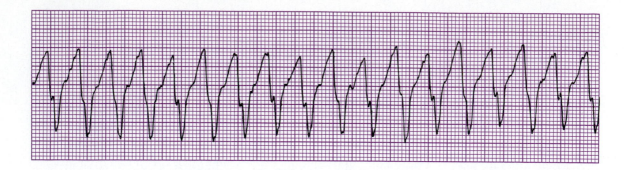

30. QRS complexes _____ Regularity _____

Heart rate _____

P waves _____

PR interval _____ QRS interval _____

Interpretation _____

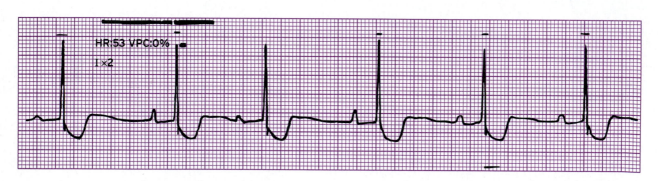

31. QRS complexes _____ Regularity _____

Heart rate _____

P waves _____

PR interval _____ QRS interval _____

Interpretation _____

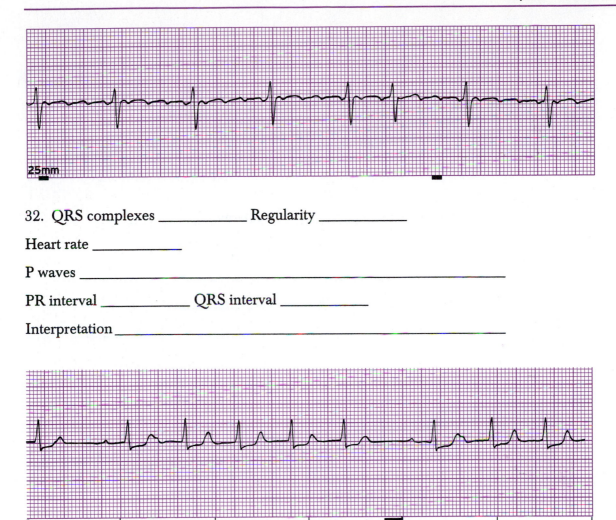

32. QRS complexes _____ Regularity _____

Heart rate _____

P waves _____

PR interval _____ QRS interval _____

Interpretation _____

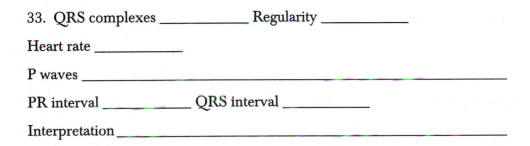

33. QRS complexes _____ Regularity _____

Heart rate _____

P waves _____

PR interval _____ QRS interval _____

Interpretation _____

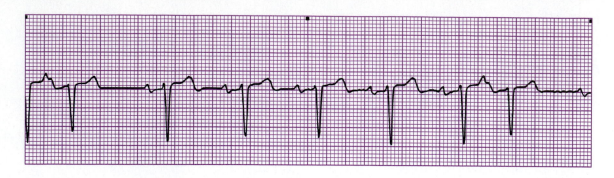

34. QRS complexes _____ Regularity _____

Heart rate _____

P waves _____

PR interval _____ QRS interval _____

Interpretation _____

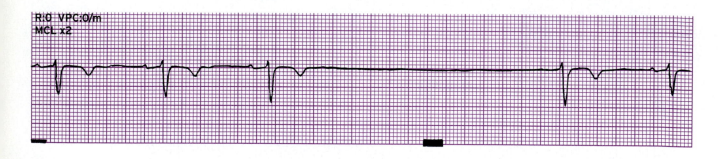

35. QRS complexes _____ Regularity _____

Heart rate _____

P waves _____

PR interval _____ QRS interval _____

Interpretation _____

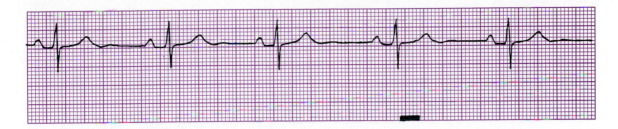

36. QRS complexes _____ Regularity _____

Heart rate _____

P waves _____

PR interval _____ QRS interval _____

Interpretation _____

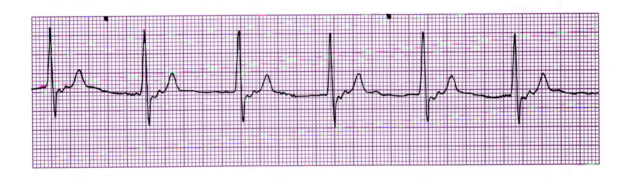

37. QRS complexes _____ Regularity _____

Heart rate _____

P waves _____

PR interval _____ QRS interval _____

Interpretation _____

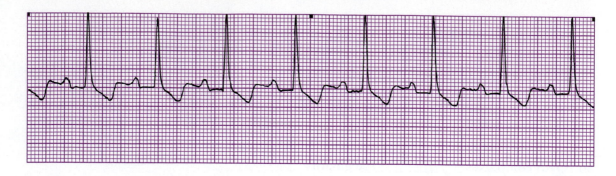

38. QRS complexes _____ Regularity _____

Heart rate _____

P waves _____

PR interval _____ QRS interval _____

Interpretation _____

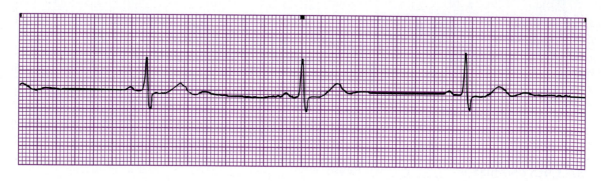

39. QRS complexes _____ Regularity _____

Heart rate _____

P waves _____

PR interval _____ QRS interval _____

Interpretation _____

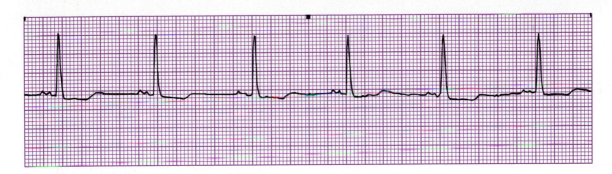

40. QRS complexes _____ Regularity _____

Heart rate _____

P waves _____

PR interval _____ QRS interval _____

Interpretation _____

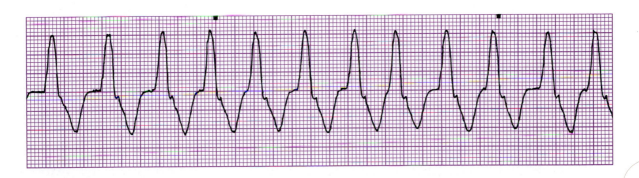

41. QRS complexes _____ Regularity _____

Heart rate _____

P waves _____

PR interval _____ QRS interval _____

Interpretation _____

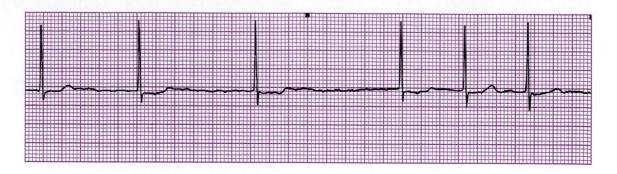

42. QRS complexes _____ Regularity _____

Heart rate _____

P waves _____

PR interval _____ QRS interval _____

Interpretation _____

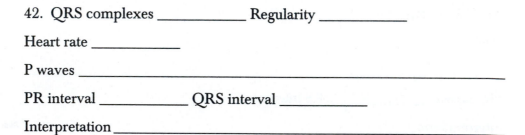

43. QRS complexes _____ Regularity _____

Heart rate _____

P waves _____

PR interval _____ QRS interval _____

Interpretation _____

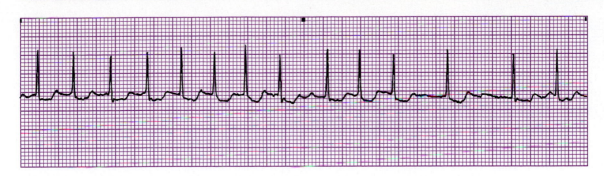

44. QRS complexes _____ Regularity _____

Heart rate _____

P waves _____

PR interval _____ QRS interval _____

Interpretation _____

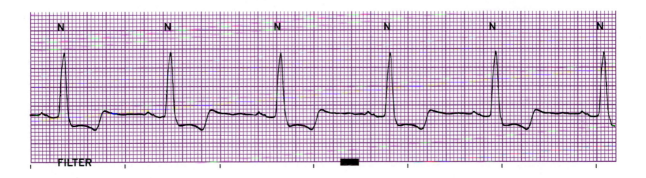

45. QRS complexes _____ Regularity _____

Heart rate _____

P waves _____

PR interval _____ QRS interval _____

Interpretation _____

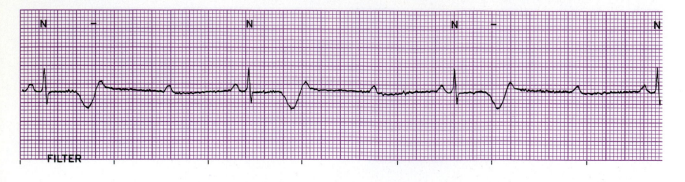

46. QRS complexes _____ Regularity _____

Heart rate _____

P waves _____

PR interval _____ QRS interval _____

Interpretation _____

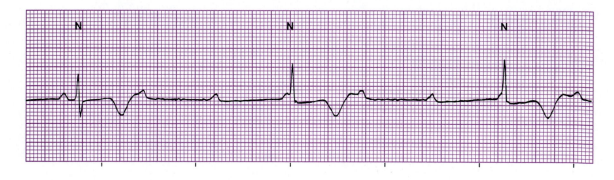

47. QRS complexes _____ Regularity _____

Heart rate _____

P waves _____

PR interval _____ QRS interval _____

Interpretation _____

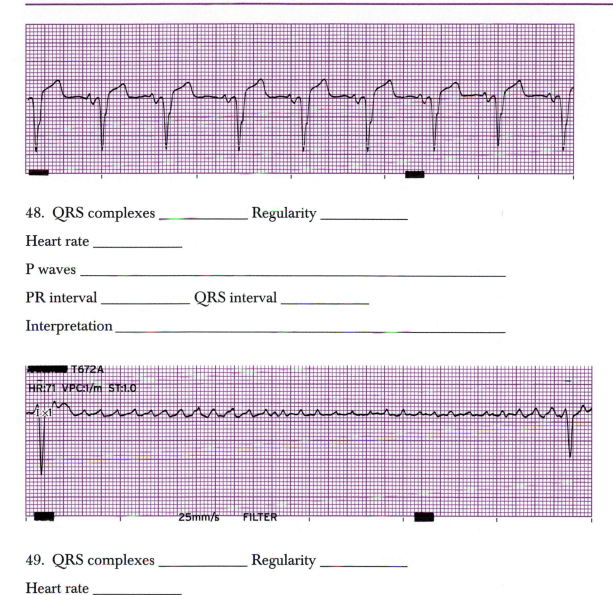

48. QRS complexes _____ Regularity _____

Heart rate _____

P waves _____

PR interval _____ QRS interval _____

Interpretation _____

49. QRS complexes _____ Regularity _____

Heart rate _____

P waves _____

PR interval _____ QRS interval _____

Interpretation _____

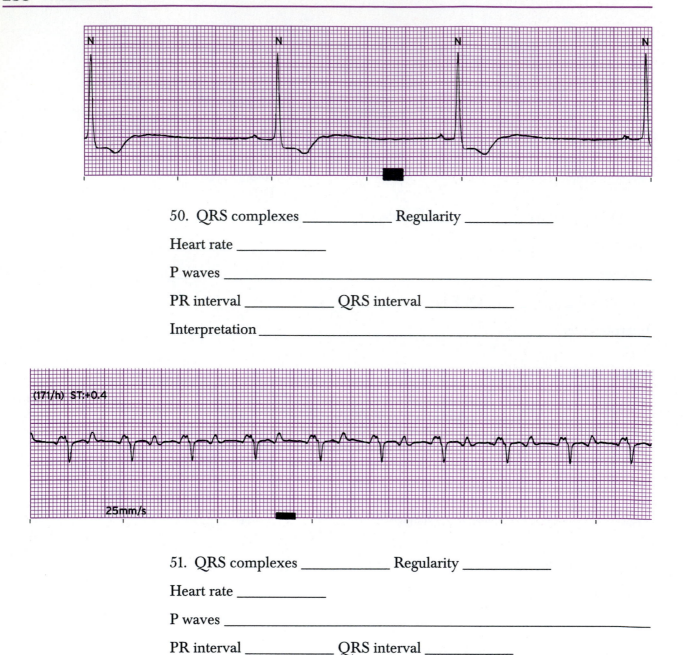

50. QRS complexes _____ Regularity _____

Heart rate _____

P waves _____

PR interval _____ QRS interval _____

Interpretation _____

51. QRS complexes _____ Regularity _____

Heart rate _____

P waves _____

PR interval _____ QRS interval _____

Interpretation _____

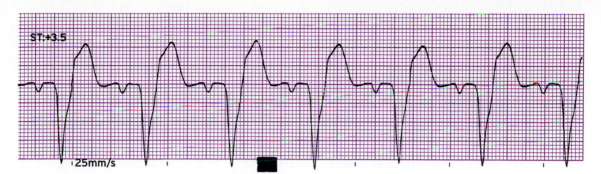

ST:+3.5

25mm/s

52. QRS complexes _____ Regularity _____

Heart rate _____

P waves _____

PR interval _____ QRS interval _____

Interpretation _____

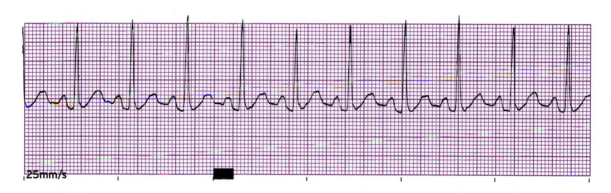

25mm/s

53. QRS complexes _____ Regularity _____

Heart rate _____

P waves _____

PR interval _____ QRS interval _____

Interpretation _____

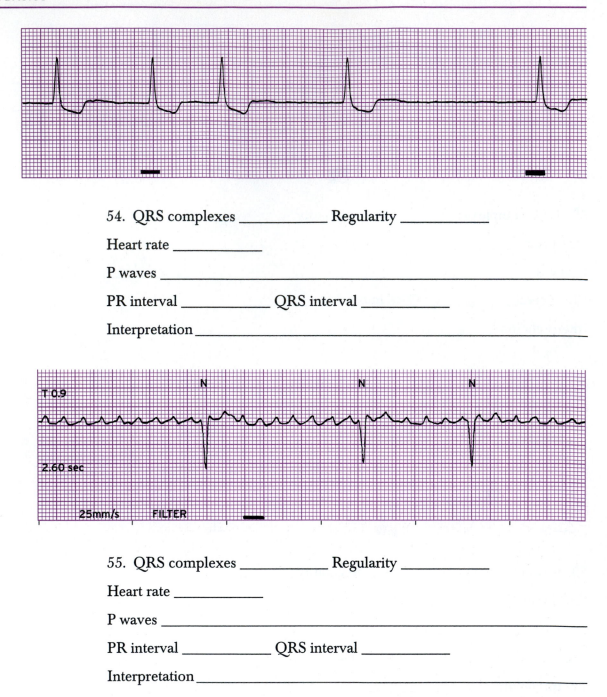

54. QRS complexes _____ Regularity _____

Heart rate _____

P waves _____

PR interval _____ QRS interval _____

Interpretation _____

55. QRS complexes _____ Regularity _____

Heart rate _____

P waves _____

PR interval _____ QRS interval _____

Interpretation _____

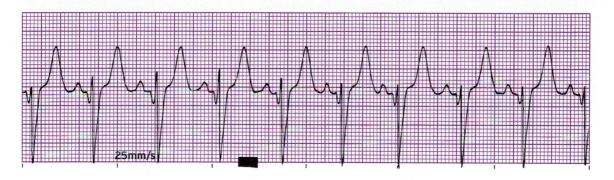

56. QRS complexes _____ Regularity _____

Heart rate _____

P waves _____

PR interval _____ QRS interval _____

Interpretation _____

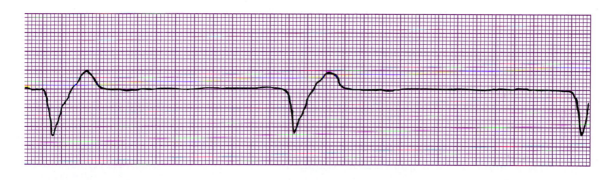

57. QRS complexes _____ Regularity _____

Heart rate _____

P waves _____

PR interval _____ QRS interval _____

Interpretation _____

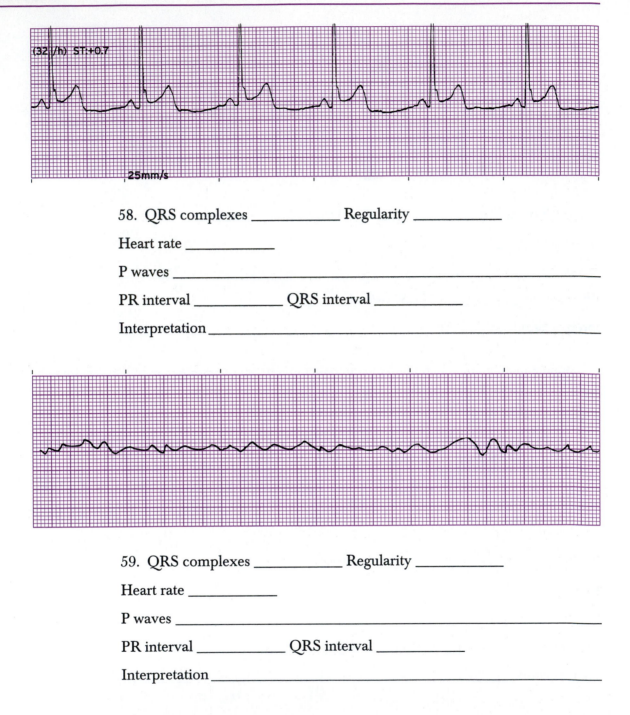

(32 /h) ST+0.7

25mm/s

58. QRS complexes _____ Regularity _____

Heart rate _____

P waves _____

PR interval _____ QRS interval _____

Interpretation _____

59. QRS complexes _____ Regularity _____

Heart rate _____

P waves _____

PR interval _____ QRS interval _____

Interpretation _____

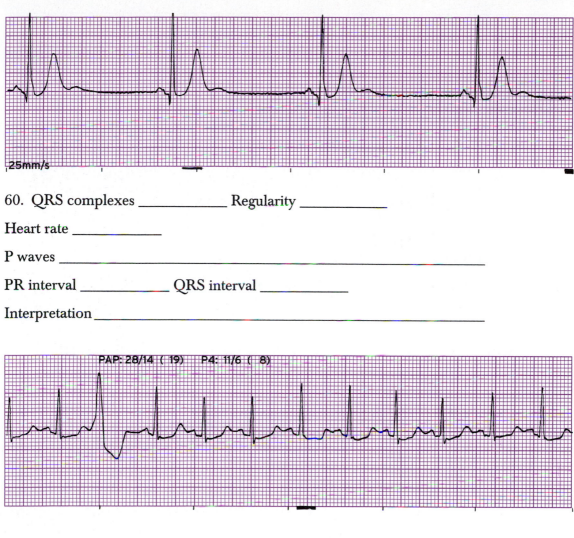

60. QRS complexes _____ Regularity _____

Heart rate _____

P waves _____

PR interval _____ QRS interval _____

Interpretation _____

61. QRS complexes _____ Regularity _____

Heart rate _____

P waves _____

PR interval _____ QRS interval _____

Interpretation _____

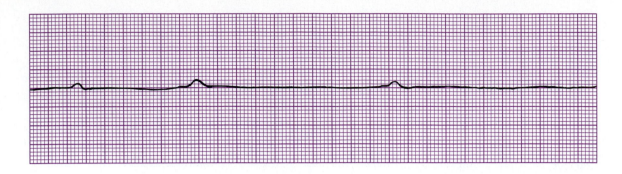

62. QRS complexes _____ Regularity _____

Heart rate _____

P waves _____

PR interval _____ QRS interval _____

Interpretation _____

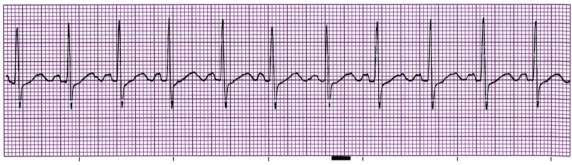

63. QRS complexes _____ Regularity _____

Heart rate _____

P waves _____

PR interval _____ QRS interval _____

Interpretation _____

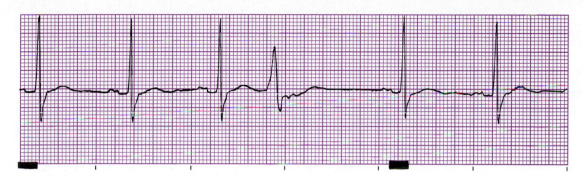

64. QRS complexes _____ Regularity _____

Heart rate _____

P waves _____

PR interval _____ QRS interval _____

Interpretation _____

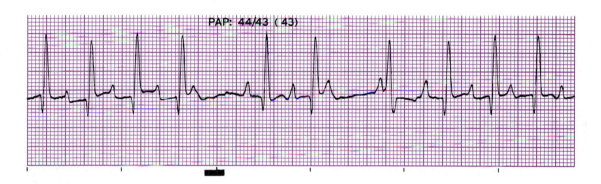

PAP: 44/43 (43)

65. QRS complexes _____ Regularity _____

Heart rate _____

P waves _____

PR interval _____ QRS interval _____

Interpretation _____

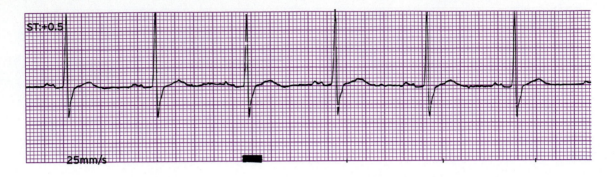

66. QRS complexes _____ Regularity _____

Heart rate _____

P waves _____

PR interval _____ QRS interval _____

Interpretation _____

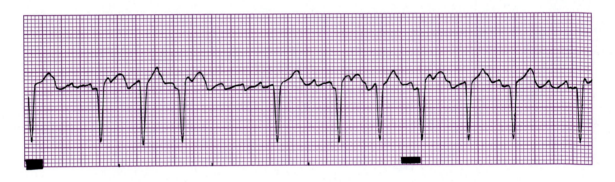

67. QRS complexes _____ Regularity _____

Heart rate _____

P waves _____

PR interval _____ QRS interval _____

Interpretation _____

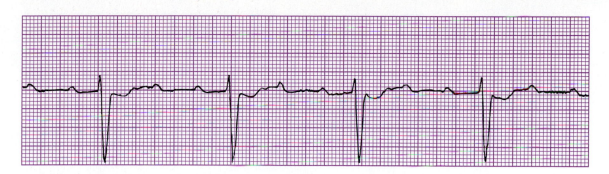

68. QRS complexes _____ Regularity _____

Heart rate _____

P waves _____

PR interval _____ QRS interval _____

Interpretation _____

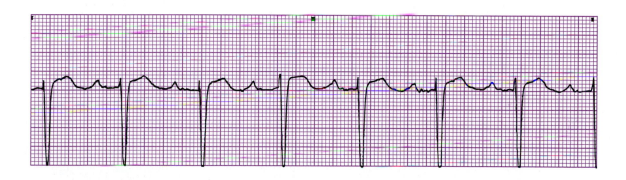

69. QRS complexes _____ Regularity _____

Heart rate _____

P waves _____

PR interval _____ QRS interval _____

Interpretation _____

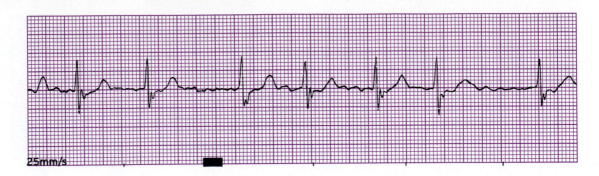

25mm/s

70. QRS complexes _____ Regularity _____

Heart rate _____

P waves _____

PR interval _____ QRS interval _____

Interpretation _____

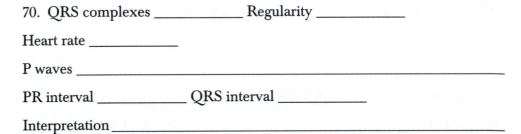

71. QRS complexes _____ Regularity _____

Heart rate _____

P waves _____

PR interval _____ QRS interval _____

Interpretation _____

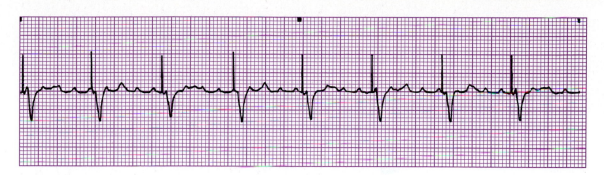

72. QRS complexes _____ Regularity _____

Heart rate _____

P waves _____

PR interval _____ QRS interval _____

Interpretation _____

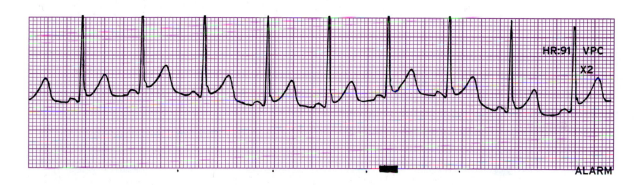

73. QRS complexes _____ Regularity _____

Heart rate _____

P waves _____

PR interval _____ QRS interval _____

Interpretation _____

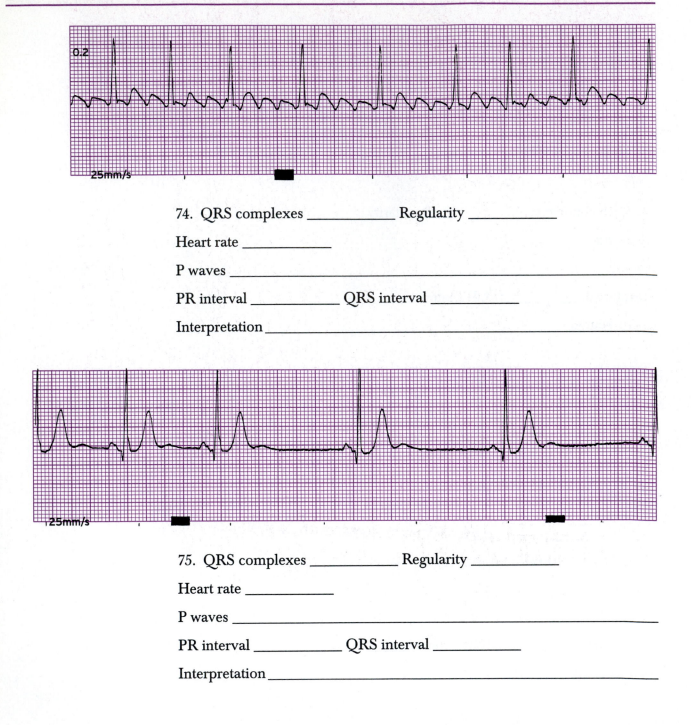

74. QRS complexes _____ Regularity _____

Heart rate _____

P waves _____

PR interval _____ QRS interval _____

Interpretation _____

75. QRS complexes _____ Regularity _____

Heart rate _____

P waves _____

PR interval _____ QRS interval _____

Interpretation _____

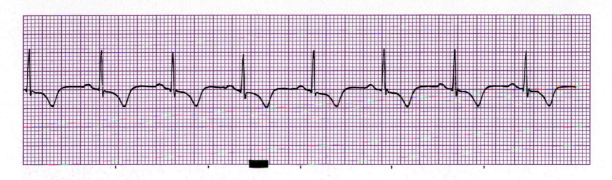

76. QRS complexes _____ Regularity _____

Heart rate _____

P waves _____

PR interval _____ QRS interval _____

Interpretation _____

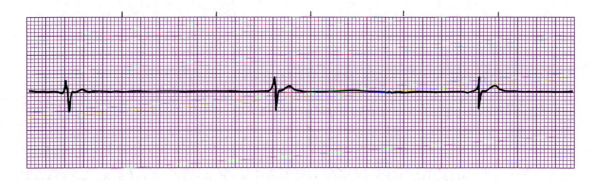

77. QRS complexes _____ Regularity _____

Heart rate _____

P waves _____

PR interval _____ QRS interval _____

Interpretation _____

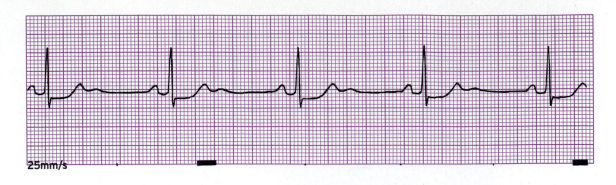

25mm/s

78. QRS complexes _____ Regularity _____

Heart rate _____

P waves _____

PR interval _____ QRS interval _____

Interpretation _____

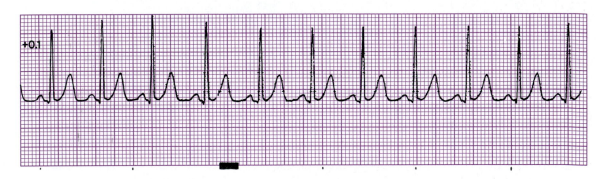

+0.1

79. QRS complexes _____ Regularity _____

Heart rate _____

P waves _____

PR interval _____ QRS interval _____

Interpretation _____

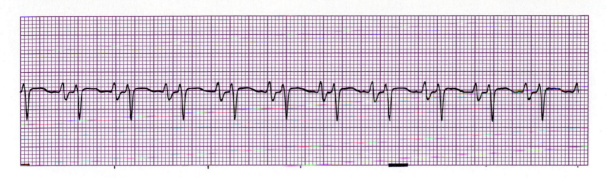

80. QRS complexes _____ Regularity _____

Heart rate _____

P waves _____

PR interval _____ QRS interval _____

Interpretation _____

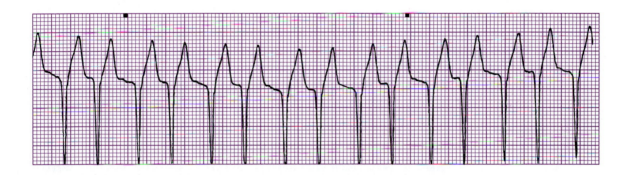

81. QRS complexes _____ Regularity _____

Heart rate _____

P waves _____

PR interval _____ QRS interval _____

Interpretation _____

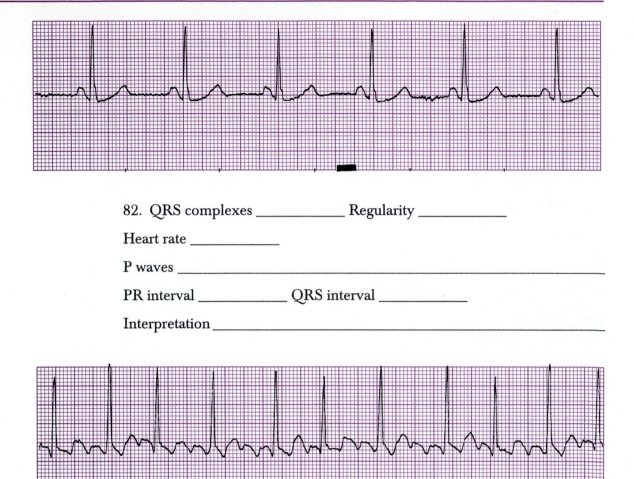

82. QRS complexes _____ Regularity _____

Heart rate _____

P waves _____

PR interval _____ QRS interval _____

Interpretation _____

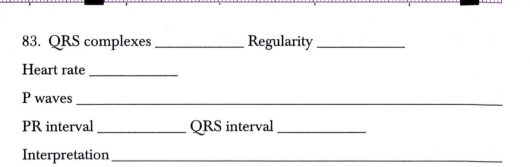

83. QRS complexes _____ Regularity _____

Heart rate _____

P waves _____

PR interval _____ QRS interval _____

Interpretation _____

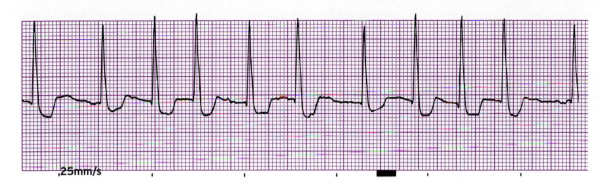

,25mm/s

84. QRS complexes _____ Regularity _____

Heart rate _____

P waves _____

PR interval _____ QRS interval _____

Interpretation _____

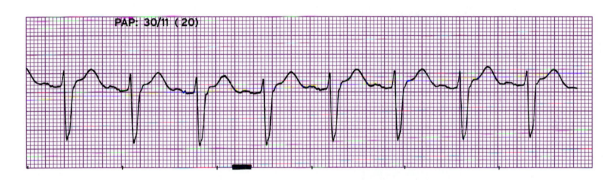

PAP: 30/11 (20)

85. QRS complexes _____ Regularity _____

Heart rate _____

P waves _____

PR interval _____ QRS interval _____

Interpretation _____

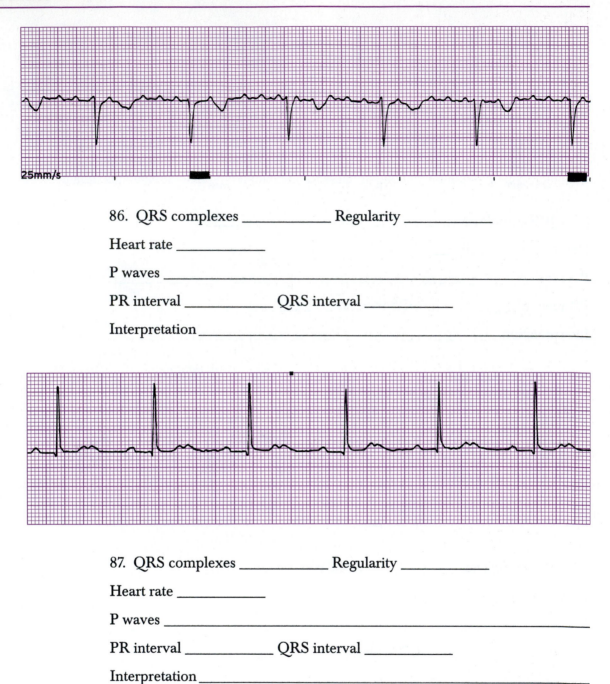

86. QRS complexes _____ Regularity _____

Heart rate _____

P waves _____

PR interval _____ QRS interval _____

Interpretation _____

87. QRS complexes _____ Regularity _____

Heart rate _____

P waves _____

PR interval _____ QRS interval _____

Interpretation _____

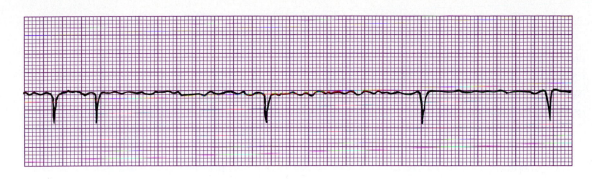

88. QRS complexes _____ Regularity _____

Heart rate _____

P waves _____

PR interval _____ QRS interval _____

Interpretation _____

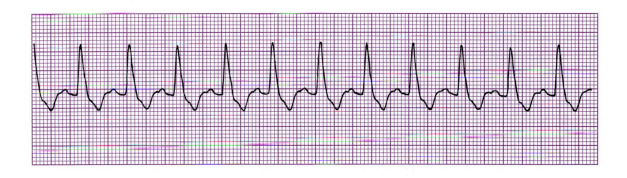

89. QRS complexes _____ Regularity _____

Heart rate _____

P waves _____

PR interval _____ QRS interval _____

Interpretation _____

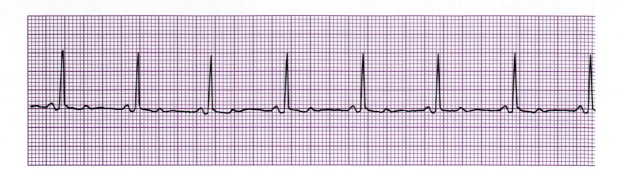

90. QRS complexes _____ Regularity _____

Heart rate _____

P waves _____

PR interval _____ QRS interval _____

Interpretation _____

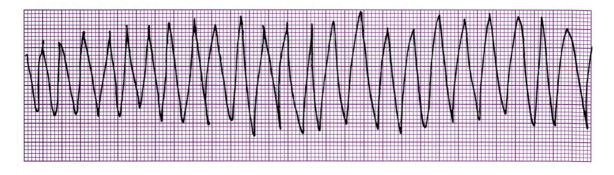

91. QRS complexes _____ Regularity _____

Heart rate _____

P waves _____

PR interval _____ QRS interval _____

Interpretation _____

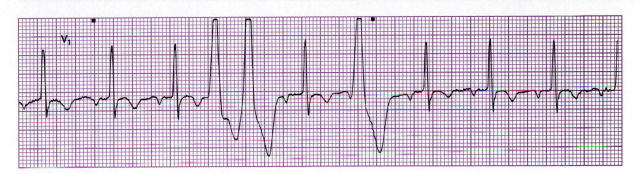

92. QRS complexes _____ Regularity _____

Heart rate _____

P waves _____

PR interval _____ QRS interval _____

Interpretation _____

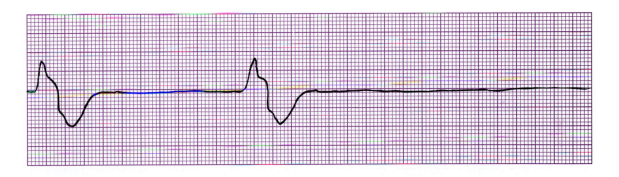

93. QRS complexes _____ Regularity _____

Heart rate _____

P waves _____

PR interval _____ QRS interval _____

Interpretation _____

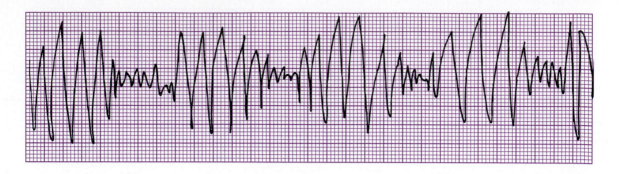

94. QRS complexes _____ Regularity _____

Heart rate _____

P waves _____

PR interval _____ QRS interval _____

Interpretation _____

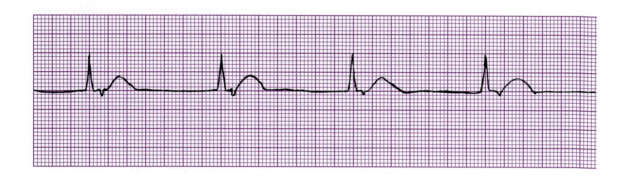

95. QRS complexes _____ Regularity _____

Heart rate _____

P waves _____

PR interval _____ QRS interval _____

Interpretation _____

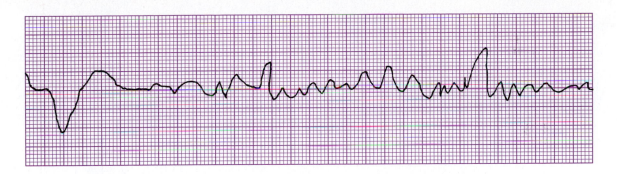

96. QRS complexes _____ Regularity _____

Heart rate _____

P waves _____

PR interval _____ QRS interval _____

Interpretation _____

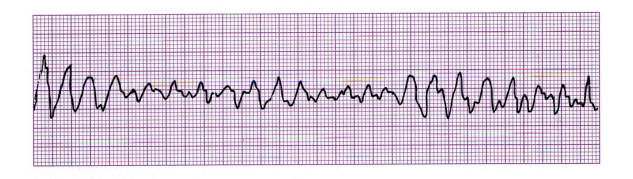

97. QRS complexes _____ Regularity _____

Heart rate _____

P waves _____

PR interval _____ QRS interval _____

Interpretation _____

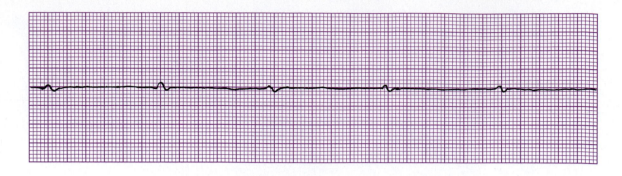

98. QRS complexes _____ Regularity _____

Heart rate _____

P waves _____

PR interval _____ QRS interval _____

Interpretation _____

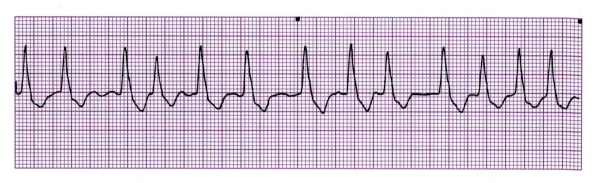

99. QRS complexes _____ Regularity _____

Heart rate _____

P waves _____

PR interval _____ QRS interval _____

Interpretation _____

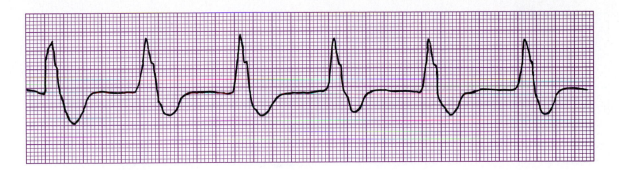

100. QRS complexes _____ Regularity _____

Heart rate _____

P waves _____

PR interval _____ QRS interval _____

Interpretation _____

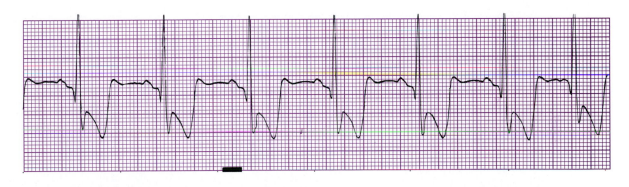

101. QRS complexes _____ Regularity _____

Heart rate _____

P waves _____

PR interval _____ QRS interval _____

Interpretation _____

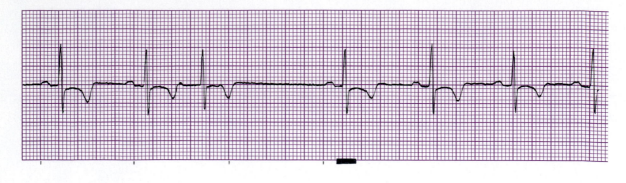

102. QRS complexes _____ Regularity _____

Heart rate _____

P waves _____

PR interval _____ QRS interval _____

Interpretation _____

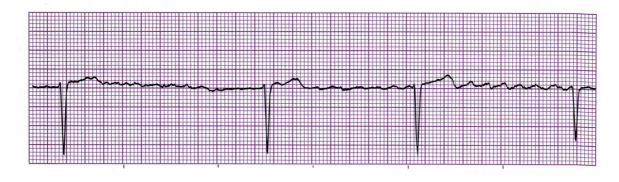

103. QRS complexes _____ Regularity _____

Heart rate _____

P waves _____

PR interval _____ QRS interval _____

Interpretation _____

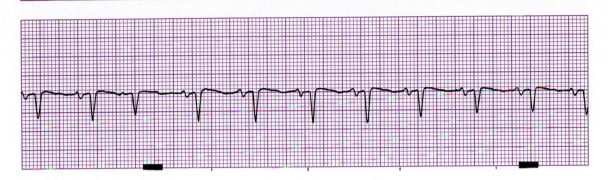

104. QRS complexes _____ Regularity _____

Heart rate _____

P waves _____

PR interval _____ QRS interval _____

Interpretation _____

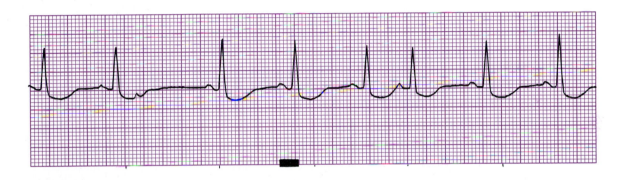

105. QRS complexes _____ Regularity _____

Heart rate _____

P waves _____

PR interval _____ QRS interval _____

Interpretation _____

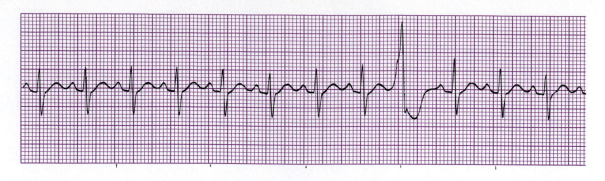

106. QRS complexes _____ Regularity _____

Heart rate _____

P waves _____

PR interval _____ QRS interval _____

Interpretation _____

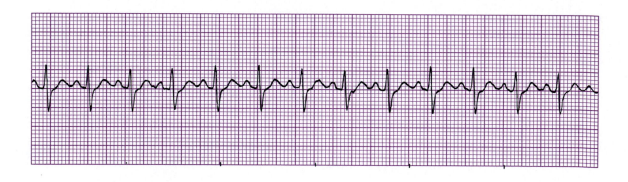

107. QRS complexes _____ Regularity _____

Heart rate _____

P waves _____

PR interval _____ QRS interval _____

Interpretation _____

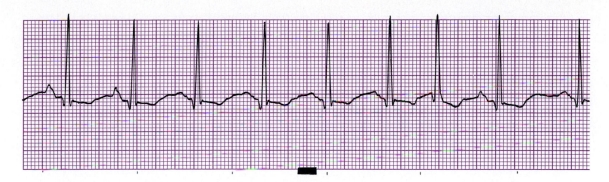

108. QRS complexes _____ Regularity _____

Heart rate _____

P waves _____

PR interval _____ QRS interval _____

Interpretation _____

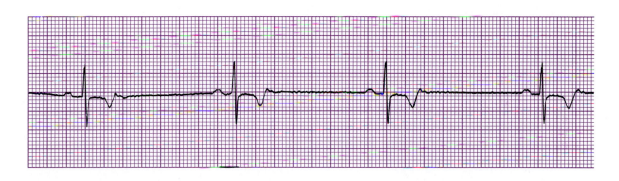

109. QRS complexes _____ Regularity _____

Heart rate _____

P waves _____

PR interval _____ QRS interval _____

Interpretation _____

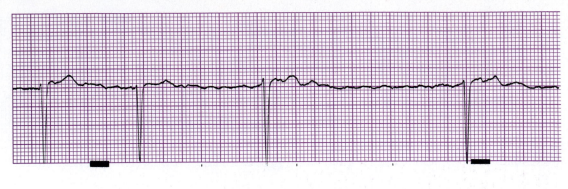

110. QRS complexes _____ Regularity _____

Heart rate _____

P waves _____

PR interval _____ QRS interval _____

Interpretation _____

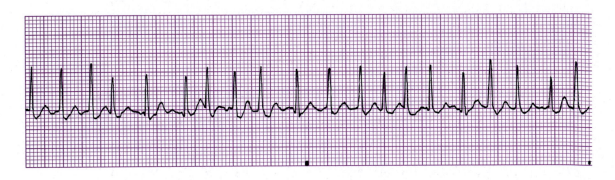

111. QRS complexes _____ Regularity _____

Heart rate _____

P waves _____

PR interval _____ QRS interval _____

Interpretation _____

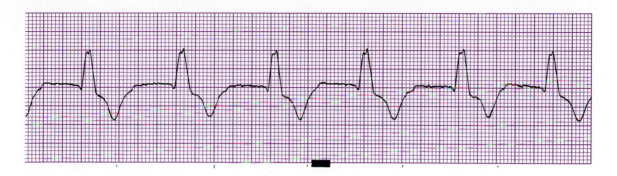

112. QRS complexes _____ Regularity _____

Heart rate _____

P waves _____

PR interval _____ QRS interval _____

Interpretation _____

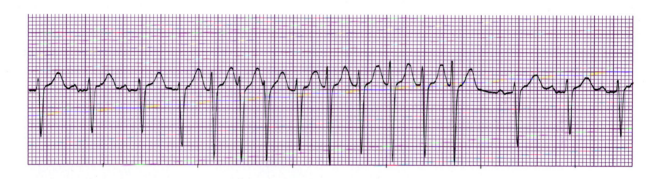

113. QRS complexes _____ Regularity _____

Heart rate _____

P waves _____

PR interval _____ QRS interval _____

Interpretation _____

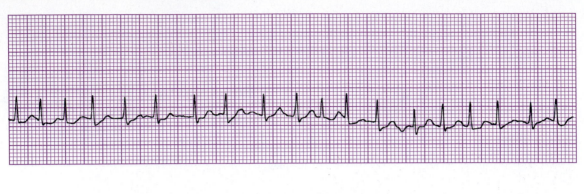

114. QRS complexes _____ Regularity _____

Heart rate _____

P waves _____

PR interval _____ QRS interval _____

Interpretation _____

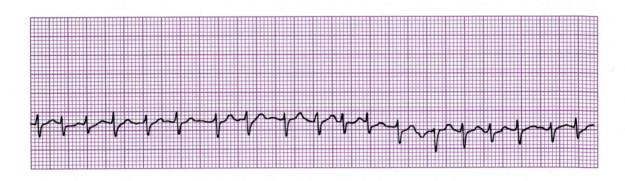

115. QRS complexes _____ Regularity _____

Heart rate _____

P waves _____

PR interval _____ QRS interval _____

Interpretation _____

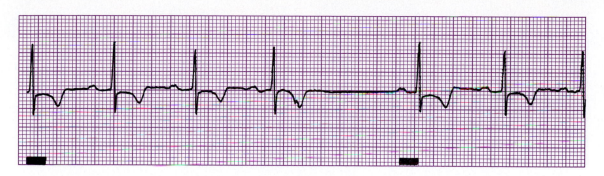

116. QRS complexes _____ Regularity _____

Heart rate _____

P waves _____

PR interval _____ QRS interval _____

Interpretation _____

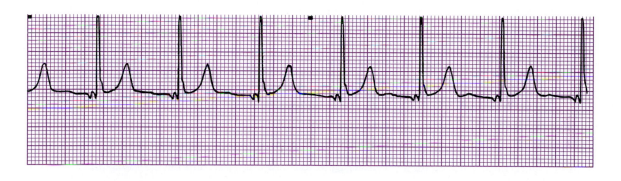

117. QRS complexes _____ Regularity _____

Heart rate _____

P waves _____

PR interval _____ QRS interval _____

Interpretation _____

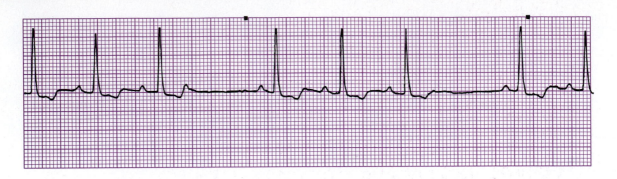

118. QRS complexes _____ Regularity _____

Heart rate _____

P waves _____

PR interval _____ QRS interval _____

Interpretation _____

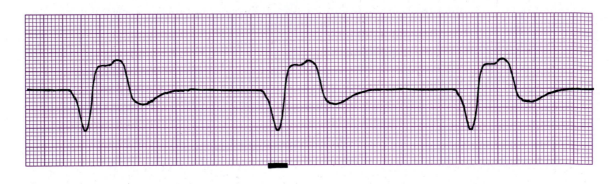

119. QRS complexes _____ Regularity _____

Heart rate _____

P waves _____

PR interval _____ QRS interval _____

Interpretation _____

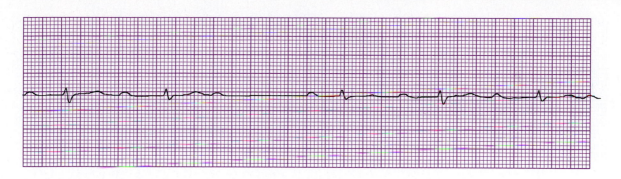

120. QRS complexes _____ Regularity _____

Heart rate _____

P waves _____

PR interval _____ QRS interval _____

Interpretation _____

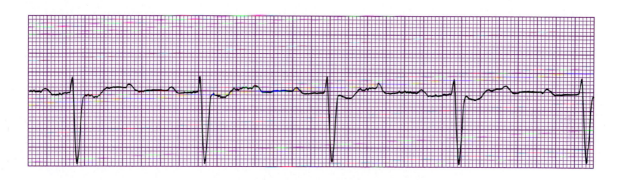

121. QRS complexes _____ Regularity _____

Heart rate _____

P waves _____

PR interval _____ QRS interval _____

Interpretation _____

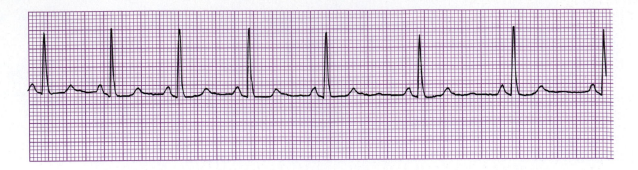

122. QRS complexes _____ Regularity _____

Heart rate _____

P waves _____

PR interval _____ QRS interval _____

Interpretation _____

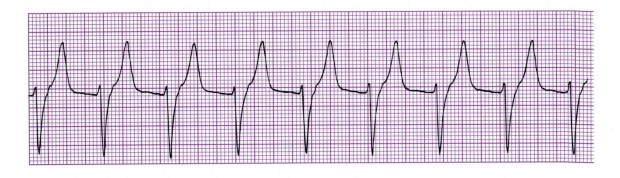

123. QRS complexes _____ Regularity _____

Heart rate _____

P waves _____

PR interval _____ QRS interval _____

Interpretation _____

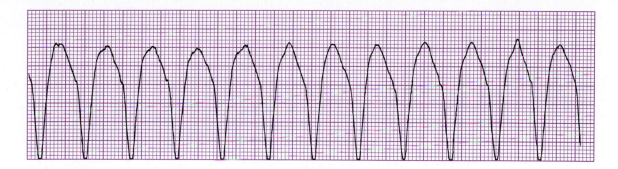

124. QRS complexes _____ Regularity _____

Heart rate _____

P waves _____

PR interval _____ QRS interval _____

Interpretation _____

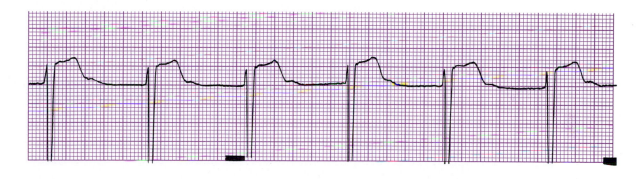

125. QRS complexes _____ Regularity _____

Heart rate _____

P waves _____

PR interval _____ QRS interval _____

Interpretation _____

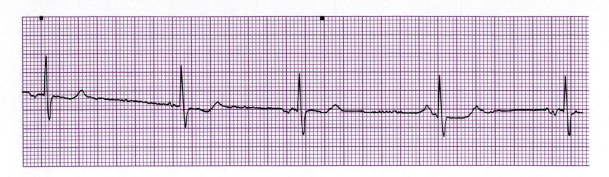

126. QRS complexes _____ Regularity _____

Heart rate _____

P waves _____

PR interval _____ QRS interval _____

Interpretation _____

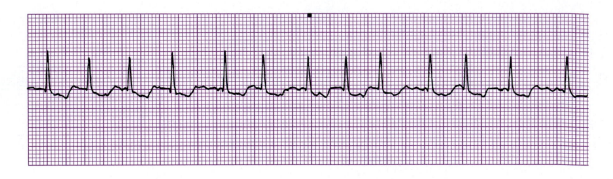

127. QRS complexes _____ Regularity _____

Heart rate _____

P waves _____

PR interval _____ QRS interval _____

Interpretation _____

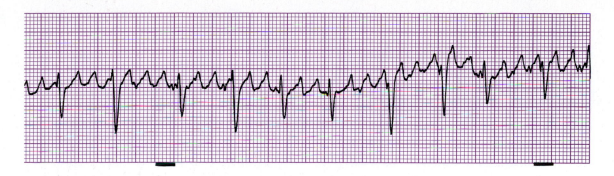

128. QRS complexes _____ Regularity _____

Heart rate _____

P waves _____

PR interval _____ QRS interval _____

Interpretation _____

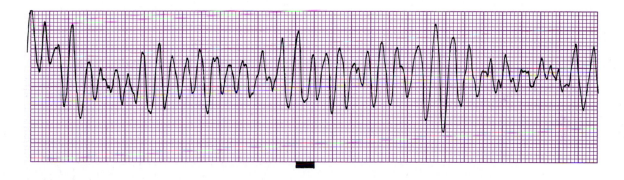

129. QRS complexes _____ Regularity _____

Heart rate _____

P waves _____

PR interval _____ QRS interval _____

Interpretation _____

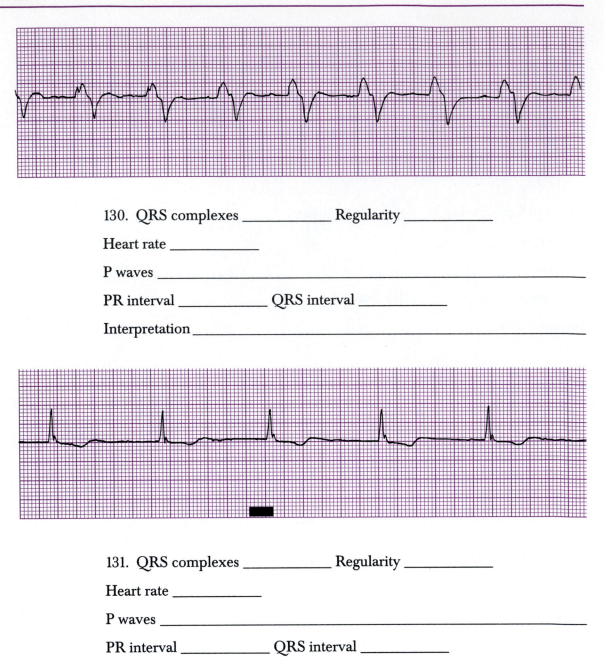

130. QRS complexes _____ Regularity _____

Heart rate _____

P waves _____

PR interval _____ QRS interval _____

Interpretation _____

131. QRS complexes _____ Regularity _____

Heart rate _____

P waves _____

PR interval _____ QRS interval _____

Interpretation _____

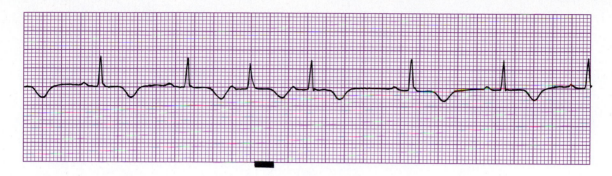

132. QRS complexes _____ Regularity _____

Heart rate _____

P waves _____

PR interval _____ QRS interval _____

Interpretation _____

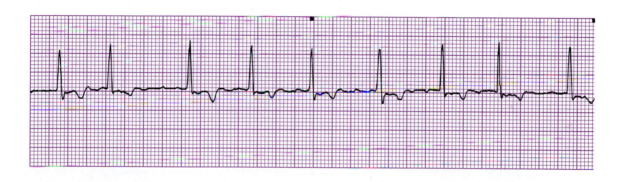

133. QRS complexes _____ Regularity _____

Heart rate _____

P waves _____

PR interval _____ QRS interval _____

Interpretation _____

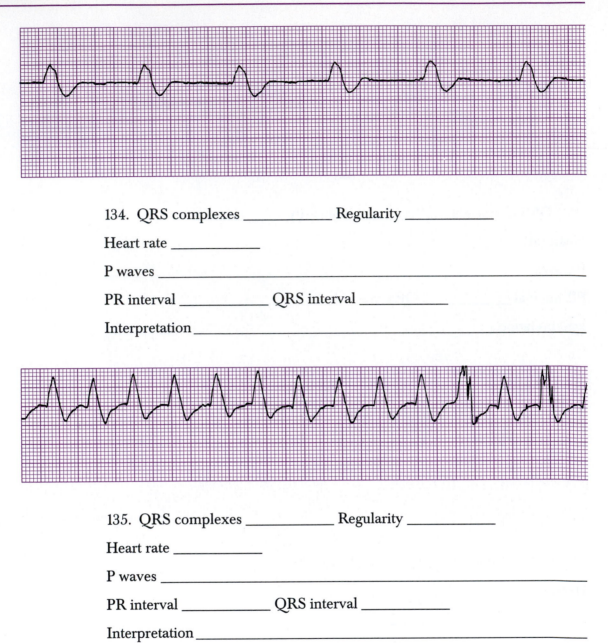

134. QRS complexes _____ Regularity _____

Heart rate _____

P waves _____

PR interval _____ QRS interval _____

Interpretation _____

135. QRS complexes _____ Regularity _____

Heart rate _____

P waves _____

PR interval _____ QRS interval _____

Interpretation _____

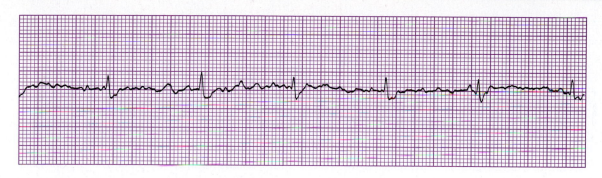

136. QRS complexes _____ Regularity _____

Heart rate _____

P waves _____

PR interval _____ QRS interval _____

Interpretation _____

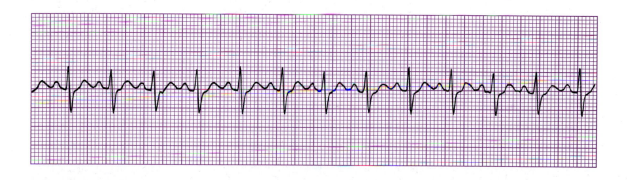

137. QRS complexes _____ Regularity _____

Heart rate _____

P waves _____

PR interval _____ QRS interval _____

Interpretation _____

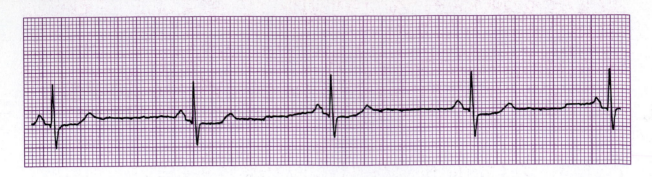

138. QRS complexes _____ Regularity _____

Heart rate _____

P waves _____

PR interval _____ QRS interval _____

Interpretation _____

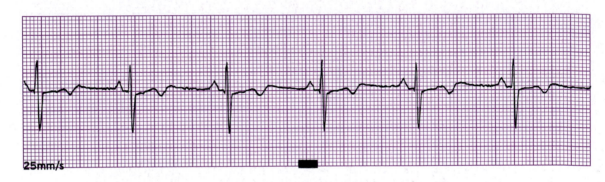

25mm/s

139. QRS complexes _____ Regularity _____

Heart rate _____

P waves _____

PR interval _____ QRS interval _____

Interpretation _____

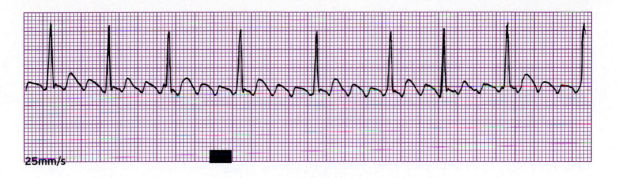

25mm/s

140. QRS complexes _____ Regularity _____

Heart rate _____

P waves _____

PR interval _____ QRS interval _____

Interpretation _____

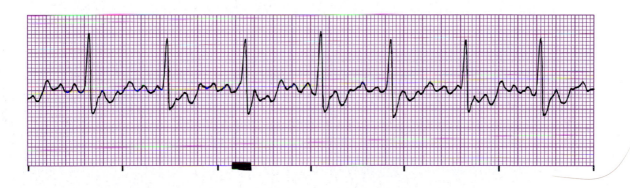

141. QRS complexes _____ Regularity _____

Heart rate _____

P waves _____

PR interval _____ QRS interval _____

Interpretation _____

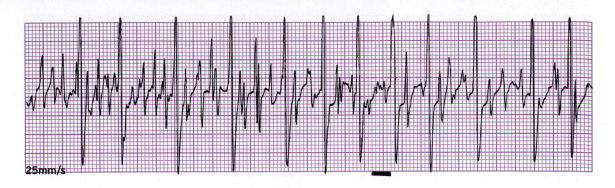

25mm/s

142. QRS complexes _____ Regularity _____

Heart rate _____

P waves _____

PR interval _____ QRS interval _____

Interpretation _____

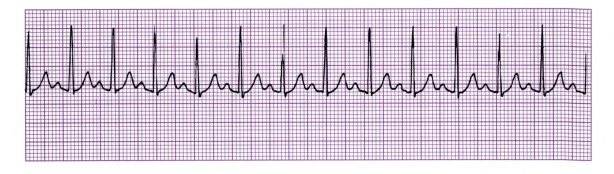

143. QRS complexes _____ Regularity _____

Heart rate _____

P waves _____

PR interval _____ QRS interval _____

Interpretation _____

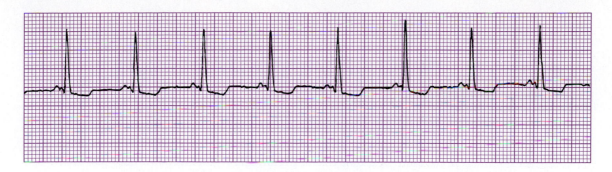

144. QRS complexes _____ Regularity _____

Heart rate _____

P waves _____

PR interval _____ QRS interval _____

Interpretation _____

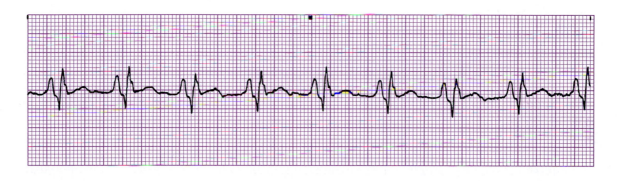

145. QRS complexes _____ Regularity _____

Heart rate _____

P waves _____

PR interval _____ QRS interval _____

Interpretation _____

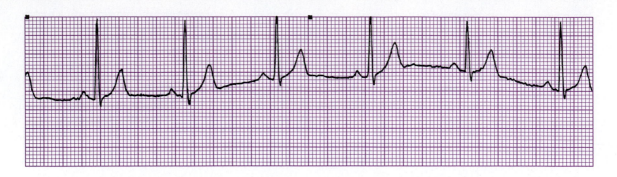

146. QRS complexes _____ Regularity _____

Heart rate _____

P waves _____

PR interval _____ QRS interval _____

Interpretation _____

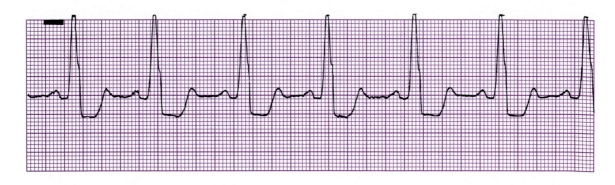

147. QRS complexes _____ Regularity _____

Heart rate _____

P waves _____

PR interval _____ QRS interval _____

Interpretation _____

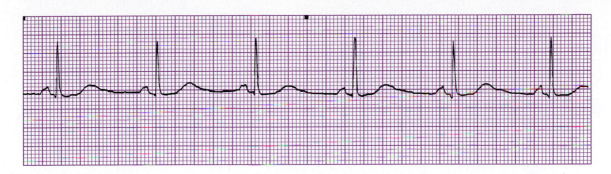

148. QRS complexes _____ Regularity _____

Heart rate _____

P waves _____

PR interval _____ QRS interval _____

Interpretation _____

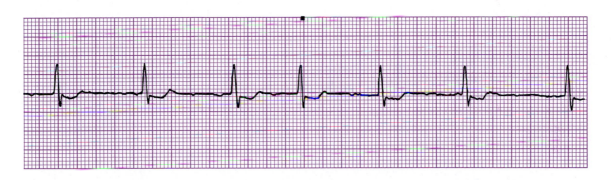

149. QRS complexes _____ Regularity _____

Heart rate _____

P waves _____

PR interval _____ QRS interval _____

Interpretation _____

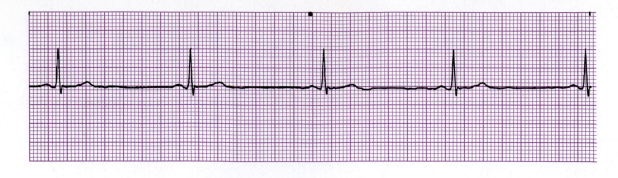

150. QRS complexes _____ Regularity _____

Heart rate _____

P waves _____

PR interval _____ QRS interval _____

Interpretation _____

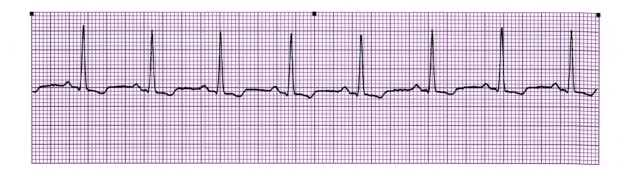

151. QRS complexes _____ Regularity _____

Heart rate _____

P waves _____

PR interval _____ QRS interval _____

Interpretation _____

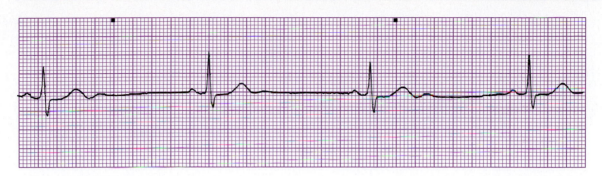

152. QRS complexes _____ Regularity _____

Heart rate _____

P waves _____

PR interval _____ QRS interval _____

Interpretation _____

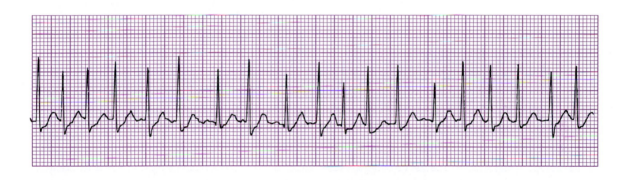

153. QRS complexes _____ Regularity _____

Heart rate _____

P waves _____

PR interval _____ QRS interval _____

Interpretation _____

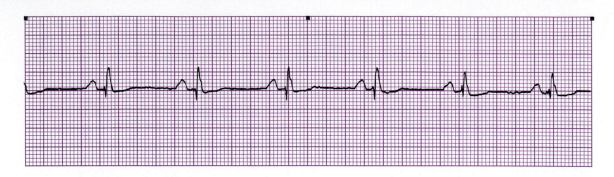

154. QRS complexes _____ Regularity _____

Heart rate _____

P waves _____

PR interval _____ QRS interval _____

Interpretation _____

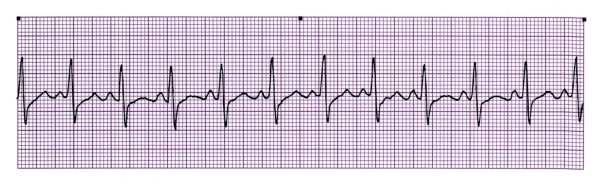

155. QRS complexes _____ Regularity _____

Heart rate _____

P waves _____

PR interval _____ QRS interval _____

Interpretation _____

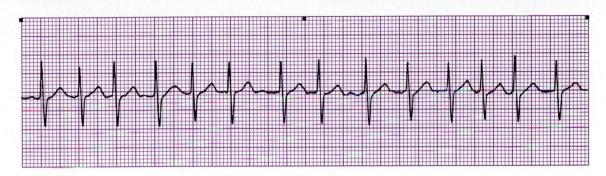

156. QRS complexes _____ Regularity _____

Heart rate _____

P waves _____

PR interval _____ QRS interval _____

Interpretation _____

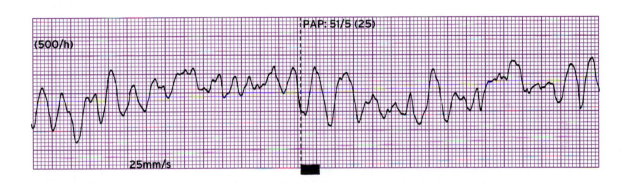

157. QRS complexes _____ Regularity _____

Heart rate _____

P waves _____

PR interval _____ QRS interval _____

Interpretation _____

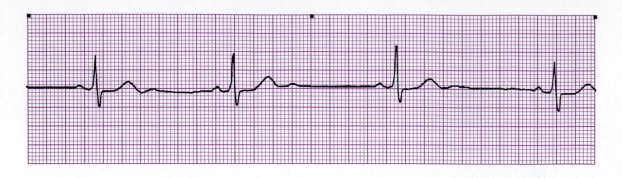

158. QRS complexes _____ Regularity _____

Heart rate _____

P waves _____

PR interval _____ QRS interval _____

Interpretation _____

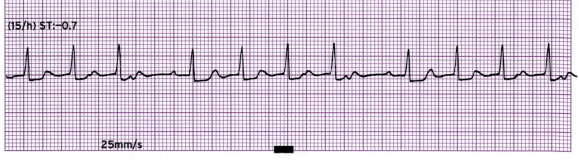

159. QRS complexes _____ Regularity _____

Heart rate _____

P waves _____

PR interval _____ QRS interval _____

Interpretation _____

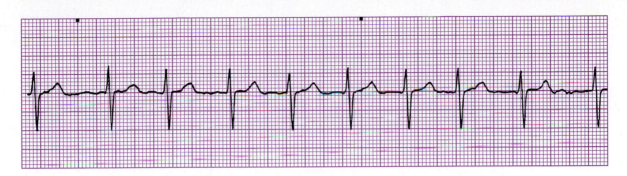

160. QRS complexes _____ Regularity _____

Heart rate _____

P waves _____

PR interval _____ QRS interval _____

Interpretation _____

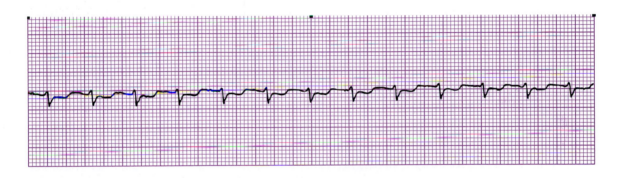

161. QRS complexes _____ Regularity _____

Heart rate _____

P waves _____

PR interval _____ QRS interval _____

Interpretation _____

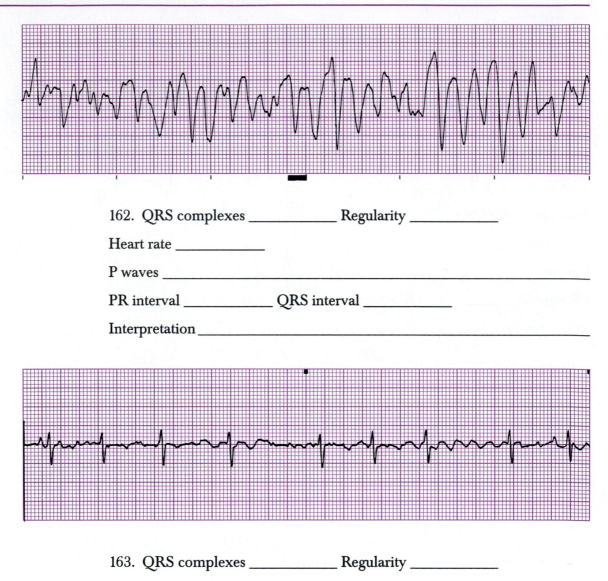

162. QRS complexes _____ Regularity _____

Heart rate _____

P waves _____

PR interval _____ QRS interval _____

Interpretation _____

163. QRS complexes _____ Regularity _____

Heart rate _____

P waves _____

PR interval _____ QRS interval _____

Interpretation _____

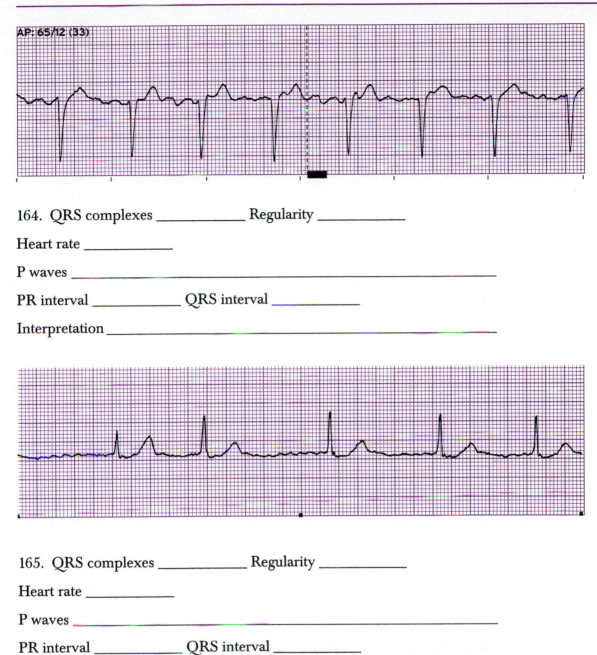

AP: 65/12 (33)

164. QRS complexes _____ Regularity _____

Heart rate _____

P waves _____

PR interval _____ QRS interval _____

Interpretation _____

165. QRS complexes _____ Regularity _____

Heart rate _____

P waves _____

PR interval _____ QRS interval _____

Interpretation _____

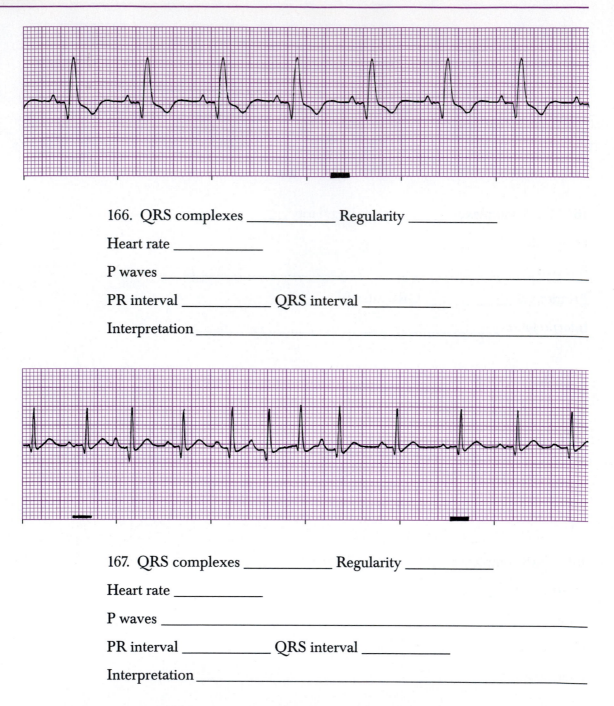

166. QRS complexes _____ Regularity _____

Heart rate _____

P waves _____

PR interval _____ QRS interval _____

Interpretation _____

167. QRS complexes _____ Regularity _____

Heart rate _____

P waves _____

PR interval _____ QRS interval _____

Interpretation _____

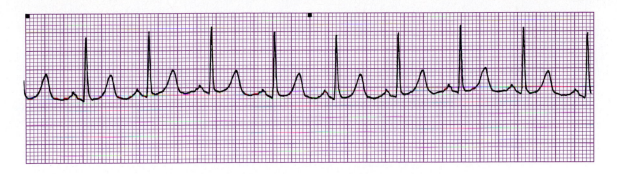

168. QRS complexes _____ Regularity _____

Heart rate _____

P waves _____

PR interval _____ QRS interval _____

Interpretation _____

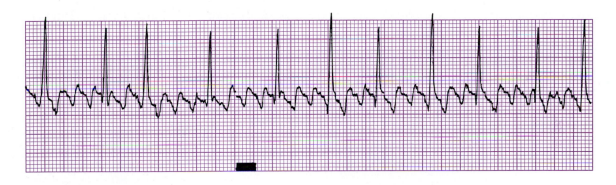

169. QRS complexes _____ Regularity _____

Heart rate _____

P waves _____

PR interval _____ QRS interval _____

Interpretation _____

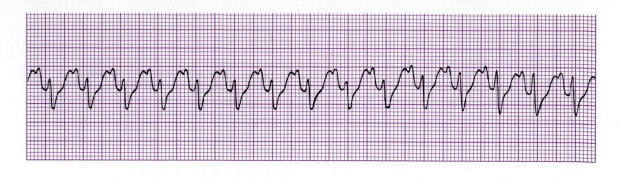

170. QRS complexes _____ Regularity _____

Heart rate _____

P waves _____

PR interval _____ QRS interval _____

Interpretation _____

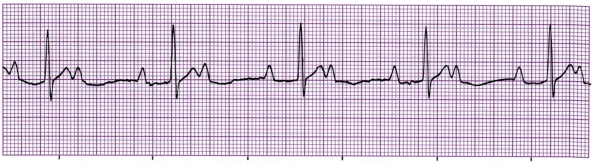

171. QRS complexes _____ Regularity _____

Heart rate _____

P waves _____

PR interval _____ QRS interval _____

Interpretation _____

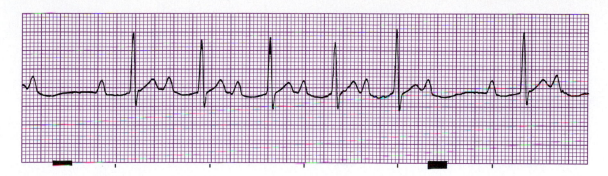

172. QRS complexes _____ Regularity _____

Heart rate _____

P waves _____

PR interval _____ QRS interval _____

Interpretation _____

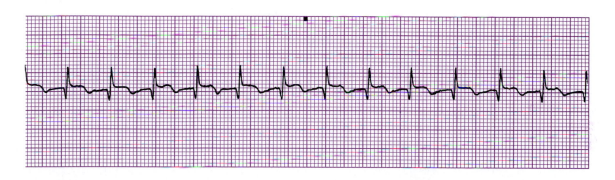

173. QRS complexes _____ Regularity _____

Heart rate _____

P waves _____

PR interval _____ QRS interval _____

Interpretation _____

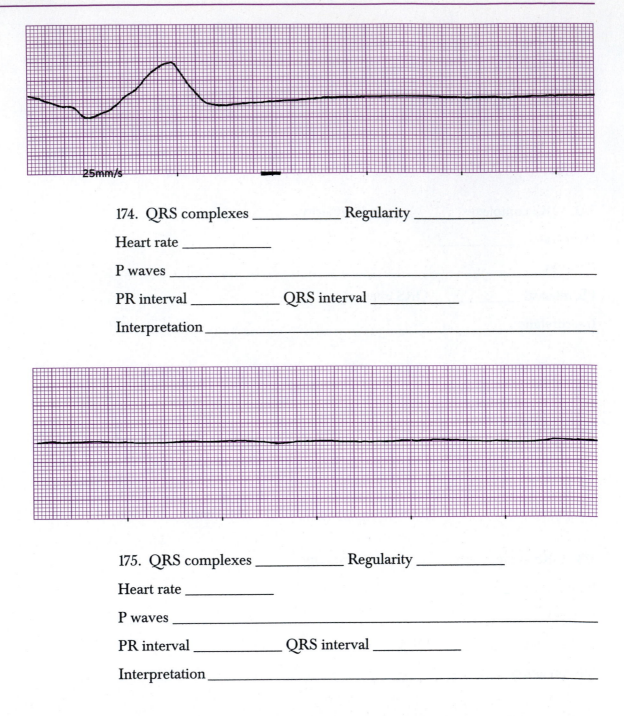

25mm/s

174. QRS complexes _____ Regularity _____

Heart rate _____

P waves _____

PR interval _____ QRS interval _____

Interpretation _____

175. QRS complexes _____ Regularity _____

Heart rate _____

P waves _____

PR interval _____ QRS interval _____

Interpretation _____

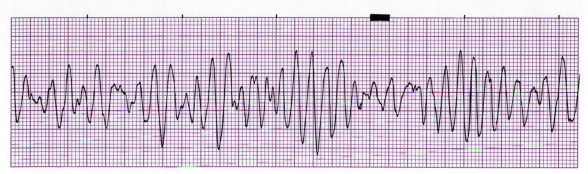

176. QRS complexes _____ Regularity _____

Heart rate _____

P waves _____

PR interval _____ QRS interval _____

Interpretation _____

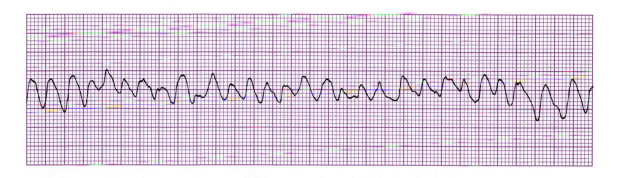

177. QRS complexes _____ Regularity _____

Heart rate _____

P waves _____

PR interval _____ QRS interval _____

Interpretation _____

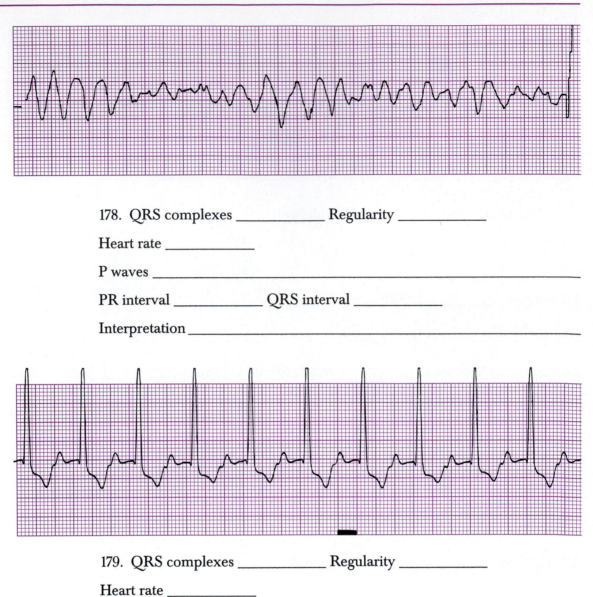

178. QRS complexes _____ Regularity _____

Heart rate _____

P waves _____

PR interval _____ QRS interval _____

Interpretation _____

179. QRS complexes _____ Regularity _____

Heart rate _____

P waves _____

PR interval _____ QRS interval _____

Interpretation _____

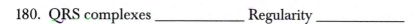

180. QRS complexes _____ Regularity _____

Heart rate _____

P waves _____

PR interval _____ QRS interval _____

Interpretation _____

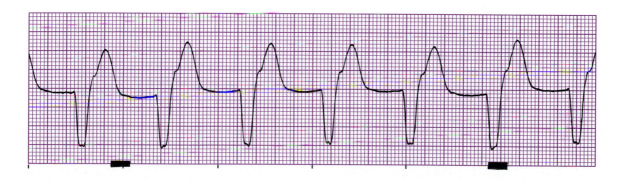

181. QRS complexes _____ Regularity _____

Heart rate _____

P waves _____

PR interval _____ QRS interval _____

Interpretation _____

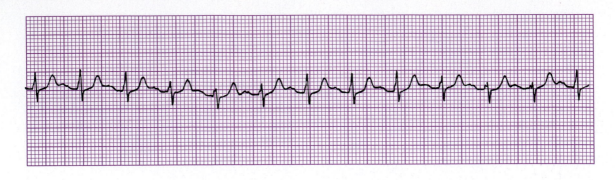

182. QRS complexes _____ Regularity _____

Heart rate _____

P waves _____

PR interval _____ QRS interval _____

Interpretation _____

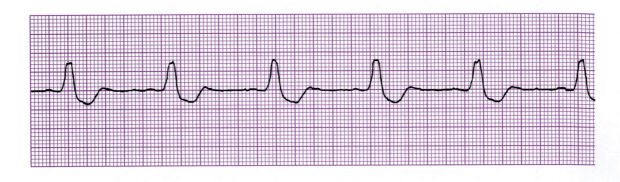

183. QRS complexes _____ Regularity _____

Heart rate _____

P waves _____

PR interval _____ QRS interval _____

Interpretation _____

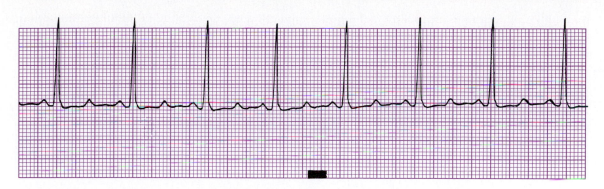

184. QRS complexes _____ Regularity _____

Heart rate _____

P waves _____

PR interval _____ QRS interval _____

Interpretation _____

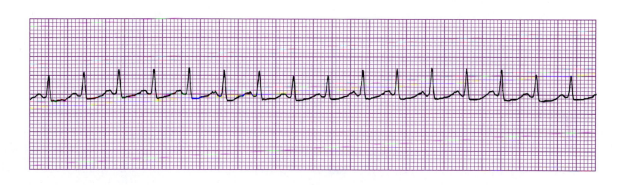

185. QRS complexes _____ Regularity _____

Heart rate _____

P waves _____

PR interval _____ QRS interval _____

Interpretation _____

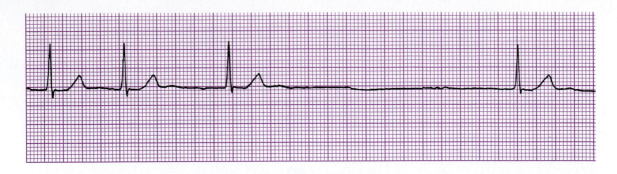

186. QRS complexes _____ Regularity _____

Heart rate _____

P waves _____

PR interval _____ QRS interval _____

Interpretation _____

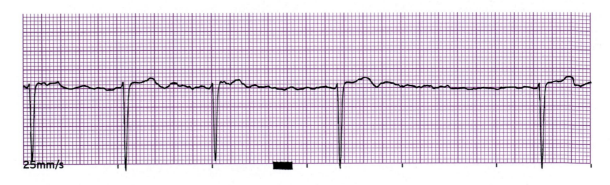

25mm/s

187. QRS complexes _____ Regularity _____

Heart rate _____

P waves _____

PR interval _____ QRS interval _____

Interpretation _____

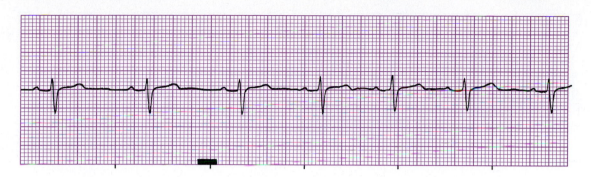

188. QRS complexes _____ Regularity _____

Heart rate _____

P waves _____

PR interval _____ QRS interval _____

Interpretation _____

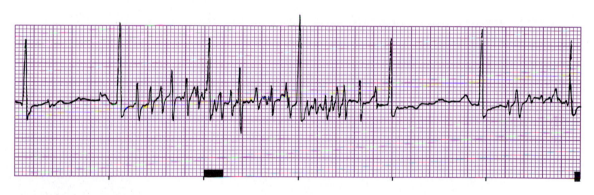

189. QRS complexes _____ Regularity _____

Heart rate _____

P waves _____

PR interval _____ QRS interval _____

Interpretation _____

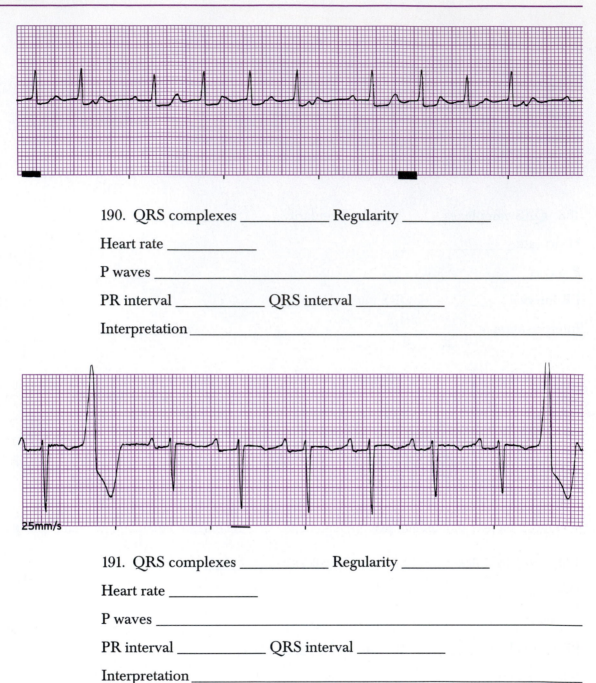

190. QRS complexes _____ Regularity _____

Heart rate _____

P waves _____

PR interval _____ QRS interval _____

Interpretation _____

191. QRS complexes _____ Regularity _____

Heart rate _____

P waves _____

PR interval _____ QRS interval _____

Interpretation _____

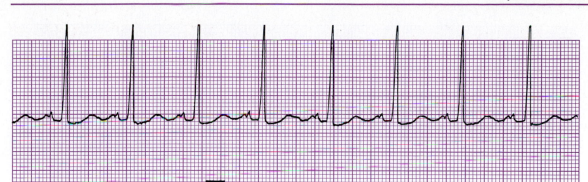

192. QRS complexes _____ Regularity _____

Heart rate _____

P waves _____

PR interval _____ QRS interval _____

Interpretation _____

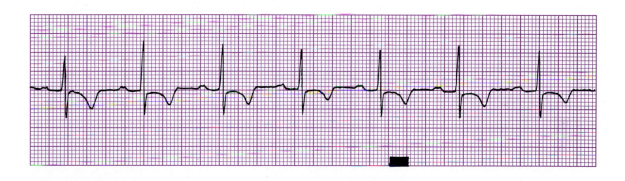

193. QRS complexes _____ Regularity _____

Heart rate _____

P waves _____

PR interval _____ QRS interval _____

Interpretation _____

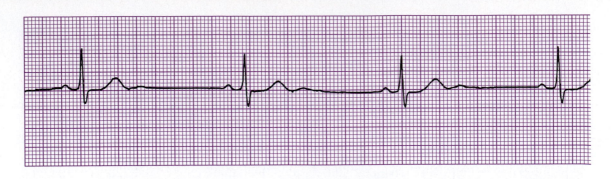

194. QRS complexes _____ Regularity _____

Heart rate _____

P waves _____

PR interval _____ QRS interval _____

Interpretation _____

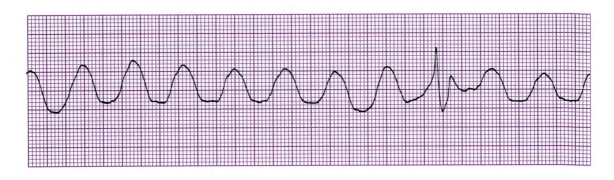

195. QRS complexes _____ Regularity _____

Heart rate _____

P waves _____

PR interval _____ QRS interval _____

Interpretation _____

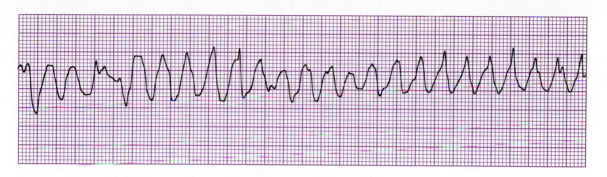

196. QRS complexes _____ Regularity _____

Heart rate _____

P waves _____

PR interval _____ QRS interval _____

Interpretation _____

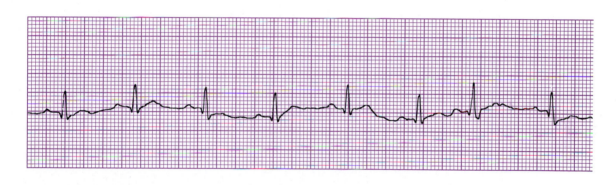

197. QRS complexes _____ Regularity _____

Heart rate _____

P waves _____

PR interval _____ QRS interval _____

Interpretation _____

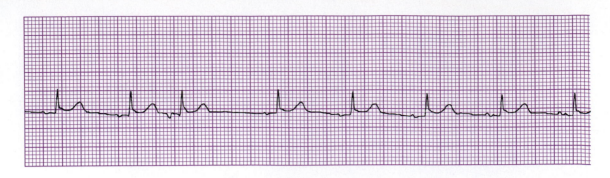

198. QRS complexes _____ Regularity _____

Heart rate _____

P waves _____

PR interval _____ QRS interval _____

Interpretation _____

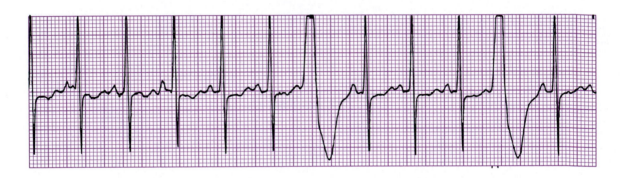

199. QRS complexes _____ Regularity _____

Heart rate _____

P waves _____

PR interval _____ QRS interval _____

Interpretation _____

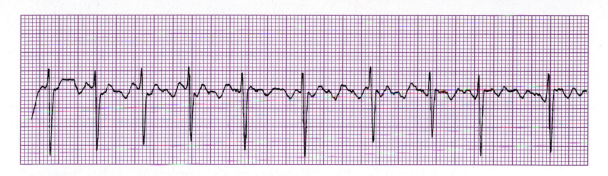

200. QRS complexes _____ Regularity _____

Heart rate _____

P waves _____

PR interval _____ QRS interval _____

Interpretation _____

Answers to Practice Rhythm Strips

1. **QRS complexes:** present, all shaped the same. **Regularity:** regular.
   Heart rate: 68. **P waves:** matching, upright, one preceding each QRS;
   P-P interval regular. **PR interval:** 0.42. **QRS interval:** 0.16. **Interpretation:** sinus rhythm with first-degree AV block and a bundle branch
   block (BBB).

2. **QRS complexes:** present, all shaped the same. **Regularity:** regular.
   Heart rate: 37. **P waves:** none seen. **PR interval:** not applicable. **QRS
   interval:** 0.12 **Interpretation:** junctional bradycardia with BBB.

3. **QRS complexes:** present, all shaped the same. **Regularity:** regular.
   Heart rate: 71. **P waves:** matching, upright, one preceding each QRS;
   P-P interval regular. **PR interval:** 0.24. **QRS interval:** 0.12. **Interpretation:** sinus rhythm with first-degree AV block and BBB.

4. **QRS complexes:** present, all shaped the same. **Regularity:** regular.
   Heart rate: 125. **P waves:** an occasional dissociated P can be seen. **PR
   interval:** cannot measure. **QRS interval:** 0.22. **Interpretation:** ventricular tachycardia.

5. **QRS complexes:** present, all shaped the same. **Regularity:** irregular.
   Heart rate: 65 to 94, with a mean rate of 80. **P waves:** none present;
   wavy, undulating baseline is present. **PR interval:** not applicable.
   QRS interval: 0.06. **Interpretation:** atrial fibrillation.

6. **QRS complexes:** Present, all shaped the same, low voltage. **Regularity:** regular. **Heart rate:** 125. **P waves:** matching, upright, one preceding each QRS, low voltage; P-P interval regular. **PR interval:** 0.16.
   QRS interval: 0.06. **Interpretation:** sinus tachycardia.

7. **QRS complexes:** present, all shaped the same. **Regularity:** regular. **Heart rate:** 32. **P waves:** upright, matching, some nonconducted; P-P interval regular; atrial rate 125. **PR interval:** varies. **QRS interval:** 0.13. **Interpretation:** sinus tachycardia with third-degree AV block and an idioventricular rhythm.

8. **QRS complexes:** present, all shaped the same. **Regularity:** regular. **Heart rate:** 150. **P waves:** none present; regular sawtooth-shaped waves between QRS complexes present instead, two to each QRS; atrial rate about 300. **PR interval:** not applicable. **QRS interval:** 0.06. **Interpretation:** atrial flutter with 2:1 conduction. Were you thinking it was something else? Look at the tail end of the QRS complex. See how it looks rounded at the bottom? That rounded part looks a lot like the other rounded wave that follows it, doesn't it? Those are both flutter waves. You'll notice these flutter waves march out—they're all the same distance from each other. Always be very suspicious when the heart rate is 150—it may be atrial flutter with 2:1 conduction.

9. **QRS complexes:** present, all shaped the same. **Regularity:** regular but interrupted (by two pauses). **Heart rate:** 44 to 75, with a mean rate of 60. **P waves:** upright, one preceding each QRS; shape varies slightly, but not enough to be significant. Don't get too hyper about the P wave shapes. Slight variability can be caused by fine baseline artifact. Different P wave shapes will be much more obvious. If you have to agonize over whether the P waves are shaped the same or are different, they're probably not different enough to be significant in terms of rhythm interpretation. **PR interval:** 0.20 to 0.22. **QRS interval:** 0.08. **Interpretation:** sinus rhythm with two sinus pauses. Why is this not a sinus arrhythmia? Sinus arrhythmia is cyclic, with slow periods, then faster periods. And it's irregular. Here the rhythm is regular, with an R-R interval of about 20 small blocks, except during the pauses. Sinus arrhythmia would be more irregular across the strip. Pay close attention to the regularity and it should lead the way.

10. **QRS complexes:** present, all shaped the same. Say what? They look different, you say? Hold on—the explanation is coming soon. **Regularity:** irregular. **Heart rate:** 100 to 150, with a mean rate of 120. **P waves:** upright and matching on the first four beats, then changes to flutter waves after that. **PR interval:** 0.16 on the first four beats, not applicable after that. **QRS interval:** 0.08. **Interpretation:** sinus tachycardia converting after four beats to atrial flutter with variable conduction. The QRS complexes in atrial flutter here are distorted by the flutter waves. That's why they look different.

11. **QRS complexes:** present, all shaped the same. **Regularity:** regular. **Heart rate:** 44. **P waves:** upright, matching, some nonconducted; P-P interval regular; atrial rate 150. **PR interval:** varies. **QRS interval:** 0.14. **Interpretation:** sinus tachycardia with third-degree AV block and an accelerated idioventricular rhythm.

12. **QRS complexes:** present, all shaped the same. **Regularity:** regular. **Heart rate:** 125. **P waves:** upright, matching, one preceding each QRS; P-P interval regular. **PR interval:** 0.16. **QRS interval:** 0.06. **Interpretation:** sinus tachycardia.

13. **QRS complexes:** present, all but three shaped the same. Three beats are wide and bizarre in shape. **Regularity:** regular but interrupted (by premature beats). **Heart rate:** 125. **P waves:** upright and matching on the narrow beats, absent on the wide beats. **PR interval:** 0.12. **QRS interval:** 0.08 on the narrow beats, 0.16 on the wide beats. **Interpretation:** sinus tachycardia with unifocal PVCs in quadrigeminy (every fourth beat is a PVC).

14. **QRS complexes:** present, all shaped the same. **Regularity:** regular. **Heart rate:** 137. **P waves:** none seen. **PR interval:** not applicable. **QRS interval:** 0.10. **Interpretation:** SVT.

15. **QRS complex:** present, all shaped the same, very low voltage. **Regularity:** regular. **Heart rate:** about 135. **P waves:** not discernible; they may be present, but can't tell for sure. **PR interval:** cannot measure. **QRS interval:** 0.08. **Interpretation:** junctional tachycardia or SVT. Since there are no P waves, it's safer to call this SVT, as the real origin of this rhythm is not clear.

16. **QRS complex:** present, all shaped the same. **Regularity:** irregular. **Heart rate:** 56 to 71, with a mean rate of 70. **P waves:** upright, matching, one preceding each QRS; P-P interval irregular. **PR interval:** 0.12. **QRS interval:** 0.10. **Interpretation:** sinus arrhythmia. Note the longest R-R interval is between the last two QRS complexes on the strip, ending with the barely–there QRS at the very end. That R-R interval is 27 small blocks. The shortest R-R is between the third and fourth QRS complexes. That R-R is 21 small blocks. Since the rhythm is irregular, the longest R-R exceeds the shortest by four or more small blocks and this is definitely sinus in origin, it's a sinus arrhythmia. If you thought there was a sinus pause here, remember that sinus pause usually interrupts an otherwise regular rhythm. This rhythm is irregular.

17. **QRS complexes:** present, all shaped the same. **Regularity:** slightly irregular. R-R intervals vary from 22 to 25 small blocks. **Heart rate:** 60 to 68, with a mean rate of 60. **P waves:** upright, matching, one preceding each QRS. **PR interval:** 0.12. **QRS interval:** 0.10. **Interpretation:** sinus rhythm versus sinus arrhythmia. This one is a bit odd. It's really not irregular enough to call it a sinus arrhythmia, since the longest R-R interval does not exceed the shortest by four or more small blocks. On the other hand, it's a bit irregular for the typical sinus rhythm. Since we're in a gray area here, it's OK to call it one versus the other. It would be nice to have a longer rhythm strip to evaluate. If, on the longer strip, the rhythm is an obvious sinus rhythm or an obvious sinus arrhythmia, then this little stretch of the total rhythm is probably also that same rhythm.

18. **QRS complexes:** present, all shaped the same. **Regularity:** regular. **Heart rate:** 75. **P waves:** none seen. **PR interval:** not applicable. **QRS interval:** around 0.20 to 0.28. This is a guesstimate, since it's hard to tell where the QRS ends and the ST segment begins. **Interpretation:** accelerated idioventricular rhythm.

19. **QRS complexes:** present, all shaped the same. **Regularity:** regular. **Heart rate:** 167. **P waves:** occasionally seen hidden in the T waves. Note the T waves between the first and second and eleventh and twelfth QRS complexes. Those T waves reveal the hidden P waves. **PR interval:** cannot measure, as cannot see the beginning of the P wave. **QRS interval:** 0.08. **Interpretation:** atrial tachycardia or SVT. It's probably more correct to call it atrial tachycardia, because the P waves are evident in places, but it's acceptable to say SVT.

20. **QRS complexes:** present, all shaped the same. **Regularity:** regular but interrupted (by premature beats). Remember it's normal to have a short pause following each premature beat. That's why this is not an irregular rhythm. **Heart rate:** about 85. Where did that heart rate come from? The first two beats on the strip are sinus beats with a rate of 85. From then on, every other beat is a PAC, so the heart rate cannot be determined accurately there. **P waves:** upright, two different shapes; almost every other P wave is premature and of a different shape. **PR interval:** 0.12 on the sinus beats, 0.16 on the premature beats. **QRS interval:** 0.08. **Interpretation:** sinus rhythm with frequent PACs, most of it in bigeminy.

21. **QRS complexes:** none present; wavy, static-looking baseline present instead. **Regularity:** not applicable. **Heart rate:** cannot measure, has no QRS complexes. **P waves:** none. **PR interval:** not applicable. **QRS interval:** not applicable. **Interpretation:** ventricular fibrillation.

22. **QRS complexes:** present, two different shapes. Some QRS complexes are narrow, others are wide. **Regularity:** regular but interrupted (by premature beats). **Heart rate:** 94. **P waves:** upright and matching preceding the narrow QRS complexes, and seen in the T wave following the premature beats. **PR interval:** 0.18 on the narrow beats; not calculated on the premature beats, as the P is retrograde. **QRS interval:** 0.08 on the narrow beats, 0.14 on the wide beats. **Interpretation:** sinus rhythm with unifocal PVCs in trigeminy.

23. **QRS complexes:** present, all shaped the same. **Regularity:** irregular. **Heart rate:** 48 to 81, with a mean rate of 60. **P waves:** upright, matching, some nonconducted; P-P interval regular. **PR interval:** varies. **QRS interval:** 0.11. **Interpretation:** sinus rhythm with type I second-degree AV block (Wenckebach). Note how the PR interval gradually prolongs, then a beat is dropped.

24. **QRS complexes:** present, all shaped the same. **Regularity:** regular. **Heart rate:** 79. **P waves:** none present; regular sawtooth-shaped waves present instead. **PR interval:** not applicable. **QRS interval:** 0.08. **Interpretation:** atrial flutter with 4:1 conduction.

25. **QRS complexes:** present, all but one having the same shape. One is very wide compared to the others. **Regularity:** regular but interrupted (by a premature beat). **Heart rate:** 107. **P waves:** upright and matching on the narrow beats, absent on the wide beat. **PR interval:** 0.12 to 0.14. **QRS interval:** 0.08 on the narrow beats, 0.16 on the wide beat. **Interpretation:** sinus tachycardia with one PVC.

26. **QRS complexes:** none. **Regularity:** not applicable, as there are no QRS complexes. **Heart rate:** zero. **P waves:** none. **PR interval:** not applicable. **QRS interval:** not applicable. **Interpretation:** asystole.

27. **QRS complexes:** present, all shaped the same. **Regularity:** regular. **Heart rate:** 50. **P waves:** upright, matching, P-P interval regular; one P wave is hidden inside the last QRS; atrial rate 88. **PR interval:** varies. **QRS interval:** 0.14. **Interpretation:** sinus rhythm with third-degree AV block and an accelerated idioventricular rhythm.

28. **QRS complexes:** present, all shaped the same. **Regularity:** regular. **Heart rate:** 79. **P waves:** matching, upright, one preceding each QRS; P-P interval regular. **PR interval:** 0.28. **QRS interval:** 0.08. **Interpretation:** sinus rhythm with first-degree AV block.

29. **QRS complexes:** present, all shaped the same. **Regularity:** regular. **Heart rate:** 68. **P waves:** none present; regular sawtooth-shaped waves present instead. **PR interval:** not applicable. **QRS interval:** about 0.10. The end of the QRS is distorted by a flutter wave, making the QRS look artificially wide. **Interpretation:** atrial flutter with 4:1 conduction. Two of the flutter waves are hidden inside the QRS and T wave. So how can we tell the flutter waves are even there if we can't see them? We can definitely see two obvious flutter waves between the QRS complexes. Since we know that flutter waves are regular, we simply note the distance between the two flutter waves we see together, then march out where the rest of them should be.

30. **QRS complexes:** present, most shaped the same. An occasional QRS is missing the notch on the downstroke. **Regularity:** regular. **Heart rate:** 187. **P waves:** an occasional dissociated P wave is seen. **PR interval:** not applicable. **QRS interval:** 0.14. **Interpretation:** ventricular tachycardia.

31. **QRS complexes:** present, all shaped the same. **Regularity:** irregular. **Heart rate:** 48 to 60, with a mean rate of 60. **P waves:** all upright, but there are at least three different shapes; P-P interval irregular. **PR interval:** 0.24 to 0.28. **QRS interval:** 0.10. **Interpretation:** wandering atrial pacemaker.

32. **QRS complexes:** present, all shaped the same. **Regularity:** regular but interrupted (by a prematurely arriving beat). **Heart rate:** 71. **P waves:** none present; regular sawtooth-shaped waves present instead. **PR interval:** not applicable. **QRS interval:** 0.10. **Interpretation:** atrial flutter with 2:1 and 4:1 conduction. The one episode of the 2:1 conduction is responsible for the interruption of this otherwise regular 4:1 conduction. This beat that comes in early because of the conduction

ratio change is not per se a premature beat in the way that PVCs are, but nevertheless it does arrive earlier than expected, given the surrounding R-R intervals. For this reason the regularity is called *regular but interrupted* rather than irregular. All R-R intervals except this short one are about the same.

33. **QRS complexes:** present, all shaped the same. **Regularity:** regular but interrupted (by pauses). **Heart rate:** 62 to 107, with a mean rate of 90. **P waves:** upright, matching, some nonconducted, others hidden inside T waves; P-P interval regular; atrial rate about 115. **PR interval:** varies. **QRS interval:** 0.08. **Interpretation:** sinus tachycardia with type I second-degree AV block (Wenckebach).

34. **QRS complexes:** present, all shaped the same. **Regularity:** regular but interrupted (by premature beats). **Heart rate:** 79. **P waves:** biphasic except for the two that are inside the T wave. There are two different shapes of P waves. P-P interval varies. **PR interval:** 0.18 on the normal beats, approximately 0.22 on the premature beats. **QRS interval:** 0.08. **Interpretation:** sinus rhythm with two PACs.

35. **QRS complexes:** present, all shaped the same, one shorter than the rest. **Regularity:** regular but interrupted (by a pause). **Heart rate:** 19 to 54, with a mean rate of 50. **P waves:** upright, matching, none present on the beat ending the pause; P-P interval irregular. **PR interval:** 0.16 to 0.18. **QRS interval:** 0.09. **Interpretation:** sinus bradycardia with a 3.28-second sinus arrest ending with a junctional escape beat. Whenever there is a pause, the length of it must be recorded. If there is a sinus arrest, the beat ending the pause will be an escape beat from a lower pacemaker. Which pacemaker takes over should also be recorded.

36. **QRS complexes:** present, all shaped the same. **Regularity:** regular; the R-R intervals vary only by two small blocks. **Heart rate:** about 50. **P waves:** upright and matching, one preceding each QRS; P-P interval regular. **PR interval:** 0.20. **QRS interval:** 0.08. **Interpretation:** sinus bradycardia. A PR interval of 0.20 is still normal. There's no first-degree AV block.

37. **QRS complexes:** present, all shaped the same. **Regularity:** regular. **Heart rate:** 61. **P waves:** inverted inside ST segment following the QRS complexes. **PR interval:** not applicable. **QRS interval:** 0.12. **Interpretation:** accelerated junctional rhythm with a BBB.

38. **QRS complexes:** present, all shaped the same. **Regularity:** regular. **Heart rate:** 88. **P waves:** upright and matching, one preceding each QRS; P-P interval regular. **PR interval:** 0.24. **QRS interval:** 0.10. **Interpretation:** sinus rhythm with first-degree AV block.

39. **QRS complexes:** present, all shaped the same. **Regularity:** regular. The R-R intervals vary by only two small blocks. **Heart rate:** about 36. **P waves:** upright and matching, one preceding each QRS; P-P interval regular. **PR interval:** 0.16. **QRS interval:** 0.12. **Interpretation:** sinus bradycardia with a BBB; there's a prominent U wave following the T waves.

40. **QRS complexes:** present, all shaped the same. **Regularity:** regular. **Heart rate:** 60. **P waves:** upright, notched, and matching, one preceding each QRS; P-P interval regular. **PR interval:** 0.16. **QRS interval:** 0.08. **Interpretation:** sinus rhythm.

41. **QRS complexes:** present, all shaped the same. **Regularity:** irregular. The R-R intervals vary from 11 to 15 small blocks. **Heart rate:** 100 to 137, with a mean rate of 120. **P waves:** none seen. **PR interval:** not applicable. **QRS interval:** 0.20. **Interpretation:** ventricular tachycardia. Remember v-tach is usually regular, but can be irregular at times.

42. **QRS complexes:** present, all shaped the same. **Regularity:** irregular. **Heart rate:** 39 to 88, with a mean rate of 60. **P waves:** none present; wavy, undulating baseline present instead. **PR interval:** not applicable. **QRS interval:** 0.06. **Interpretation:** atrial fibrillation.

43. **QRS complexes:** present, all shaped the same. **Regularity:** regular. **Heart rate:** 115. **P waves:** upright and matching, one preceding each QRS; P-P interval regular. **PR interval:** 0.12. **QRS interval:** 0.10. **Interpretation:** sinus tachycardia.

44. **QRS complexes:** present, all shaped the same. **Regularity:** irregular. **Heart rate:** 83 to 167, with a mean rate of 140. **P waves:** none present; wavy, undulating baseline present instead. **PR interval:** not applicable. **QRS interval:** 0.04. **Interpretation:** atrial fibrillation.

45. **QRS complexes:** present, all shaped the same. **Regularity:** regular. **Heart rate:** about 52. **P waves:** upright, matching, one preceding each QRS. **PR interval:** 0.18. **QRS interval:** 0.13. **Interpretation:** sinus bradycardia with a BBB.

46. **QRS complexes:** present, all shaped the same. **Regularity:** regular. **Heart rate:** 28. **P waves:** upright, matching, some nonconducted. P-P interval regular. Atrial rate 83. **PR interval:** 0.16. **QRS interval:** 0.06. **Interpretation:** sinus rhythm with type II second-degree AV block.

47. **QRS complexes:** present, all but one shaped the same. **Regularity:** regular. **Heart rate:** 26. **P waves:** matching, upright, some nonconducted; P-P interval regular; atrial rate 75. **PR interval:** varies. **QRS interval:** 0.04 to 0.08. **Interpretation:** sinus rhythm with third-degree AV block and a junctional bradycardia. This heart rate is extremely slow for the junction. Remember, it normally escapes at a rate of 40 to 60. This patient not only has an AV block, but also a sick AV node in terms of its pacemaking ability. Also of concern is the ventricle as a pacemaker. It normally escapes at a rate of 20 to 40. Where is it? Why didn't it kick in as the pacemaker at a faster rate than we have here? This rhythm indicates a very sick heart.

48. **QRS complexes:** present, all shaped the same. **Regularity:** regular. The R-R intervals vary by only two small blocks. **Heart rate:** 88. **P waves:** biphasic, matching, one preceding each QRS; P-P interval regular. **PR interval:** 0.12. **QRS interval:** 0.10. **Interpretation:** sinus rhythm.

49. **QRS complexes:** present, all shaped the same, though one is shorter than the other. **Regularity:** cannot assess as only two QRS complexes are present (at least three QRS complexes are needed to determine regularity). **Heart rate:** about 11. **P waves:** none present; wavy, undulating baseline present instead. **PR interval:** not applicable. **QRS interval:** 0.12. **Interpretation:** atrial fibrillation with a BBB. This could also be called atrial fib-flutter, as it does look quite fluttery in places. It is best not to call this an outright atrial flutter, though, as the waves dampen out in the middle of the strip, causing the waves to look different throughout the strip. This is a drastic representation of how slow the heart rate can go with atrial fibrillation. This is a 5.6-second pause, erroneously labeled on the strip as 5.52 seconds. This patient was lucky to be asleep and had no problems. A pause this long could easily have caused serious symptoms of low cardiac output.

50. **QRS complexes:** present, all shaped the same. **Regularity:** slightly irregular. The R-R intervals vary by three small blocks. **Heart rate:** 30 to 32. **P waves:** upright, three different shapes, one preceding each QRS; P-P interval slightly irregular. **PR interval:** 0.16 to 0.20. **QRS interval:** 0.10. **Interpretation:** wandering atrial pacemaker.

51. **QRS complexes:** present, all shaped the same. **Regularity:** regular. **Heart rate:** 94. **P waves:** matching, biphasic, two to each QRS; atrial rate 187. **PR interval:** 0.06. **QRS interval:** 0.08. **Interpretation:** atrial tachycardia with 2:1 block. One P wave is easy to see between the QRS complexes. The other is right *on* the QRS, distorting the shape of the QRS and the P a little. It wouldn't be correct to call this atrial flutter, since there is an obvious flat baseline between the P waves. You'll recall atrial flutter has no flat isoelectric line—flutter waves all zigzag one after the other.

52. **QRS complexes:** present, all shaped the same. **Regularity:** regular. **Heart rate:** 68. **P waves:** negative, one preceding each QRS; P-P interval regular. **PR interval:** 0.24. **QRS interval:** 0.20. **Interpretation:** sinus rhythm with first-degree AV block and a BBB. Though the lead is not recorded on this strip, it's probably V_1. Sinus rhythms can have a negative P wave in V_1 This is a very sick heart. The AV node is sick, as evidenced by the first-degree block, but also the bundle branches are sick, as evidenced by the width of the QRS complexes. Many cardiologists feel that to some extent a patient's ventricular function can be predicted by the QRS interval. This patient was predicted to have a very low functioning heart, and that was borne out by further studies.

53. **QRS complexes:** present, all shaped the same. **Regularity:** regular. **Heart rate:** about 103. **P waves:** upright, matching, one preceding each QRS. **PR interval:** 0.16. **QRS interval:** 0.08. **Interpretation:** sinus tachycardia.

54. **QRS complexes:** present, all shaped the same. **Regularity:** irregular. **Heart rate:** 29 to 83, with a mean rate of 50. **P waves:** none present; *very* low voltage wavy, undulating baseline present instead. **PR inter-**

val: not applicable. **QRS interval:** 0.08. **Interpretation:** atrial fibrillation. This is an example of what's sometimes called *straight-line* atrial fibrillation. There is barely a bobble of the baseline between QRS complexes. The most obvious feature that suggests atrial fibrillation is the irregularity of the rhythm. Then you notice the very fine fibrillatory waves. This patient has probably been in atrial fibrillation for years.

55. **QRS complexes:** present, all shaped the same. **Regularity:** irregular. **Heart rate:** 37 to 52, with a mean rate of 30. The strip starts in the middle of a 2.6-second pause, though, so we know the heart rate actually gets much slower at times. **P waves:** none present. Regular sawtooth-shaped waves present instead. **PR interval:** not applicable. **QRS interval:** 0.08. **Interpretation:** atrial flutter with variable conduction.

56. **QRS complexes:** present, all shaped the same. **Regularity:** regular. **Heart rate:** 94. **P waves:** upright, matching, one preceding each QRS. **PR interval:** 0.16. **QRS interval:** 0.14. **Interpretation:** sinus rhythm with BBB.

57. **QRS complexes:** present, all shaped the same. **Regularity:** irregular. **Heart rate:** about 19 to 23, with a mean rate of 30. **P waves:** none present. **PR interval:** not applicable. **QRS interval:** 0.28. **Interpretation:** dying heart (agonal rhythm). Though the heart rate is a little fast for dying heart, it must be called this because it is so irregular. Idioventricular rhythm is usually more regular.

58. **QRS complexes:** present, all shaped the same. **Regularity:** regular. R-R intervals vary by only one small block. **Heart rate:** 60. **P waves:** upright, matching, one preceding each QRS; P-P interval regular. **PR interval:** 0.12. **QRS interval:** 0.10. **Interpretation:** sinus rhythm.

59. **QRS complexes:** none present; wavy, static-looking baseline present instead. **Regularity:** not applicable. **Heart rate:** cannot measure. **P waves:** none present. **PR interval:** not applicable. **QRS interval:** not applicable. **Interpretation:** ventricular fibrillation.

60. **QRS complexes:** present, all shaped the same. **Regularity:** irregular. The R-R intervals vary by four small blocks. **Heart rate:** about 37 to 40, with a mean rate of 40. **P waves:** upright, matching, one preceding each QRS; P-P interval slightly irregular. **PR interval:** 0.13. **QRS interval:** 0.09. **Interpretation:** sinus arrhythmia.

61. **QRS complexes:** present, all but one having the same shape. One is much wider than the others. **Regularity:** regular but interrupted (by a premature beat). **Heart rate:** 115. **P waves:** upright, matching, one preceding all QRS complexes except the wide one. **PR interval:** 0.14. **QRS interval:** 0.06 on the narrow beats, 0.14 on the wide beat. **Interpretation:** sinus tachycardia with a PVC.

62. **QRS complexes:** none present. **Regularity:** cannot determine since there are no QRS complexes. **Heart rate:** zero. **P waves:** upright and matching; P-P interval irregular. **PR interval:** not applicable. **QRS interval:** not applicable. **Interpretation:** ventricular asystole.

63. **QRS complexes:** present, all shaped the same. **Regularity:** regular. **Heart rate:** about 110. **P waves:** upright, matching, one preceding each QRS; P-P interval regular. **PR interval:** 0.16. **QRS interval:** 0.08. **Interpretation:** sinus tachycardia.

64. **QRS complexes:** present, all but one shaped the same. One is wider than the others. **Regularity:** regular but interrupted (by a premature beat). **Heart rate:** 62. **P waves:** upright, matching, one preceding all QRS complexes except the premature one. There is a P wave in the premature beat's ST segment. **PR interval:** 0.20. **QRS interval:** 0.10 on the narrow beats, 0.18 on the wide beat. **Interpretation:** sinus rhythm with a PVC.

65. **QRS complexes:** present, all shaped the same. **Regularity:** irregular. **Heart rate:** 68 to 125, with a mean rate of 100. **P waves:** upright, matching, some nonconducted; P-P interval regular; atrial rate 115. **PR interval:** varies. **QRS interval:** 0.10. **Interpretation:** sinus tachycardia with type I second-degree AV block (Wenckebach).

66. **QRS complexes:** present, all shaped the same. **Regularity:** regular. **Heart rate:** 65. **P waves:** upright, matching, one preceding each QRS; P-P interval regular. **PR interval:** 0.22. **QRS interval:** 0.10. **Interpretation:** sinus rhythm with first-degree AV block.

67. **QRS complexes:** present, all shaped the same. **Regularity:** irregular. **Heart rate:** 62 to 137, with a mean rate of 110. **P waves:** none present; wavy, undulating baseline present instead. **PR interval:** not applicable. **QRS interval:** 0.08. **Interpretation:** atrial fib-flutter. Though this may indeed be a true atrial flutter, the flutter waves are not as obvious at the beginning of the strip as they are later on, so it's possible this may be a combination of fib and flutter.

68. **QRS complexes:** present, all shaped the same. **Regularity:** regular. **Heart rate:** 44. **P waves:** upright, matching, some nonconducted; P-P interval regular; atrial rate 137. **PR interval:** 0.28 to 0.40. **QRS interval:** 0.14. **Interpretation:** sinus tachycardia with third-degree AV block and accelerated idioventricular rhythm. There are three P waves to each QRS. If you counted only two, look again. Note the distance between two consecutive P waves. Now march out where the rest of them are. There's more here than first meets the eye. Always march out the P waves!

69. **QRS complexes:** present, all shaped the same. **Regularity:** regular. **Heart rate:** 71. **P waves:** upright, matching, one preceding each QRS; P-P interval regular. **PR interval:** 0.28. **QRS interval:** 0.10. **Interpretation:** sinus rhythm with first-degree AV block.

70. **QRS complexes:** present, all shaped the same. **Regularity:** irregular. **Heart rate:** 60 to 94, with a mean rate of 70. **P waves:** none present; wavy, undulating baseline present instead. **PR interval:** not applicable. **QRS interval:** 0.10. **Interpretation:** atrial fibrillation.

71. **QRS complexes:** present, all shaped the same. **Regularity:** regular. **Heart rate:** 56. **P waves:** upright, matching, one preceding each QRS;

P-P interval regular. **PR interval:** 0.14. **QRS interval:** 0.10. **Interpretation:** sinus bradycardia.

72. **QRS complexes:** present, all shaped the same. **Regularity:** regular. **Heart rate:** 79. **P waves:** none present; regular, sawtooth-shaped waves present instead. Also note the pacemaker spike preceding each QRS. **PR interval:** not applicable. **QRS interval:** 0.12. **Interpretation:** ventricular pacing with underlying atrial flutter.

73. **QRS complexes:** present, all shaped the same. **Regularity:** regular. **Heart rate:** 94. **P waves:** upright, matching, one preceding each QRS; P-P interval regular. **PR interval:** 0.12. **QRS interval:** 0.08. **Interpretation:** sinus rhythm. Baseline sway artifact is present.

74. **QRS complexes:** present, all shaped the same. **Regularity:** irregular. **Heart rate:** 75 to 107, with a mean rate of 90. **P waves:** none present; regular sawtooth-shaped waves present instead. **PR interval:** not applicable. **QRS interval:** 0.08. **Interpretation:** atrial flutter with variable conduction.

75. **QRS complexes:** present, all shaped the same. **Regularity:** irregular. **Heart rate:** 37 to 62, with a mean rate of 60. **P waves:** upright, matching, one preceding each QRS complex; P-P interval irregular. **PR interval:** 0.12. **QRS interval:** 0.10. **Interpretation:** sinus arrhythmia. If you count out the R-R intervals, you'll note they grow steadily longer throughout the strip.

76. **QRS complexes:** present, all shaped the same. **Regularity:** regular. **Heart rate:** 79. **P waves:** upright, matching, one preceding each QRS complex; P-P interval regular. **PR interval:** 0.14. **QRS interval:** 0.08. **Interpretation:** sinus rhythm.

77. **QRS complexes:** present, all shaped the same. **Regularity:** regular. **Heart rate:** 27. **P waves:** none present. **PR interval:** not applicable. **QRS interval:** 0.08. **Interpretation:** junctional bradycardia.

78. **QRS complexes:** present, all shaped the same. **Regularity:** regular. **Heart rate:** 45. **P waves:** upright, matching, one preceding each QRS; P-P interval regular. **PR interval:** 0.20. **QRS interval:** 0.08. **Interpretation:** sinus bradycardia. Note also a very prominent U wave.

79. **QRS complexes:** present, all shaped the same. **Regularity:** regular. **Heart rate:** 115. **P waves:** upright, matching, one preceding each QRS; P-P interval regular. **PR interval:** 0.12. **QRS interval:** 0.06. **Interpretation:** sinus tachycardia.

80. **QRS complexes:** present, all shaped the same. **Regularity:** regular. **Heart rate:** 107. **P waves:** biphasic, matching, one preceding each QRS; P-P interval regular. **PR interval:** 0.14. **QRS interval:** 0.10. **Interpretation:** sinus tachycardia.

81. **QRS complexes:** present, all shaped the same. **Regularity:** irregular. **Heart rate:** 137 to 167, with a mean rate of 150. **P waves:** none seen. **PR interval:** not applicable. **QRS interval:** 0.08. **Interpretation:** atrial fibrillation. If you thought it was ventricular tachycardia, look

again. The QRS complexes are not wide enough to be ventricular. Since it's irregular, it can't be called SVT. Though there are no obvious fibrillatory waves visible, it's prudent to call this rhythm atrial fibrillation because of its pronounced irregularity and lack of P waves.

82. **QRS complexes:** present, all shaped the same. **Regularity:** regular. **Heart rate:** 60. **P waves:** upright, matching, one preceding each QRS; P-P interval regular. **PR interval:** 0.12. **QRS interval:** 0.10. **Interpretation:** sinus rhythm.

83. **QRS complexes:** present, all shaped the same. **Regularity:** irregular. **Heart rate:** 88 to 115, with a mean rate of 110. **P waves:** none present; regular sawtooth-shaped waves present instead. **PR interval:** not applicable. **QRS interval:** 0.08. **Interpretation:** atrial flutter with variable conduction.

84. **QRS complexes:** present, all shaped the same. **Regularity:** irregular. **Heart rate:** 79 to 137, with a mean rate of 110. **P waves:** none present; way, undulating baseline present instead. **PR interval:** not applicable. **QRS interval:** 0.10. **Interpretation:** atrial fibrillation.

85. **QRS complexes:** present, all shaped the same. **Regularity:** regular. **Heart rate:** 88. **P waves:** upright, matching, one preceding each QRS; P-P interval regular. **PR interval:** 0.22. **QRS interval:** 0.12. **Interpretation:** sinus rhythm with first-degree AV block and BBB.

86. **QRS complexes:** present, all shaped the same. **Regularity:** regular. **Heart rate:** 60. **P waves:** none present; regular sawtooth-shaped waves present instead. **PR interval:** not applicable. **QRS interval:** 0.10. **Interpretation:** atrial flutter with variable conduction. Many of the flutter waves are lost inside the big inverted T wave.

87. **QRS complexes:** present, all shaped the same. **Regularity:** regular. **Heart rate:** 59. **P waves:** upright, matching, two to each QRS. The T wave has a double hump—do you see it? The first hump is the first P wave. The second P is right in front of the QRS. P-P interval regular. Atrial rate 115. **PR interval:** 0.24. **QRS interval:** 0.08. **Interpretation:** sinus tachycardia with 2:1 AV block, probably type I.

88. **QRS complexes:** present, all shaped the same. **Regularity:** irregular. **Heart rate:** 33 to 137, with a mean rate of 50. **P waves:** none present; wavy, undulating baseline present instead. **PR interval:** not applicable. **QRS interval:** 0.08. **Interpretation:** atrial fibrillation.

89. **QRS complexes:** present, all shaped the same. **Regularity:** regular. **Heart rate:** 115. **P waves:** upright, matching, one preceding each QRS; P-P interval regular. **PR interval:** 0.16. **QRS interval:** 0.12. **Interpretation:** sinus tachycardia with a BBB.

90. **QRS complexes:** present, all shaped the same. **Regularity:** regular. **Heart rate:** 75. **P waves:** upright, matching, one preceding each QRS; P-P interval regular. **PR interval:** 0.12. **QRS interval:** 0.06. **Interpretation:** sinus rhythm.

91. **QRS complexes:** present, sawtooth-shaped. **Regularity:** irregular.

Heart rate: 187 to 300. **P waves:** none seen. **PR interval:** not applicable. **QRS interval:** cannot measure, as cannot tell where QRS ends and T wave begins. **Interpretation:** ventricular flutter.

92. **QRS complexes:** present. **Regularity:** regular but interrupted (by premature beats). **Heart rate:** about 85. **P waves:** inverted, matching, one preceding all the narrow QRS complexes. **PR interval:** 0.16. **Interpretation:** sinus rhythm with a unifocal ventricular couplet and a PVC. Wait a minute. The P wave here is negative. Why is this not a junctional rhythm? This is V$_1$—see the notation at the top of the strip? Recall the P wave can be normally inverted in V$_1$. So that doesn't necessarily imply a junctional pacemaker. Also, a junctional rhythm would have had a shorter PR interval, less than 0.12.

93. **QRS complexes:** present, all shaped the same. **Regularity:** irregular. **Heart rate:** 29, then slower. **P waves:** none present. **PR interval:** not applicable. **QRS interval:** 0.24 to 0.28. **Interpretation:** dying heart.

94. **QRS complexes:** present, different shapes. **Regularity:** irregular. **Heart rate:** >300 in places. **P waves:** none seen. **PR interval:** not applicable. **QRS interval:** cannot measure, as cannot tell where QRS ends and T wave begins. **Interpretation:** torsades de pointes. Remember torsades is identified more by its classic shape than by any other criteria.

95. **QRS complexes:** present, all shaped the same. **Regularity:** regular. **Heart rate:** 43. **P waves:** inverted following each QRS complex in the ST segment. **PR interval:** not applicable. **QRS interval:** 0.08. **Interpretation:** junctional rhythm.

96. **QRS complexes:** only one present—at the beginning of the strip. Then a wavy, static-looking baseline is seen. **Regularity:** not applicable. **Heart rate:** zero after that first beat. **P waves:** none present. **PR interval:** not applicable. **QRS interval:** 0.28 on the only QRS complex on the strip. **Interpretation:** one ventricular beat, then ventricular fibrillation.

97. **QRS complexes:** none present; wavy, static-looking baseline present instead. **Regularity:** not applicable. **Heart rate:** cannot measure. **P waves:** none present. **PR interval:** not applicable. **QRS interval:** not applicable. **Interpretation:** ventricular fibrillation.

98. **QRS complexes:** none present. **Regularity:** not applicable, as there are no QRS complexes. **Heart rate:** zero. **P waves:** biphasic, matching; P-P interval regular. **PR interval:** not applicable. **QRS interval:** not applicable. **Interpretation:** ventricular asystole.

99. **QRS complexes:** present, all shaped the same. **Regularity:** irregular. **Heart rate:** 100 to 177. **P waves:** none present; wavy, undulating baseline present instead. **PR interval:** not applicable. **QRS interval:** 0.12. **Interpretation:** atrial fibrillation with a BBB.

100. **QRS complexes:** present, all shaped the same. **Regularity:** regular. **Heart rate:** 60. **P waves:** none present. **PR interval:** not applicable. **QRS interval:** 0.16 to 0.22. **Interpretation:** accelerated idioventricular rhythm.

101. **QRS complexes:** present, all shaped the same. **Regularity:** regular but interrupted (by a premature beat). **Heart rate:** 68. **P waves:** upright and matching except for the very last beat, which has a tiny inverted P wave. One P wave precedes each QRS. P-P interval is irregular. **PR interval:** 0.14 on all but the last beat. The PR interval of the last beat is 0.12. **QRS interval:** 0.12. **Interpretation:** sinus rhythm with a PJC and BBB.

102. **QRS complexes:** present, all shaped the same. **Regularity:** regular but interrupted (by a premature beat and also a pause). **Heart rate:** 39 to 100, with a mean rate of 70. **P waves:** upright and matching on all but the third beat, which has a tiny upright P wave at the end of the preceding T wave. There is also a tiny upright P wave just before the downstroke of the third T wave (inside the pause). P-P interval is irregular. **PR interval:** 0.18 on the normal beats; 0.22 on the premature beat. **QRS interval:** 0.06. **Interpretation:** sinus rhythm with a PAC and a nonconducted PAC. The third beat is the PAC. The P wave at the downstroke of the third beat's T wave is the nonconducted PAC. If you called this an AV block of some kind, remember that in AV blocks the P-P interval is regular. Here we have two premature P waves.

103. **QRS complexes:** present, all shaped the same. **Regularity:** irregular. **Heart rate:** 28 to 38, with a mean rate of 40. **P waves:** none present; wavy, undulating baseline present instead. **PR interval:** not applicable. **QRS interval:** 0.08. **Interpretation:** atrial fibrillation.

104. **QRS complexes:** present, all shaped the same. **Regularity:** regular but interrupted (by a premature beat). **Heart rate:** 100. **P waves:** biphasic and matching on all but the third beat, which is premature and has a different shape P wave. **PR interval:** 0.14 on the normal beats; 0.12 on the premature beat. **QRS interval:** 0.06. **Interpretation:** sinus rhythm with a PAC.

105. **QRS complexes:** present, all shaped the same. **Regularity:** regular but interrupted (by premature beats and pauses). **Heart rate:** 38 to 125, with a mean rate of 80. **P waves:** upright and matching on all but the P wave following the second QRS and also the P wave preceding the sixth QRS. Those P waves have a different shape. P-P interval is irregular. **PR interval:** 0.14 on the normal beats; 0.12 on the sixth beat. **QRS interval:** 0.08. **Interpretation:** sinus rhythm with a PAC (the sixth beat) and a nonconducted PAC (the premature P after the second QRS).

106. **QRS complexes:** present, all but one shaped the same. One is wider and taller than the others. **Regularity:** regular but interrupted (by a premature beat). **Heart rate:** 125. **P waves:** upright and matching on all but the wide QRS beat, which has no P wave. **PR interval:** 0.16. **QRS interval:** 0.08 on the normal beats, 0.14 on the premature beat. **Interpretation:** sinus tachycardia with a PVC.

107. **QRS complexes:** present, all shaped the same. **Regularity:** regular. **Heart rate:** about 130. **P waves:** upright, matching, one preceding

each QRS; P-P interval regular. **PR interval:** 0.14. **QRS interval:** 0.08. **Interpretation:** sinus tachycardia.

108. **QRS complexes:** present, all shaped the same. **Regularity:** irregular. **Heart rate:** 68 to 125, with a mean rate of 90. **P waves:** at least three different shapes; P-P interval irregular. **PR interval:** varies. **QRS interval:** 0.10. **Interpretation:** wandering atrial pacemaker. Since the mean rate is less than 100, it is better to call this WAP than MAT.

109. **QRS complexes:** present, all shaped the same. **Regularity:** regular. **Heart rate:** 38. **P waves:** upright and matching directly preceding the QRS. There is an extra premature P wave at the end of each T wave. That P has a different shape—it's pointy. **PR interval:** 0.20. **QRS interval:** 0.08. **Interpretation:** sinus bradycardia with bigeminal nonconducted PACs. This was a stinky strip, you say. It just looks like sinus bradycardia. That's right. But do you see the premature P wave now that it's been pointed out? Always be suspicious of T waves with humps on their ends. That hump might just be a P wave.

110. **QRS complexes:** present, all shaped the same. **Regularity:** irregular. **Heart rate:** 29 to 60, with a mean rate of 40. **P waves:** none present; wavy, undulating baseline present instead. **PR interval:** not applicable. **QRS interval:** 0.08. **Interpretation:** atrial fibrillation.

111. **QRS complexes:** present; most but not all shaped the same. **Regularity:** irregular. **Heart rate:** 167 to 250, with a mean rate of 200. **P waves:** none present; wavy, undulating baseline present instead. **PR interval:** not applicable. **QRS interval:** 0.06 to 0.08. **Interpretation:** atrial fibrillation. If you were tempted to call this SVT, remember that SVT is a regular rhythm. This strip is not regular.

112. **QRS complexes:** present, all shaped the same. **Regularity:** regular. **Heart rate:** 62. **P waves:** none seen. **PR interval:** not applicable. **QRS interval:** 0.20. **Interpretation:** accelerated idioventricular rhythm.

113. **QRS complexes:** present, all shaped the same, though some are deeper than others. **Regularity:** regular but interrupted (by a run of premature beats). **Heart rate:** 88 when in sinus tachycardia, about 187 when in atrial tachycardia. **P waves:** upright and matching on all but the very rapid beats, whose P waves are inside the preceding T wave. **PR interval:** 0.20 on the normal beats, unable to measure on the rapid beats, as the P is inside the T wave. **QRS interval:** 0.08. **Interpretation:** sinus tachycardia with a 10-beat run of PAT. We know this is PAT, as we see that the run of PAT begins with a PAC (the fourth beat).

114. **QRS complexes:** present, all shaped the same. **Regularity:** irregular. **Heart rate:** 150 to 250, with a mean rate of 190. **P waves:** none present; wavy, undulating baseline present instead. **PR interval:** not applicable. **QRS interval:** 0.06. **Interpretation:** atrial fibrillation.

115. **QRS complexes:** present, all shaped the same. **Regularity:** irregular. **Heart rate:** 150 to 250, with a mean rate of 190. **P waves:** none present; wavy, undulating baseline present instead. **PR interval:** not applicable. **QRS interval:** 0.06. **Interpretation:** atrial fibrillation.

116. **QRS complexes:** present, all shaped the same. **Regularity:** regular but interrupted (by a pause). **Heart rate:** 37 to 72. **P waves:** upright and matching except for the premature P wave inside the fourth T wave. **PR interval:** 0.24. **QRS interval:** 0.08. **Interpretation:** sinus rhythm with a nonconducted PAC.

117. **QRS complexes:** present, all shaped the same. **Regularity:** regular. **Heart rate:** 71. **P waves:** tiny inverted P waves present preceding the QRS complexes. **PR interval:** about 0.06. **QRS interval:** 0.10. **Interpretation:** accelerated junctional rhythm.

118. **QRS complexes:** present, all shaped the same. **Regularity:** regular but interrupted (by pauses). **Heart rate:** 48 to 88, with a mean rate of 80. **P waves:** upright and matching except for the premature P waves inside the third and sixth T waves. **PR interval:** 0.18. **QRS interval:** 0.08. **Interpretation:** sinus rhythm with two nonconducted PACs.

119. **QRS complexes:** present, all shaped the same. **Regularity:** regular. **Heart rate:** 29. **P waves:** none present. **PR interval:** not applicable. **QRS interval:** 0.28. **Interpretation:** idioventricular rhythm.

120. **QRS complexes:** present, all shaped the same. **Regularity:** regular but interrupted (by a pause). **Heart rate:** 32 to 58, with a mean rate of 50. **P waves:** upright, matching, sometimes more than one per QRS; atrial rate 60. **PR interval:** varies. **QRS interval:** 0.10. **Interpretation:** sinus rhythm with type I second-degree AV block. (Wenckebach) See how the PR interval gradually prolongs until a P wave is blocked (not followed by a QRS)?

121. **QRS complexes:** present, all shaped the same. **Regularity:** regular. **Heart rate:** 45. **P waves:** upright, matching, some nonconducted; atrial rate 137. **PR interval:** varies. **QRS interval:** 0.16. **Interpretation:** sinus tachycardia with third-degree AV block and an accelerated idioventricular rhythm. Did you think this was type II second-degree AV block? The differentiating factor here is the changing PR intervals. Type II has constant PR intervals. Did you think it was type I second-degree AV block? Type I does not have regular R-R intervals. So it could only be third-degree AV block.

122. **QRS complexes:** present, all shaped the same. **Regularity:** irregular. **Heart rate:** 60 to 83, with a mean rate of 80. **P waves:** upright, matching, one per QRS. P-P interval irregular. **PR interval:** 0.14. **QRS interval:** 0.08. **Interpretation:** sinus arrhythmia.

123. **QRS complexes:** present, all shaped the same. **Regularity:** regular. **Heart rate:** 83. **P waves:** none noted. **PR interval:** not applicable. **QRS interval:** 0.16. **Interpretation:** accelerated idioventricular rhythm.

124. **QRS complexes:** present, all shaped the same. **Regularity:** regular. **Heart rate:** 125. **P waves:** none seen. **PR interval:** not applicable. **QRS interval:** 0.20. **Interpretation:** ventricular tachycardia.

125. **QRS complexes:** present, all shaped the same. **Regularity:** regular. **Heart rate:** 58. **P waves:** none seen. There's a U wave immediately

following the T waves—don't confuse those with P waves. **PR interval:** not applicable. **QRS interval:** 0.10. **Interpretation:** junctional rhythm.

126. **QRS complexes:** present, all shaped the same. **Regularity:** irregular. **Heart rate:** 42 to 47, with a mean rate of 50. **P waves:** at least three different shapes, one preceding each QRS. **PR interval:** varies. **QRS interval:** 0.10. **Interpretation:** wandering atrial pacemaker.

127. **QRS complexes:** present, all shaped the same. **Regularity:** irregular. **Heart rate:** 100 to 150, with a mean ate of 130. **P waves:** none noted; wavy, undulating baseline present instead. **PR interval:** not applicable. **QRS interval:** 0.06. **Interpretation:** atrial fibrillation.

128. **QRS complexes:** present, all shaped the same. **Regularity:** irregular. **Heart rate:** 85 to 137, with a mean rate of 100. **P waves:** none present; sawtooth-shaped waves present between QRS complexes. **PR interval:** not applicable. **QRS interval:** 0.10. **Interpretation:** atrial flutter with variable conduction.

129. **QRS complexes:** present with differing shapes, if indeed those are real QRS complexes and not just spiked fibrillatory waves. **Regularity:** irregular. **Heart rate:** around 300 to 375, but difficult to count as QRS shapes change. **P waves:** none seen. **PR interval:** not applicable. **QRS interval:** cannot measure at times. **Interpretation:** torsades de pointes versus ventricular fibrillation. This is a judgment call, as this rhythm might well be ventricular fibrillation. You will find that torsades and v-fib can be easily mistaken for each other.

130. **QRS complexes:** present, all shaped the same. **Regularity:** regular. **Heart rate:** 79. **P waves:** upright, matching, one preceding each QRS; P-P interval regular. **PR interval:** 0.14. **QRS interval:** 0.12. **Interpretation:** sinus rhythm.

131. **QRS complexes:** present, all shaped the same. **Regularity:** regular. **Heart rate:** 51. **P waves:** none seen. **PR interval:** not applicable. **QRS interval:** 0.10. **Interpretation:** junctional rhythm.

132. **QRS complexes:** present, all shaped the same. **Regularity:** regular but interrupted (by premature beats). **Heart rate:** 65. **P waves:** upright, all except the third and fourth P waves matching. The third and fourth P waves are premature and shaped a bit differently. P-P interval irregular. **PR interval:** 0.16 to 0.20. **QRS interval:** 0.06. **Interpretation:** sinus rhythm with two PACs (the third and fourth beats).

133. **QRS complexes:** present, all shaped the same. **Regularity:** irregular. **Heart rate:** 71 to 110, with a mean rate of 90. **P waves:** none present; wavy, undulating baseline present instead. **PR interval:** not applicable. **QRS interval:** 0.08. **Interpretation:** atrial fibrillation. In places it looks pretty fluttery, doesn't it? You might have been tempted to call this atrial flutter. The problem is that the fluttery pattern is not consistent. Its waves could never be marched out, as the waves dampen out so much in places. It's safer to call this atrial fibrillation.

134. **QRS complexes:** present, all shaped the same. **Regularity:** regular. **Heart rate:** 60. **P waves:** none noted. **PR interval:** not applicable. **QRS interval:** 0.20. **Interpretation:** accelerated idioventricular rhythm.

135. **QRS complexes:** present, all shaped the same, though two are distorted by artifact. **Regularity:** regular. **Heart rate:** 137. **P waves:** none seen. **PR interval:** not applicable. **QRS interval:** 0.18. **Interpretation:** ventricular tachycardia.

136. **QRS complexes:** present, all shaped the same. **Regularity:** regular. **Heart rate:** 60. **P waves:** none seen; wavy, undulating baseline present instead. **PR interval:** not applicable. **QRS interval:** 0.10. **Interpretation:** atrial fibrillation. Though normally atrial fibrillation is a very irregular rhythm, you can see that it may look regular at times. This is not common, but you should be aware it does happen sometimes.

137. **QRS complexes:** present, all shaped the same. **Regularity:** regular. **Heart rate:** 137. **P waves:** upright, matching, one preceding each QRS; P-P interval regular. **PR interval:** 0.16. **QRS interval:** 0.08. **Interpretation:** sinus tachycardia.

138. **QRS complexes:** present, all shaped the same. **Regularity:** regular. **Heart rate:** 42. **P waves:** upright, matching (some a little distorted by artifact), one preceding each QRS; P-P interval regular. **PR interval:** 0.16. **QRS interval:** 0.10. **Interpretation:** sinus bradycardia.

139. **QRS complexes:** present, all shaped the same. **Regularity:** regular. **Heart rate:** 60. **P waves:** upright, matching, one preceding each QRS; P-P interval regular. **PR interval:** 0.14. **QRS interval:** 0.08. **Interpretation:** sinus rhythm.

140. **QRS complexes:** present, all shaped the same. **Regularity:** irregular. **Heart rate:** 71 to 107, with a mean rate of 90. **P waves:** none present; sawtooth waves present instead. **PR interval:** not applicable. **QRS interval:** 0.06. **Interpretation:** atrial flutter with variable conduction.

141. **QRS complexes:** present, all shaped the same. **Regularity:** regular. **Heart rate:** about 73. **P waves:** none noted; sawtooth waves present instead. **PR interval:** not applicable. **QRS interval:** 0.12, though difficult to measure as QRS is distorted by flutter waves. **Interpretation:** atrial flutter with variable conduction and a possible BBB.

142. **QRS complexes:** cannot distinguish. **Regularity:** can't tell. **Heart rate:** can't tell. **P waves:** can't distinguish. **PR interval:** not applicable. **QRS interval:** not applicable. **Interpretation:** unknown rhythm with artifact. Why is this strip even in here if you can't possibly tell what it is? Because it's important for you to know *not to even try to interpret a rhythm this obscured by artifact*. There is no way to tell what the underlying rhythm is here. Check the patient's monitor lead wires and electrode patches or change the lead the patient is being monitored in to get a better tracing, and try again with a clearer strip.

143. **QRS complexes:** present, all shaped the same. **Regularity:** regular. **Heart rate:** about 130. **P waves:** upright, matching, one preceding each QRS; P-P interval regular. **PR interval:** 0.16. **QRS interval:** 0.06. **Interpretation:** sinus tachycardia.

144. **QRS complexes:** present, all shaped the same. **Regularity:** regular. **Heart rate:** 83. **P waves:** upright, matching, one preceding each QRS; P-P interval regular. **PR interval:** 0.10. **QRS interval:** 0.08. **Interpretation:** sinus rhythm with accelerated AV conduction. If the PR interval is this short, we know the impulse blasts through the AV node faster than normal.

145. **QRS complexes:** present, all shaped the same. **Regularity:** regular. **Heart rate:** 88. **P waves:** upright, matching, one preceding each QRS; P-P interval regular. **PR interval:** 0.12. **QRS interval:** 0.12. **Interpretation:** sinus rhythm with BBB.

146. **QRS complexes:** present, all shaped the same. **Regularity:** regular. **Heart rate:** 60. **P waves:** upright, matching, one preceding each QRS; P-P interval regular. **PR interval:** 0.16. **QRS interval:** 0.08. **Interpretation:** sinus rhythm.

147. **QRS complexes:** present, all shaped the same. **Regularity:** regular. **Heart rate:** 68. **P waves:** upright, matching, one preceding each QRS; P-P interval regular. **PR interval:** 0.18. **QRS interval:** 0.14. **Interpretation:** sinus rhythm with a BBB.

148. **QRS complexes:** present, all shaped the same. **Regularity:** regular. **Heart rate:** about 57. **P waves:** upright, matching, one preceding each QRS; P-P interval regular. **PR interval:** 0.16. **QRS interval:** 0.08. **Interpretation:** sinus bradycardia.

149. **QRS complexes:** present, all shaped the same. **Regularity:** irregular. **Heart rate:** 56 to 83, with a mean rate of 70. **P waves:** none noted; wavy, undulating baseline present instead. **PR interval:** not applicable. **QRS interval:** 0.10. **Interpretation:** atrial fibrillation.

150. **QRS complexes:** present, all shaped the same. **Regularity:** regular. **Heart rate:** 43. **P waves:** upright, matching, one preceding each QRS; P-P interval regular. **PR interval:** 0.16. **QRS interval:** 0.08. **Interpretation:** sinus bradycardia.

151. **QRS complexes:** present, all shaped the same. **Regularity:** regular. **Heart rate:** 83. **P waves:** upright, matching, one preceding each QRS; P-P interval regular. **PR interval:** 0.14. **QRS interval:** 0.10. **Interpretation:** sinus rhythm.

152. **QRS complexes:** present, all shaped the same. **Regularity:** regular. **Heart rate:** about 35. **P waves:** upright, matching, one preceding each QRS; P-P interval regular. **PR interval:** 0.16. **QRS interval:** 0.10. **Interpretation:** sinus bradycardia.

153. **QRS complexes:** present, most but not all shaped the same. Some have an S wave, while others do not. **Regularity:** irregular. **Heart rate:**

150 to 250, with a mean rate of 190. **P waves:** none noted; wavy, undulating baseline present instead. **PR interval:** not applicable. **QRS interval:** 0.06 to 0.08. **Interpretation:** atrial fibrillation.

154. **QRS complexes:** present, all shaped the same. **Regularity:** regular. **Heart rate:** 62. **P waves:** upright, matching, one preceding each QRS; P-P interval regular. **PR interval:** 0.20. **QRS interval:** 0.08. **Interpretation:** sinus rhythm.

155. **QRS complexes:** present, all shaped the same. **Regularity:** regular. **Heart rate:** 115. **P waves:** upright, matching, one preceding each QRS; P-P interval regular. **PR interval:** 0.12. **QRS interval:** 0.10. **Interpretation:** sinus tachycardia.

156. **QRS complexes:** present, all shaped the same. **Regularity:** irregular. **Heart rate:** 107 to 167, with a mean rate of 140. **P waves:** none seen; wavy, undulating baseline present instead. **PR interval:** not applicable. **QRS interval:** 0.08. **Interpretation:** atrial fibrillation.

157. **QRS complexes:** one present; wavy, static-looking baseline present instead. **Regularity:** not applicable. **Heart rate:** cannot determine, as there are no QRS complexes. **P waves:** none seen. **PR interval:** not applicable. **QRS interval:** not applicable. **Interpretation:** ventricular fibrillation.

158. **QRS complexes:** present, all shaped the same. **Regularity:** irregular. **Heart rate:** 36 to 42, with a mean rate of 40. **P waves:** upright, matching, one preceding each QRS; P-P interval irregular. **PR interval:** 0.16. **QRS interval:** 0.10. **Interpretation:** sinus arrhythmia.

159. **QRS complexes:** present, all shaped the same. **Regularity:** regular but interrupted (by pauses). **Heart rate:** 75 to 125, with a mean rate of 110. **P waves:** upright, many hidden in T waves. Some P waves are nonconducted. P-P interval regular. Atrial rate 137. **PR interval:** varies. **QRS interval:** 0.06. **Interpretation:** sinus tachycardia with type I second-degree AV block (Wenckebach). This is not a very obvious Wenckebach, is it? See the pause between the third and fourth QRS complexes? Note the P wave preceding the fourth QRS. Now back up to the T wave of the third beat. See how deformed the shape is? That's because there's a P wave inside it. Note the P-P interval between those two P waves and you can march out where the rest of the P waves are. You'll find the P-P intervals are all regular and the PR intervals gradually prolong until a beat is dropped.

160. **QRS complexes:** present, all shaped the same. **Regularity:** irregular. **Heart rate:** 75 to 107, with a mean rate of 100. **P waves:** none noted; wavy, undulating baseline present instead. **PR interval:** not applicable. **QRS interval:** 0.10. **Interpretation:** atrial fibrillation.

161. **QRS complexes:** present, all shaped the same. **Regularity:** regular. **Heart rate:** about 130. **P waves:** none seen. **PR interval:** not applicable. **QRS interval:** 0.08. **Interpretation:** SVT.

162. **QRS complexes:** can't be sure if there are QRS complexes of varying

shapes or if it is just a static-looking baseline without QRS complexes. **Regularity:** irregular. **Heart rate:** 250 to 300. **P waves:** none seen. **PR interval:** not applicable. **QRS interval:** 0.12 or greater. **Interpretation:** either torsades de pointes or ventricular fibrillation. It oscillates like torsades but looks more uncoordinated, like v-fib. The treatment for these is very similar, thankfully, so calling it either torsades or v-fib would still get appropriate treatment for the patient.

163. **QRS complexes:** present, all shaped the same. **Regularity:** irregular. **Heart rate:** 60 to 107, with a mean rate of 90. **P waves:** none seen; wavy, undulating baseline present instead. **PR interval:** not applicable. **QRS interval:** 0.06. **Interpretation:** atrial fibrillation.

164. **QRS complexes:** present, all shaped the same. **Regularity:** regular. **Heart rate:** about 80. **P waves:** none seen; wavy, undulating baseline present instead. **PR interval:** not applicable. **QRS interval:** 0.10. **Interpretation:** atrial fibrillation. This is another example of a regular spell of atrial fibrillation.

165. **QRS complexes:** present, all but one shaped the same. One is shorter than the rest. **Regularity:** irregular. **Heart rate:** 45 to 65, with a mean rate of 50. **P waves:** none noted; wavy, undulating baseline present instead. **PR interval:** not applicable. **QRS interval:** 0.08. **Interpretation:** atrial fibrillation.

166. **QRS complexes:** present, all shaped the same. **Regularity:** regular. **Heart rate:** 75. **P waves:** upright, matching, one preceding each QRS; P-P interval regular. **PR interval:** 0.16. **QRS interval:** 0.14. **Interpretation:** sinus rhythm with a BBB.

167. **QRS complexes:** present, all shaped the same. **Regularity:** irregular. **Heart rate:** 88 to 187, with a mean rate of 120. **P waves:** present, at least three different shapes; P-P interval irregular. **PR interval:** varies. **QRS interval:** 0.08. **Interpretation:** multifocal atrial tachycardia.

168. **QRS complexes:** present, all shaped the same. **Regularity:** regular. **Heart rate:** around 90. **P waves:** upright, matching, one preceding each QRS; P-P interval regular. **PR interval:** 0.14. **QRS interval:** 0.08. **Interpretation:** sinus rhythm.

169. **QRS complexes:** present, all shaped the same. **Regularity:** irregular. **Heart rate:** 83 to 137, with a mean rate of 110. **P waves:** none noted; sawtooth waves present instead. **PR interval:** not applicable. **QRS interval:** 0.08. **Interpretation:** atrial flutter with variable conduction.

170. **QRS complexes:** present, all shaped the same. **Regularity:** regular. **Heart rate:** 150. **P waves:** upright, matching, one preceding each QRS; P-P interval regular. **PR interval:** 0.10. **QRS interval:** 0.10. **Interpretation:** sinus tachycardia with accelerated AV conduction.

171. **QRS complexes:** present, all shaped the same. **Regularity:** regular. **Heart rate:** 45. **P waves:** upright, matching, two preceding each QRS; P-P interval regular; atrial rate 88. **PR interval:** 0.36. **QRS interval:** 0.08. **Interpretation:** sinus rhythm with 2:1 AV block.

172. **QRS complexes:** present, all shaped the same. **Regularity:** regular but interrupted (by pauses). **Heart rate:** 44 to 83, with a mean rate of 60. **P waves:** upright, matching, some nonconducted; P-P interval regular; atrial rate 88. **PR interval:** 0.36. **QRS interval:** 0.08. **Interpretation:** sinus rhythm with type II second-degree AV block.

173. **QRS complexes:** present, all shaped the same. **Regularity:** regular. **Heart rate:** 137. **P waves:** none seen. **PR interval:** not applicable. **QRS interval:** 0.06. **Interpretation:** SVT.

174. **QRS complexes:** only one mammoth QRS on the strip. Believe it or not, that huge wave at the beginning of the strip is a QRS and T wave. **Regularity:** cannot determine. **Heart rate:** cannot determine. **P waves:** none seen. **PR interval:** not applicable. **QRS interval:** about 0.60, but that's a guesstimate. **Interpretation:** dying heart (agonal rhythm). It is unusual for dying heart's QRS complexes to be this wide. It's likely this patient has an *extremely elevated* potassium level in his or her bloodstream, which can cause the QRS to widen out more than usual.

175. **QRS complexes:** none seen. **Regularity:** not applicable. **Heart rate:** zero. **P waves:** none seen. **PR interval:** not applicable. **QRS interval:** not applicable. **Interpretation:** asystole.

176. **QRS complexes:** present, differing shapes. **Regularity:** irregular. **Heart rate:** about 375. **P waves:** none seen. **PR interval:** not applicable. **QRS interval:** 0.12 or greater. **Interpretation:** torsades de pointes.

177. **QRS complexes:** none; wavy, static-looking baseline present instead. **Regularity:** not applicable. **Heart rate:** cannot measure. **P waves:** none seen. **PR interval:** not applicable. **QRS interval:** not applicable. **Interpretation:** ventricular fibrillation.

178. **QRS complexes:** none; wavy, static-looking baseline present instead. **Regularity:** not applicable. **Heart rate:** cannot measure. **P waves:** none seen. **PR interval:** not applicable. **QRS interval:** not applicable. **Interpretation:** ventricular fibrillation.

179. **QRS complexes:** present, all shaped the same. **Regularity:** regular. **Heart rate:** just a hair over 100. **P waves:** upright, matching, one preceding each QRS; P-P interval regular. **PR interval:** 0.22. **QRS interval:** 0.10. **Interpretation:** sinus tachycardia with a first-degree AV block.

180. **QRS complexes:** present, all shaped the same. **Regularity:** irregular. **Heart rate:** 80 to 167, with a mean rate of 110. **P waves:** present, at least three different shapes. **PR interval:** not applicable. **QRS interval:** 0.06. **Interpretation:** multifocal atrial tachycardia. If you thought it was atrial fibrillation, remember that *atrial fibrillation has no P waves.* There are obvious P waves on this strip.

181. **QRS complexes:** present, all shaped the same. **Regularity:** regular. **Heart rate:** 68. **P waves:** none seen. **PR interval:** not applicable.

QRS interval: 0.18. **Interpretation:** accelerated idioventricular rhythm.

182. **QRS complexes:** present, all shaped the same. **Regularity:** regular. **Heart rate:** 125. **P waves:** upright, matching, one preceding each QRS; P-P interval regular. **PR interval:** 0.16. **QRS interval:** 0.06. **Interpretation:** sinus tachycardia. You may recognize this strip. It's the same as number 6. Did you come up with the same answer on this strip as on number 6? You should have.

183. **QRS complexes:** present, all shaped the same. **Regularity:** regular. **Heart rate:** 56. **P waves:** upright, matching, one preceding each QRS; P-P interval regular; P waves are very small. **PR interval:** 0.16. **QRS interval:** 0.16. **Interpretation:** sinus bradycardia with a BBB. Look again at this strip if you thought this was atrial fibrillation. There are obvious, though tiny, P waves. And if you thought this was a ventricular rhythm of some kind because of the QRS width, note the matching upright P waves. Ventricular rhythms don't have that. Remember—the width of the QRS does not determine whether a rhythm can be sinus. The P waves are the key criterion.

184. **QRS complexes:** present, all shaped the same. **Regularity:** regular. **Heart rate:** 83. **P waves:** upright, matching, one preceding each QRS; P-P interval regular. **PR interval:** 0.13. **QRS interval:** 0.10. **Interpretation:** sinus rhythm. Did you think this was a 2:1 AV block? The T wave does look an awful lot like the P wave, doesn't it? Remember AV blocks have regular P-P intervals. If this T wave were hiding a P wave, the P-P intervals would not be regular. So it's not an AV block.

185. **QRS complexes:** present, all shaped the same. **Regularity:** regular. **Heart rate:** 167. **P waves:** upright, matching, one preceding each QRS; P-P interval regular. **PR interval:** 0.12. **QRS interval:** 0.06. **Interpretation:** atrial tachycardia. Remember, the sinus node does not usually fire at rates above 160 in supine resting adults. Since this rate is above 160, we must call it atrial tachycardia.

186. **QRS complexes:** present, all shaped the same. **Regularity:** irregular. **Heart rate:** 20 to 75, with a mean rate of 50. **P waves:** none seen; very fine wavy, undulating baseline present instead. **PR interval:** not applicable. **QRS interval:** 0.08. **Interpretation:** atrial fibrillation.

187. **QRS complexes:** present, all shaped the same. **Regularity:** irregular. **Heart rate:** 28 to 62, with a mean rate of 50. **P waves:** none seen; wavy, undulating baseline present instead. **PR interval:** not applicable. **QRS interval:** 0.10. **Interpretation:** atrial fibrillation.

188. **QRS complexes:** present, all shaped the same. **Regularity:** irregular. **Heart rate:** 60 to 79, with a mean rate of 70. **P waves:** upright, matching, one preceding each QRS; P-P interval regular. **PR interval:** 0.18. **QRS interval:** 0.08. **Interpretation:** sinus arrhythmia.

189. **QRS complexes:** present, all shaped the same. **Regularity:** regular. **Heart rate:** 60. **P waves:** upright, matching (the ones that can be seen),

one preceding each QRS; P-P interval regular, as far as can be seen. **PR interval:** 0.18. **QRS interval:** 0.08. **Interpretation:** sinus rhythm partially obscured by artifact. Unlike strip number 142, which had so much artifact that the underlying rhythm could not be determined, this strip has measurable waves and complexes. Since we can pick out the QRS complexes throughout the strip, we can deduce that the P waves continue as well during the artifact spells. Even so, it would be better not to mount a strip like this in the patient's chart, since one cannot be entirely sure what is happening during the periods of artifact.

190. **QRS complexes:** present, all shaped the same. **Regularity:** regular but interrupted (by pauses). **Heart rate:** 75 to 125. **P waves:** upright, some hidden in T waves, some nonconducted; P-P interval regular; atrial rate 137. **PR interval:** varies. **QRS interval:** 0.06. **Interpretation:** sinus tachycardia with type I second-degree AV block.

191. **QRS complexes:** present, all but two shaped the same (two are taller and wider). **Regularity:** regular but interrupted (by premature beats). **Heart rate:** 88. **P waves:** upright and matching on the narrow beats, none on the wide beats; P-P regular. **PR interval:** 0.24. **QRS interval:** 0.08 on the narrow beats, 0.14 on the wide beats. **Interpretation:** sinus rhythm with PVCs and a first-degree AV block.

192. **QRS complexes:** present, all shaped the same. **Regularity:** regular. **Heart rate:** 88. **P waves:** notched, matching, one preceding each QRS; P-P interval regular. **PR interval:** 0.20. **QRS interval:** 0.08. **Interpretation:** sinus rhythm.

193. **QRS complexes:** present, all shaped the same. **Regularity:** regular. **Heart rate:** 71. **P waves:** upright, matching, one preceding each QRS; P-P interval regular. **PR interval:** 0.22. **QRS interval:** 0.08. **Interpretation:** sinus rhythm with a first-degree AV block.

194. **QRS complexes:** present, all shaped the same. **Regularity:** regular. **Heart rate:** 36. **P waves:** upright, matching, one preceding each QRS; P-P interval regular. **PR interval:** 0.16. **QRS interval:** 0.10. **Interpretation:** sinus bradycardia.

195. **QRS complexes:** only one seen on the strip. **Regularity:** cannot determine. **Heart rate:** cannot determine from just one QRS complex. **P waves:** cannot distinguish due to artifact. **PR interval:** not applicable. **QRS interval:** cannot measure, as it's distorted by artifact. **Interpretation:** probably agonal rhythm obscured by CPR artifact. This strip looks a lot like the example of CPR artifact in Chapter 17, doesn't it? In order to know for sure what this rhythm is, CPR would need to be stopped briefly to allow a strip without artifact to be analyzed.

196. **QRS complexes:** none present; wavy, static-looking baseline present instead. **Regularity:** not applicable. **Heart rate:** not applicable. **P waves:** none seen. **PR interval:** not applicable. **QRS interval:** not applicable. **Interpretation:** ventricular fibrillation.

197. **QRS complexes:** present, all shaped the same. **Regularity:** regular but interrupted (by a premature beat). **Heart rate:** 71 to 107. **P waves:** upright and matching except for the premature P wave on the seventh beat; P-P interval irregular because of this premature beat. **PR interval:** 0.16. **QRS interval:** 0.10. **Interpretation:** sinus rhythm with a PAC.

198. **QRS complexes:** present, all shaped the same. **Regularity:** regular but interrupted (by a premature beat). **Heart rate:** about 77. **P waves:** tiny, biphasic and matching except for the third beat, which is premature. The P-P interval is irregular because of this premature beat. **PR interval:** 0.14 to 0.16. **QRS interval:** 0.06. **Interpretation:** sinus rhythm with a PAC. This premature beat is not a PJC because the PR interval of that beat is greater than 0.12.

199. **QRS complexes:** present, two different shapes. **Regularity:** regular but interrupted (by premature beats). **Heart rate:** 115. **P waves:** upright and matching on the narrow beats, none on the wide beats. **PR interval:** 0.14. **QRS interval:** 0.08 on the narrow beats, 0.16 on the wide beats. **Interpretation:** sinus tachycardia with two PVCs.

200. **QRS complexes:** present, all shaped the same. **Regularity:** irregular. **Heart rate:** 79 to 125, with an atrial rate of 100. **P waves:** none present; sawtooth waves present instead. **PR interval:** not applicable. **QRS interval:** 0.08. **Interpretation:** atrial flutter with variable conduction.

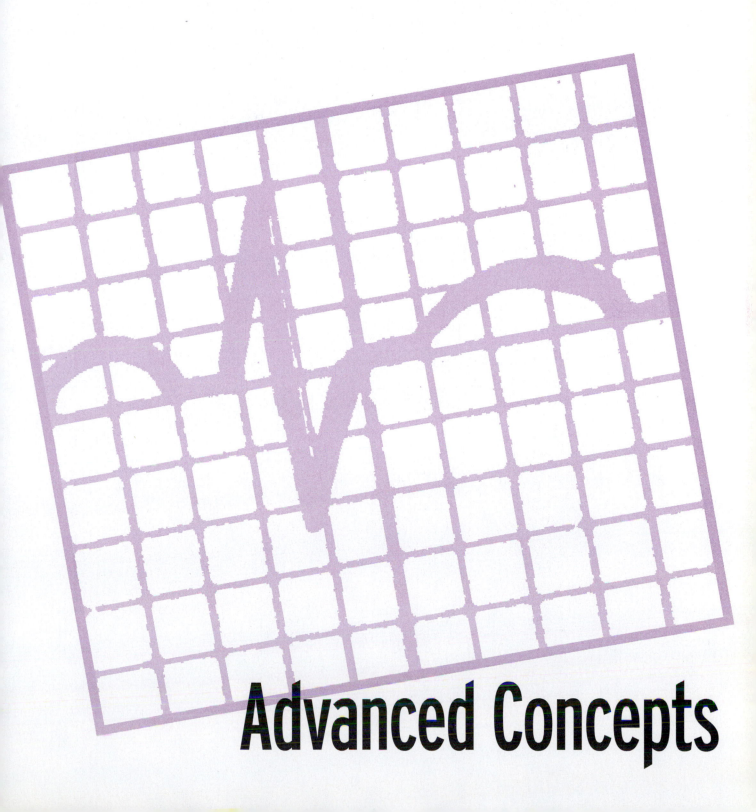

PART TWO

Advanced Concepts

Rhythm Odds and Ends

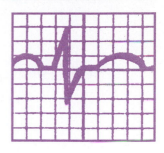

Chapter 19 Objectives

Upon completion of this chapter, the student will be able to:

- State the criteria for fusion beats, Wolff-Parkinson-White (WPW), and AV dissociation.
- Differentiate between fusion beats and PVCs.
- Differentiate between AV dissociation and third-degree AV block.
- Correctly identify fusion beats, WPW, and AV dissociation.
- State the causes, adverse effects, and treatment for each rhythm.

Chapter 19 Outline

I.   Fusion beats

II.   Wolff-Parkinson-White syndrome

III.   AV dissociation

IV.   Practice quiz

V.   Practice quiz answers

Chapter 19 Glossary

Ablation: Destruction of an accessory conductive pathway in the heart.

Fusion beat: A beat that results when a sinus impulse arrives to depolarize the ventricle at the same time a PVC was activating the same tissue.

Preexcitation: Depolarizing tissue earlier than normal.

Fusion Beats

What are they? Fusion beats are a combination of a sinus beat and a PVC. The sinus impulse arrives to depolarize the ventricle *at the same time* that a premature ventricular impulse was starting to depolarize the same tissue. The resultant QRS complex is intermediate in shape and size between the sinus beat and the PVC. Imagine the sinus beat as the mother and the PVC as the father. Fusion beats are their offspring. Just as in humans, where some children look more like their mother and others resemble the father, some fusion beats will look more like the sinus beat and others will look more like the PVC.

Rate	Can occur at any rate
Regularity	Regular but interrupted (by premature beats)
P waves	May or may not be present on the fusion beats. If present, P waves will be sinus Ps.
PR	Usually shorter than the PR of the surrounding sinus beats (if P waves present)
QRS	Usually shaped like a narrowed PVC or a widened sinus beat. QRS interval may be normal (<0.12 s) or prolonged (>0.12 s), depending on whether the sinus or the ventricular impulse contributed more to the depolarization of the ventricle.
Cause	Fusions are caused by the same things that cause PVCs.
Adverse effects	Same as PVCs
Treatment	Same as PVCs

In Figure 19-1, the dotted QRS complexes represent fusion beats. Note the shape of the PVC and the sinus beats. Look at fusion beat 1. It looks like a narrowed PVC, doesn't it? The ventricle obviously contributed more to its shape than the sinus node did. Now look at fusion 2. It looks more like the sinus beats, with a thicker R wave. Its shape was contributed mostly by the sinus impulse, with a little contribution from the ventricle.

Wolff-Parkinson-White Syndrome (WPW)

What is it? WPW is a syndrome in which there is an accessory conductive pathway between the atrium and the ventricle. This accessory pathway, called the **Kent bundle,** allows impulses to bypass the AV node—and its resultant slowing of the impulse—and arrive at the ventricle earlier than if they had gone down the normal conduction pathway. For this reason, WPW is known as a **preexcitation syndrome.** The ventricle is excited (depolarized) earlier than usual.

Here's how it works: The sinus node or the atrium (whichever is the pacemaker) sends out its impulse as usual. The atria are depolarized, and a P wave is written on the EKG. Part of the impulse then heads down the Kent bundle toward the ventricle, while the rest travels the normal conduction system. The Kent bundle impulses arrive at the ventricle first, since they do

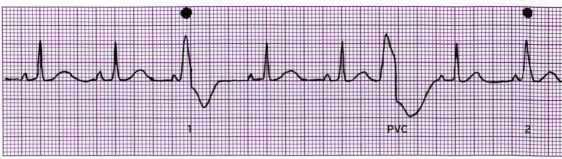

Figure 19-1 Fusion beats.

not have the AV node to slow them down, and they write a delta wave (a slurred upstroke to the QRS complex) on the EKG. These impulses arrive so early that the PR interval is shortened. The rest of the impulses then arrive via the normal conduction pathway and contribute the remainder of the QRS complex. The QRS will be wider than normal due to the delta wave. On occasion, *all* the impulses will travel the Kent bundle and result in a very wide QRS complex that resembles ventricular beats. Figure 19-2 reveals the bypass tract in WPW.

There are several conductive possibilities in WPW. See Figure 19-3.

Rate	Can occur at any rate
Regularity	Depends on the underlying rhythm
P waves	Normal if the sinus node is the pacemaker, shaped differently if the atrium is the pacemaker
PR interval	Shorter than normal (<0.12 s)
QRS	Wider than normal (>0.12 s). The QRS complex has a slurred upstroke to the R wave, called a *delta wave.*
Cause	Usually congenital
Adverse effects	Patients with WPW have a tendency to have supraventricular arrhythmias, which can look deceptively like

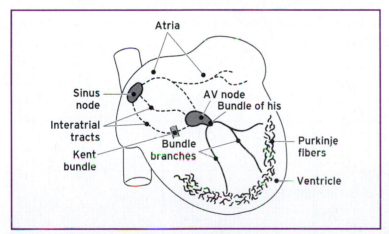

Figure 19-2   The bypass tract in WPW.

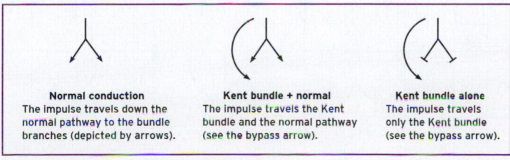

Figure 19-3   Conductive possibilities in WPW.

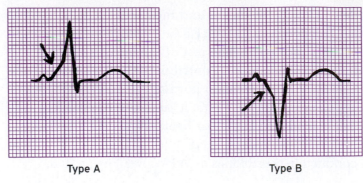

Type A   Type B

Figure 19-4   WPW types A and B.

v-tach because of the wide QRS complex. Decreased cardiac output can result if tachycardia occurs. No adverse effects at normal heart rates.

Treatment   Surgical or radiofrequency ablation (destruction of the accessory pathway) may be necessary if tachycardias become a problem.

There are two types of WPW. Type A has an upright QRS in V_1. Type B has a downward QRS in V_1. Figure 19-4 shows both types. Note the short PR interval and the delta wave (indicated by arrow).

Figure 19-5 shows an EKG with type A WPW. Note how subtle the delta waves are (seen best here in the precordial leads). This subtlety of delta waves makes WPW easy to miss.

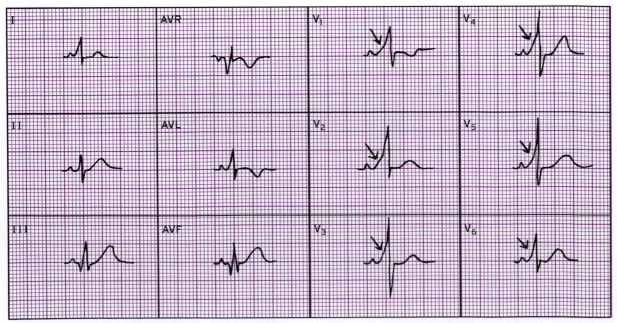

Figure 19-5   Type A WPW.

AV Dissociation

What is it? AV dissociation is a mismatch between the atrial rate and the ventricular rate, which results in independent beating of atria and ventricles. Though it is a hallmark of third-degree AV block, AV dissociation can exist without AV block. In third-degree AV block, the atrial rate is faster than the ventricular rate. In other kinds of AV dissociation, the ventricular rate is faster than the atrial rate. In either case, the sinus node fires out its P waves and depolarizes the atria, but a lower pacemaker controls the ventricle. In third-degree AV block, this dissociation is caused by a block in the conduction pathway, which requires a lower pacemaker to **escape.** In other kinds of AV dissociation, the lower pacemaker **usurps** the sinus node to control the ventricle.

Rate	Can occur any rate
Regularity	Atrial rate and P-P interval are regular, ventricular rate and R-R interval are regular, but the atrial and ventricular rates are different.
P waves	Normal sinus P waves
PR	Varies. The varying PR in the face of differing atrial and ventricular rates and regular P-P and R-R intervals proves dissociation.
QRS	Narrow (<0.12) if the AV node is the pacemaker of the ventricles, wide (>0.12) if the ventricle is the pacemaker of the ventricles
Cause	Medications such as digitalis; heart disease; or it can be a normal variant
Adverse effects	No ill effects unless the heart rate is too slow or too fast
Treatment	If caused by medication, remove or decrease the dose of the medication. Treat the cause.

In Figure 19-6, note the dots under the P waves and the lines under the QRS complexes. Note that the atrial rate is slower than the ventricular rate, the P-P and R-R intervals are all regular, and the PR interval varies. This is *not* third-degree AV block! The ventricular rate is faster than the atrial rate. This rhythm would be sinus rhythm with AV dissociation and an accelerated junctional rhythm. Sinus rhythm? Where does that come from, you wonder?

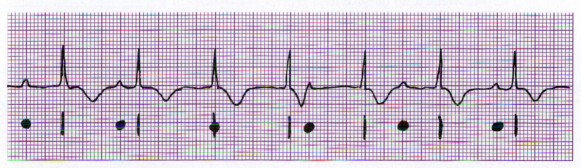

Figure 19-6   AV dissociation.

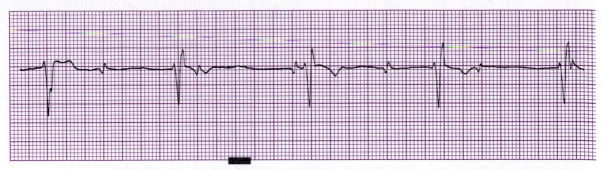

Figure 19-7 Third-degree AV block.

The P waves are all upright and matching, with an atrial rate of 60, so that is sinus rhythm. But the QRS complexes are not obeying the sinus node—they are marching to their own drummer, in this case the AV junction. We know the junction is the pacemaker of the ventricles because the QRS interval is <0.12 second. Had the ventricle been the pacemaker, the QRS would have been wider, >0.12 second. Now see Figure 19-7, which shows third-degree AV block. Note the atrial rate is faster than the ventricular rate, the P-P and R-R intervals are regular though different, and the PR intervals vary.

Keep in mind that AV dissociation does not necessarily imply third-degree AV block.

Practice Quiz

1. A fusion beat is a combination of which two kinds of beats? _____

   _____

2. What are the three conductive possibilities in WPW? _____

   _____

3. What is a delta wave? _____

4. Explain why the PR interval is shorter than normal in WPW. _____

   _____

5. WPW can cause supraventricular tachycardias that can look deceptively like which life-threatening rhythm? _____

6. What kind of QRS does type A WPW have in V_1? _____

7. In third-degree AV block, are there more P waves or more QRS complexes? _____

   _____

8. True or false: AV dissociation can exist without third-degree AV block.

9. True or false: The P waves in third-degree AV block and AV dissociation are sinus P waves.

10. True or false: AV dissociation can occur because a lower pacemaker usurps control from the sinus node to control the ventricles.

Practice Quiz Answers

1. A fusion beat is a combination of **a sinus beat and a PVC.**

2. The three conductive possibilities in WPW are **conduction down the normal pathway, conduction via the bypass tract plus the normal pathway,** or **conduction down the bypass tract alone.**

3. A delta wave is **a slurred upstroke to the QRS complex. The delta wave is a hallmark of WPW.**

4. The PR interval in WPW is shorter than normal because **the impulse progresses rapidly down the bypass tract, arriving at the ventricle sooner. Thus the impulse doesn't take as long to go from point A to point B because it bypasses the AV node.**

5. WPW can cause supraventricular tachycardias that can look deceptively like **ventricular tachycardia.**

6. Type A WPW has **an upward QRS in V_1.**

7. In third-degree AV block **there are more P waves than QRS complexes.**

8. **True.** AV dissociation can exist without third-degree AV block.

9. **True.** The P waves in third-degree AV block and AV dissociation are sinus P waves.

10. **True.** AV dissociation can occur because a lower pacemaker usurps control of the ventricle from the sinus node.

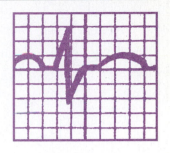

The Six Steps to 12-Lead EKG Interpretation

Chapter 20 Objectives

Upon completion of this chapter, the student will be able to:

- List the six steps to 12-lead interpretation.
- Define *axis.*
- Define *hypertrophy.*
- Define *IVCD.*
- Explain how elevated potassium level in the bloodstream can cause EKG changes.

Chapter 20 Outline

I. Introduction
II. The six steps
III. The basics
IV. Electrical axis
V. IVCDs
VI. Hypertrophy
VII. Infarction/ischemia
VIII. Miscellaneous effects
IX. Practice quiz
X. Practice quiz answers

Chapter 20 Glossary

Axis: The mean direction of the heart's current flow.
Hypertrophy: Overgrowth of myocardial tissue.

Introduction

It's true that 12-lead EKGs can be intimidating to evaluate, so it's important to have a plan of attack. Using the steps in this chapter can help uncover significant abnormalities and can help answer the following questions: What are the rhythm and heart rate? Is the patient having a heart attack? Has the patient had a heart attack in the past? Does the patient have atrial or ventricular hypertrophy? Does the patient have electrolyte abnormalities? Does he or she show signs of toxic medication levels in the bloodstream? The answers to these questions are important in order to provide appropriate treatment to the patient.

The Six Steps to 12-Lead EKG Interpretation

Use these steps in order:

1. *Interpret the basics—rhythm, heart rate, and intervals (PR, QRS, QT).* If the EKG has a rhythm strip at the bottom, assess the basics here. Otherwise, pick any lead (leads II and V_1 are the best ones to evaluate for rhythm.) Do the intervals fall within normal limits or are they abnormally shortened or prolonged? Prolonged PR intervals imply a block in conduction between atria and ventricles. Shortened PR intervals imply a change in the heart's pacemaker or a preexcitation syndrome such as WPW. Prolonged QRS intervals imply a block of one of the bundle branches, a ventricular rhythm, WPW, or severe electrolyte abnormalities. Prolonged QT intervals can herald the potential for lethal arrhythmias and can imply medication side effects.

2. *Calculate the electrical axis.* Is it normal or is there axis deviation? *Axis* is simply a degree marking given to the mean direction of current flow in the heart. Axis will be covered in the next chapter.

3. *Determine the presence of intraventricular conduction defects (IVCDs).* These are bundle branch blocks and hemiblocks.

4. *Check for hypertrophy, both atrial and ventricular.* Use leads II and V_1 to check the P waves for signs of atrial hypertrophy, and use V_1 and V_{5-6} to check the QRS complexes for signs of ventricular hypertrophy.

5. *Check for infarction/ischemia.* For this you'll look at all leads except aVR. You'll look for ST elevation or depression, inverted T waves, and significant Q waves. You'll also note R wave progression in the precordial leads.

6. *Determine the presence of miscellaneous effects.* Examine all leads for disturbances in calcium or potassium levels in the bloodstream and for various medication effects.

Step 1: The Basics

Since rhythm, heart rate, and intervals were covered in earlier chapters, we'll not repeat that information here. There is one very important issue about the QRS interval that we did not discuss yet, however—a wide QRS complex.

You'll recall that the most common causes for a QRS interval greater than 0.12 second are ventricular beats, bundle branch blocks, and WPW. But there is another ominous cause for the QRS to widen out—a very high potassium (K) level in the bloodstream. This is seen most often with patients suffering from chronic renal failure, where the kidneys are unable to filter poisons, including potassium, from the bloodstream. Normal potassium level is about 3.5 to 5 mEq/L. Potassium levels above 6 can cause very wide QRS complexes, much wider than a ventricular beat or a bundle branch block. If the potassium level is not lowered quickly, the QRS can widen out so much that it resembles a sine wave (remember sine waves from high school math?), and the heart becomes paralyzed by the potassium. The patient then suffers cardiac arrest and possibly death. See Figure 20-1.

Step 2: Electrical Axis

The electrical axis is a reference to the general direction that the heart's current is flowing. You'll recall that the heart's current normally starts in the sinus node up in the right atrium and finishes in the left ventricle. The general direction is thus top to bottom, right to left. We use the hexiaxial diagram to determine the angle, in degrees, of this direction. Axis is covered in detail in Chapter 21.

Step 3: IVCDs

Intraventricular conduction defects (IVCDs) result from abnormal conduction of cardiac impulses through the bundle branches. As a result, the QRS complexes are abnormally shaped and may be wider than normal. IVCDs include bundle branch blocks and hemiblocks. They are covered in detail in Chapter 22.

Step 4: Hypertrophy

Hypertrophy is an excessive growth of tissue of the atrium or ventricle. To determine if atrial hypertrophy is present, we examine the size and shape of the P waves. For ventricular hypertrophy, we look at QRS complexes. Hypertrophy produces a larger-than-normal current in the tissue and thus produces larger P waves and QRS complexes. Hypertrophy is covered in Chapter 24.

Step 5: Infarction/Ischemia

Myocardial ischemia and infarction produces changes in the ST segment, T wave, and/or QRS complex. It is covered in Chapter 25.

Step 6: Miscellaneous Effects

EKG changes can occur because of electrolyte disturbances and medications. These EKG effects are covered in Chapter 26.

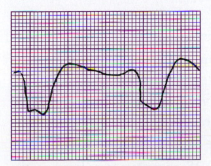 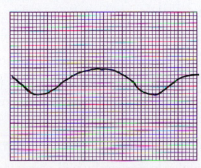

Figure 20-1 Wide QRS and sine wave pattern caused by severe hyperkalemia.

Practice Quiz

1. List the six steps to follow in 12-lead EKG interpretation.

   _____

   _____

   _____

   _____

   _____

   _____

2. A wide QRS can be a sign of excessive _____ in the blood-stream.

3. Define *IVCD*. _____

   _____

4. Define *hypertrophy*. _____

   _____

5. Atrial hypertrophy will cause which structure on the EKG to become enlarged? _____

   _____

6. Ventricular hypertrophy will cause which structure on the EKG to become enlarged? _____

   _____

7. The heart's current flows in which direction? _____

8. What kind of diagram is used to calculate the electrical axis? _____

   _____

9. True or false: Electrolyte disturbances and certain medications can have an effect on the EKG.

10. True or false: To look for myocardial ischemia and infarction, one should examine the QRS complex, the T waves, and the ST segments.

Practice Quiz Answers

1. The six steps are: **the basics (rhythm, rate, and intervals), electrical axis, IVCDs, hypertrophy, infarction/ischemia, and miscellaneous effects.**

2. A wide QRS can be a sign of excessive **potassium** in the bloodstream.

3. IVCD is **intraventricular conduction defect (a bundle branch block or a hemiblock).**

4. Hypertrophy is **excessive growth of tissue of the atrium or ventricle.**

5. Atrial hypertrophy will cause the **P wave** to enlarge on the EKG.

6. Ventricular hypertrophy will cause the **QRS complex** to enlarge on the EKG.

7. The heart's current flows **top to bottom, right to left.**

8. To calculate the electrical axis, the **hexiaxial diagram** is used.

9. **True.** Electrolyte disturbances and certain medications can have an effect on the EKG.

10. **True.** To look for myocardial ischemia and infarction, one should examine the QRS complex, the T waves, and the ST segments.

Electrical Axis

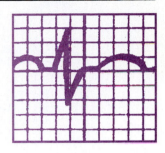

Chapter 21 Objectives

Upon completion of this chapter, the student will be able to:

- State the degree boundaries for normal axis, left axis deviation, right axis deviation, and indeterminate axis.
- State some causes of axis deviation. List the four steps to axis calculation.
- Correctly determine the axis quadrant by using leads I and aVF.
- Correctly determine the most isoelectric QRS complex.
- Correctly determine which lead is perpendicular to the isoelectric lead.
- State which leads are perpendiculars.
- Draw the perpendicular rainbow.
- Correctly calculate the axis on a variety of practice EKGs.

Chapter 21 Outline

Chapter 21 Glossary

Deviation   Going in a direction away from the normal.

Perpendicular   At a right angle to.

Introduction

The electrical axis is a degree marking given to the mean (average) direction of the heart's electrical current flow. We know that the heart's current normally starts in the sinus node and ends in the left ventricle. Thus the current travels top to bottom, right to left. We now want to assign a degree marking to this direction of current flow. Since the axis is concerned with direction, we need a compass. On a compass there are lines delineating north, south, east, and west. In axis calculation, our compass is the hexiaxial diagram superimposed on the heart, as seen in Figure 21-1. On the hexiaxial diagram are lines depicting the frontal leads—I, II, III, aVR, aVL, and aVF. Lead I runs east-west and aVF runs north-south. The other leads are points in between. The leads are separated from each other by 30° increments. The **axis circle** is made by joining the ends of these lead lines. Note the degree markings in Figure 21-1. Current of the heart flowing from the sinus node to the left ventricle would yield an axis of about 60°. That's a normal axis.

Quadrants

If we use leads I and aVF to divide the axis circle into four quadrants, **normal axis** would be between 0 to +90°. **Left axis deviation** is between 0 to −90°. **Right axis deviation** is between +90 to ±180°. **Indeterminate axis** (so-called because it cannot be determined whether it is an extreme left axis deviation or an extreme right axis deviation) is between −90 and ±180°. Note the axis quadrants in Figure 21-1. It's important to note that *right and left here are the right and left sides of the heart, not your right and left.* The 0° marking is thus on the left side and ±180° is on the right.

Axis Deviations

Axis deviations can be a normal variant. What are some other causes of axis deviations?

- Axis shifts away from infarcted tissue and toward hypertrophied tissue. Infarcted tissue does not conduct electrical current, so the current trav-

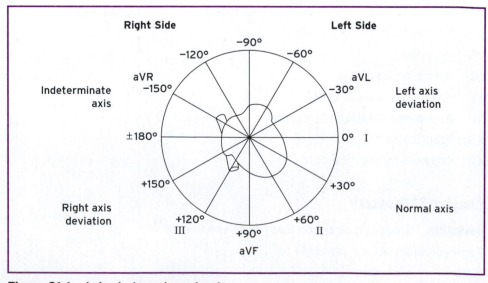

Figure 21-1 Axis circle and quadrants.

els away from this dead tissue, shifting the axis away. Hypertrophied tissue needs more current to depolarize it, so the current shifts toward it.

- Arrhythmias can cause axis deviation. Ventricular rhythms, for example, start in the ventricle and send their current upward toward the atria. The axis would then point upward rather than downward.

- Advanced pregnancy or obesity pushes the diaphragm and the heart upward, causing the axis to shift upward to the left.

- Chronic lung disease and pulmonary embolism cause a rightward axis shift because they enlarge the right ventricle.

Now let's learn how to calculate axis. There are four steps to axis calculation:

1. Determine the axis quadrant. Shade it in on the axis circle.
2. Find the lead with the most isoelectric QRS complexes.
3. Go to the perpendicular lead in the shaded quadrant.
4. Write down the degree marking at that lead. That's the axis.

How to Determine the Axis Quadrant

Think of the top half of the axis circle as the right and left arms and the entire bottom half of the circle as the left foot. Remember, the right foot is the ground electrode, so it doesn't count. Look at the QRS in leads I and aVF to determine the axis quadrant. Since lead I connects right and left arms, it tells us whether the axis is on the right or left side of the axis circle. If lead I's QRS is positive, the axis will be on the positive side of the lead I line, which is on the left half of the circle. (Remember, lead I is positive on the left arm.) Again, left and right refer to the left and right side of the heart as imagined inside the axis circle. If lead I's QRS is negative, the axis will be on the negative side of lead I, which is on the right side of the circle. Shade in the right or left half of the circle. See Figure 21-2.

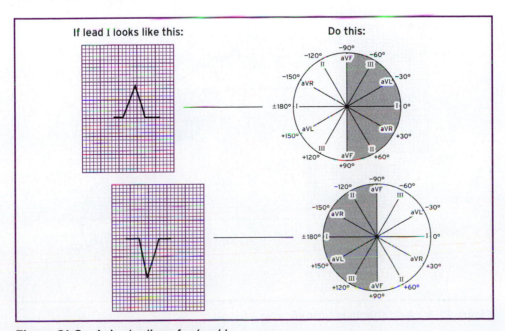

Figure 21-2 Axis shadings for lead I.

Lead aVF's positive pole is on the foot, so if aVF's QRS is positive, the axis will be on the lower half of the axis circle. A negative QRS in aVF will yield an axis on the top half of the circle. Shade in the top or bottom half of the circle. See Figure 21-3.

By combining the shadings for leads I and aVF, we find the axis quadrant. See Figure 21-4. If leads I and AVF's QRS complexes are both positive, shade in the left side and the bottom half of the axis circle. The shadings overlap in the lower left quadrant—the normal axis quadrant. If lead I is positive and aVF is negative, shade in the left side and the top half. The shadings overlap in the top left quadrant—the left axis deviation quadrant. If lead I is negative and aVF is positive, shade in the right side and the bottom half. The shadings overlap in the bottom right quadrant—the right axis deviation quadrant. If leads I and aVF are both negative, shade in the right side and the top half of the circle. The shadings overlap in the top right quadrant—the indeterminate axis quadrant.

How to Find the Lead with the Most Isoelectric QRS Complexes

The most **isoelectric** QRS complex is the one with the smallest mathematical difference between positive and negative deflections. The axis will be on the lead perpendicular to this isoelectric lead. Review the electrocardiographic truths from Chapter 7 if you need to. Examine leads I, II, III, aVR, aVL, and aVF to determine which is the most isoelectric. See Figure 21-5.

For each lead, count the positive deflection in millimeters. Then count the negative deflection. Subtract the smaller number from the larger. The one with the smallest difference between positive and negative deflections is the most isoelectric. In Figure 21-5,

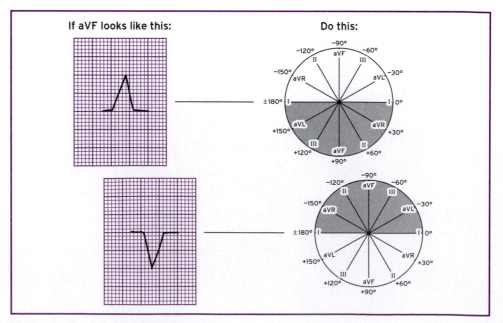

Figure 21-3 Axis shadings for aVF.

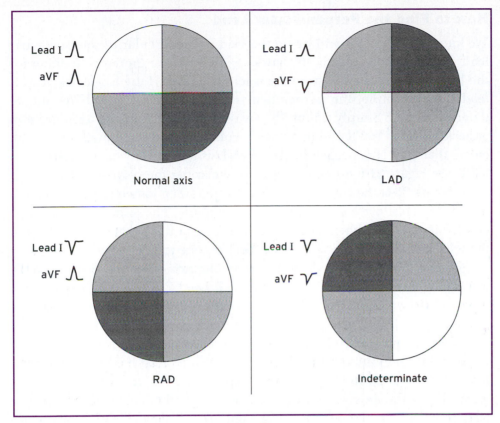

Figure 21-4 Determining the axis quadrant.

Lead I is 15 mm positive and 10 mm negative, giving a difference of 5 mm.

Lead II is 10 mm positive and 6 mm negative, with a difference of 4 mm.

Lead III is 10 mm positive and 9 mm negative, with a difference of 1 mm.

aVR is 5 mm positive and 15 mm negative, with a difference of 10 mm.

aVL is 15 mm positive and 13 mm negative, with a difference of 2 mm.

aVF is 3 mm positive and 0 mm negative, with a difference of 3 mm.

Lead III has the smallest difference between positive and negative; therefore it is the most isoelectric lead.

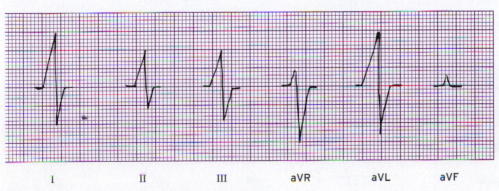

Figure 21-5 Which is the most isoelectric?

How to Find the Perpendicular Lead

We know that the axis will be on the lead perpendicular to the isoelectric lead. Perpendicular means "90° away from." We are therefore looking for the lead 90 degrees away from the isoelectric lead. If the isoelectric lead is lead I, for example, the perpendicular lead would be aVF. How did we determine that? Simply count 90° away from lead I on the axis circle in either direction. You'll end up on aVF. Following the same method, we calculate that lead II is perpendicular to aVL and lead III is perpendicular to aVR. See Figure 21-6 for an easy way to remember the perpendiculars.

In Figure 21-6, the leads are written in order, then joined in pairs from the outside in. This forms the perpendicular rainbow. The joined leads are perpendicular to each other. The degree marking at the perpendicular lead in the selected axis quadrant is the axis. Let's do one together. See Figure 21-7.

The first thing we must do is determine the axis quadrant. See Figure 21-8. We look at leads I and aVF in figure 21-7. Lead I's QRS is mostly positive (upward), so we know the axis will be on the left side of the axis circle. We shade that in. AVF is also positive, so we shade in the bottom half of the circle. From the quadrant selected, we know the axis will be normal.

Next, let's find the most isoelectric lead. Which lead has the smallest difference between positive and negative deflections? It's lead III.

We know the axis will be on the lead perpendicular to this isoelectric lead, so we look at the perpendicular rainbow and see that aVR is perpendicular to lead III. Our axis will be somewhere along aVR. But which end of aVR–the end that is −150° or the end that's +30°? That's easy. Our axis has to fall inside our selected quadrant. So the axis is +30°.

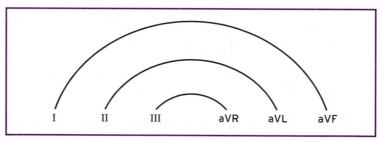

Figure 21-6 The perpendicular rainbow.

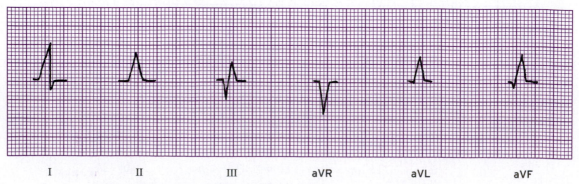

Figure 21-7 Axis practice EKG.

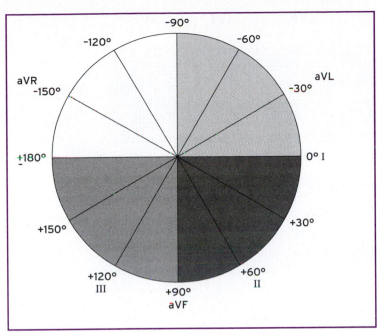

Figure 21-8 Axis circle for practice EKG.

Now you're ready for some more practice on your own.

Axis Practice EKGs

Calculate the axis on the following EKGs. Go step by step.

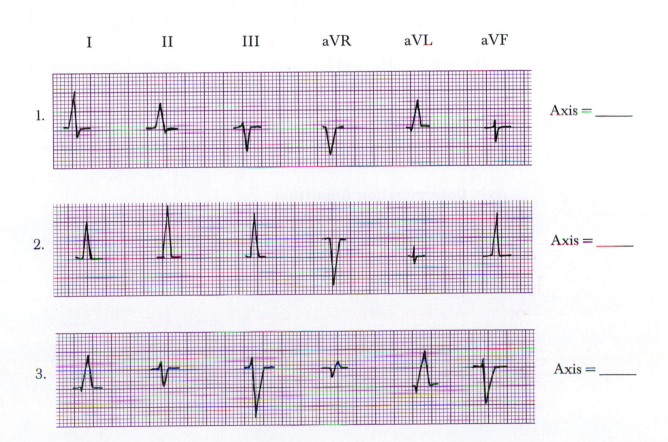

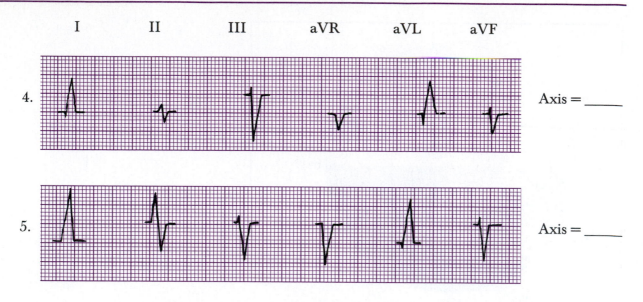

Answers to Axis Practice EKGs

1. **The axis is 0°.** Lead I is positive and aVF is negative, so there is a left axis deviation. The most isoelectric lead is aVF. Perpendicular to aVF is lead I. Lead I in our axis quadrant is 0°.

2. **The axis is +60°.** Lead I and aVF are both positive, so the axis is in the normal quadrant. The most isoelectric lead is aVL. Perpendicular to aVL is lead II. Lead II in our axis quadrant is at +60°.

3. **The axis is −60°.** Lead I is positive and aVF is negative, so we have a left axis deviation. The most isoelectric lead is aVR. Perpendicular to aVR is lead III. Lead III in our axis quadrant is at −60°.

4. **The axis is −30°.** Lead I is positive and aVF is negative, giving us a left axis deviation. The most isoelectric lead is lead II. Perpendicular to lead II is aVL. aVL in our axis quadrant is at −30°.

5. **The axis is −30°.** Lead I is positive and aVF is negative. There is a left axis deviation. The most isoelectric lead is lead II. Perpendicular to lead II is aVL. aVL in our axis quadrant is at −30°.

Axis Determination Algorithm

Now that you're proficient at calculating axis, here is a quick-and-dirty way to determine the axis when you're in a hurry. Just answer the questions and follow the arrows to the axis.

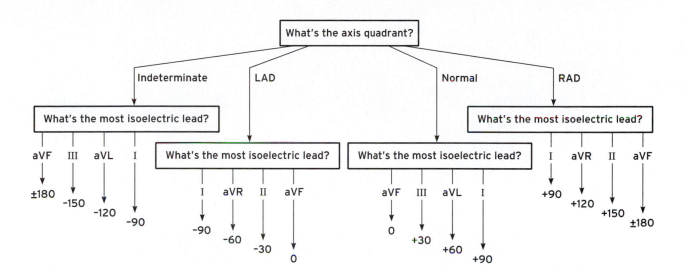

Practice Quiz

1. True or false: Axis deviation can be a normal variant.

2. Axis shifts toward _____ and away from _____

3. List the four steps in calculating the electrical axis. _____

    _____

    _____

    _____

4. True or false: If lead I's QRS complex is positive and aVF's is negative, the axis quadrant is in the indeterminate axis quadrant.

5. What effect would chronic lung disease have on the axis? _____

    _____

Practice Quiz Answers

1. **True.** Axis deviation can be a normal variant.

2. Axis shifts toward **hypertrophy** and away from **infarction.**

3. The four steps in calculating electrical axis are the following: **Determine the axis quadrant; find the most isoelectric lead; find the perpendicular lead in the axis quadrant; finally, write down the lead marking at that lead.**

4. **False.** If lead I is positive and aVF is negative, there is left axis deviation, not an indeterminate axis.

5. Chronic lung disease would **cause the axis to shift rightward.**

Intraventricular Conduction Defects

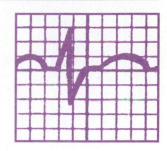

Chapter 22 Objectives

Upon completion of this chapter, the student will be able to:

- Draw the anatomy of the bundle branch system.
- Recognize normal QRS configuration in V_1 and V_6.
- Describe ventricular depolarization in V_1. Include septal and right ventricular depolarization as well as left ventricular depolarization.
- Recognize the RBBB pattern in V_1 and V_6.
- State the criteria for all bundle branch blocks (QRS interval, QRS configuration, T wave shape).
- Recognize the LBBB pattern in V_1 and V_6.
- Describe the clinical implications of BBB.
- State the causes of BBB.
- Define *rate-related BBB.*
- Define *critical rate.*
- Identify BBB on a variety of rhythm strips and EKGs.
- Define *hemiblock.*
- Recognize the LAHB pattern in leads I and III.
- Recognize the LPHB pattern in leads I and III.
- State the type of axis deviation associated with each type of hemiblock.
- Identify hemiblocks on a variety of EKGs.
- Correctly use the BBB/HB algorithm to identify BBBs and hemiblocks.
- Draw where the block is in the different kinds of bifascicular and trifascicular blocks.
- Relate the rhythm disturbances that can be a result of bifascicular and trifascicular blocks.

Chapter 22 Outline

I.   Introduction
II. Bundle branch blocks
    A. right bundle branch block, left bundle branch block
III. Summary of criteria for bundle branch blocks
IV. Clinical implications of bundle branch blocks

Chapter 22 Glossary

Bifascicular: Referring to two of the fascicles of the bundle branch system.

Critical rate: The heart rate at which a bundle branch block appears.

Fascicle: A branch of the left bundle branch; in a broader sense, can mean any of the branches of the bundle branch system.

Intermittent: Off and on.

Rate-related bundle branch block: A bundle branch block that appears at a certain critical rate.

Trifascicular: Referring to three of the fascicles of the bundle branch system, or to two fascicles plus a first-degree AV block.

Introduction

Intraventricular conduction defects (IVCDs) result from complete or partial blocks in the bundle branch system and result in abnormally shaped QRS complexes and often prolonged QRS intervals. IVCDs are seen only in supraventricular rhythms.

In Figure 22-1, note the normal anatomy of the bundle branch system. The right bundle branch is located on the right side of the interventricular septum. The left bundle branch is on the left side of the septum. The right bundle branch is all one main piece. The left bundle branch splits off into two branches called **fascicles.**

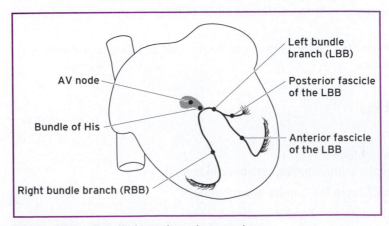

Figure 22-1 Bundle branch system anatomy.

Bundle Branch Blocks

Bundle branch blocks are interruptions in conduction through either the right or the left bundle branch. In order to understand the QRS complexes produced by bundle branch blocks, let's first review normal conduction through the bundle branch system. We'll look at leads V_1 and V_6, since those leads are the best for interpreting bundle branch blocks. See Figure 22-2.

Normally, the septum depolarizes left to right and the ventricles right to left. This means that although both ventricles begin activation simultaneously, the left ventricle completes its depolarization last because of its larger muscle bulk. In Figure 22-2, normal septal and right ventricular depolarization send the current toward the V_1 electrode, resulting in a small positive deflection. The rest of the current then travels toward the left ventricle, away from V_1's electrode. This results in a large negative deflection. Why is V_1 more negative than positive? Because most of the heart's current is traveling away from V_1's positive electrode toward the left ventricle, since that's where the larger muscle bulk is. You'll recall that an impulse traveling away from a positive electrode writes a negative deflection. V_1's QRS complex should therefore have a small R wave and a deeper S wave. It should be a predominantly negative QRS complex.

In V_6, just the opposite is seen. Septal and right ventricular depolarization send the current away from the V_6 electrode, resulting in a small negative deflection, a Q wave. Then the current travels toward the left ventricle and toward the V_6 electrode, thus writing a large positive deflection, an R wave. V_6 should be primarily positive. The other precordial leads show a gradual transition from negative to positive complexes.

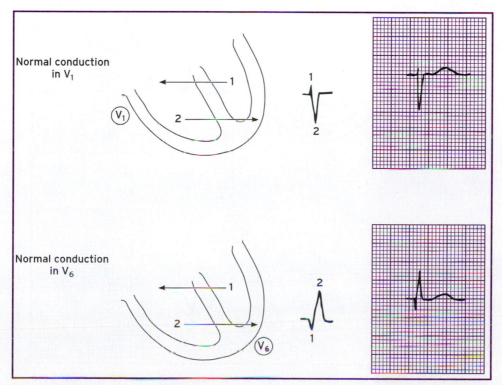

Figure 22-2 Normal conduction in V_1 and V_6: (1) septal and right ventricular activation, (2) left ventricular activation.

Right Bundle Branch Block (RBBB)

See Figure 22-3. In right bundle branch block (RBBB), septal depolarization begins normally, but, finding the right bundle branch blocked, the impulses must travel very slowly, cell by cell, through the right ventricle. Meanwhile, the healthy left bundle branch propels its impulses through the left ventricle as rapidly as usual. When left ventricular activation is complete, the impulses in the right ventricle are still trudging through the tissue, resulting in a large amount of unopposed current traveling toward the V_1 electrode. Thus, in V_1, an RBBB will have the normal R and S waves, but in addition will also have another R wave, signifying the final unopposed right ventricular forces heading toward the V_1 electrode. V_1 thus has an RSR' configuration. You'll recall a second R wave is called **R prime.** In V_6, the opposite is seen. Instead of an RSR', we see a QRS configuration with a wide terminal S wave. Since V_6 is on the opposite side of the heart as V_1, it sees the current moving in the opposite direction.

On occasion with RBBB, the initial R wave in V_1 may be missing because of a previous MI.

All bundle branch blocks will have a QRS interval of ≥0.12 and a T wave that slopes off opposite the terminal wave of the QRS complex. If the terminal wave of the QRS is upward, for example, the T wave will be inverted. If the terminal wave of the QRS is downward, the T wave will be upright. See Figure 22-3. In V_1, the QRS interval is 0.14 second and the terminal wave of the QRS is upright, so the T wave is inverted. In V_6, the QRS interval is 0.14 second and the terminal wave of the QRS is downward. The T is therefore upright. It is important to recognize these bundle-related T waves so as not to misinter-

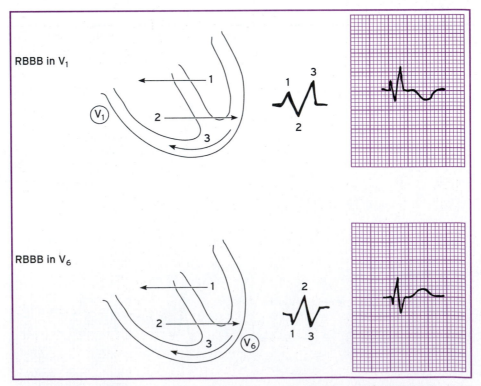

Figure 22-3 RBBB in V_1 and V_6: (1) septal and beginning right ventricular activation, (2) left ventricular activation, (3) final right ventricular activation.

pret them as signs of ischemia. An RBBB configuration with a QRS interval of 0.10 to 0.11 second is considered an *incomplete RBBB*. See Figure 22-4 for a RBBB on a 12-lead EKG.

Left Bundle Branch Block (LBBB)

See Figure 22-5. In left bundle branch block (LBBB), septal depolarization cannot occur normally. It must go backward, right to left, sending its current away from V_1's positive electrode. When the current reaches the left ventricle, it finds the bundle branch blocked and must traverse the left ventricular tissue very slowly, one cell at a time. Meanwhile, right ventricular activation occurs normally, thanks to the healthy right bundle branch. This sends the current toward V_1's electrode. Soon, right ventricular depolarization is complete, while the left ventricular forces still march slowly away from V_1's electrode. Thus in theory, an LBBB in V_1 should have a QRS configuration. However, since the left ventricular forces create such a large amount of current, the QR waves are swallowed up by the huge final S wave. LBBB in V_1 thus presents as a large, deep QS complex in V_1. On occasion, there may be a small R wave preceding the deep S wave. V_6 will show the opposite—a large, monophasic R wave. The QS and the R waves in an LBBB may be notched.

As with an RBBB, the QRS interval of an LBBB will be ≥0.12 second and the T wave will be opposite the terminal wave of the QRS complex. An LBBB configuration with a QRS interval of 0.10 to 0.11 second is considered an *incomplete LBBB*.

See Figure 22-6 for an LBBB on a 12-lead EKG.

See Figure 22-7 for a summary of the criteria for bundle branch blocks.

Rate Related BBB

Bundle branch blocks are not necessarily permanent. Sometimes they are intermittent, seen only at certain heart rates. This is known as a **rate-related bundle branch block,** and the rate at which the BBB appears is called the **critical rate.** In this disorder, conduction through the bundle branches is normal at heart rates below the critical rate. Once the critical rate is reached, however, one of the bundle branches becomes incapable of depolarizing rapidly enough to allow normal conduction, resulting in a BBB. When the heart rate falls below the critical rate, bundle branch depolarization returns to normal and the BBB disappears.

Clinical Implications of BBB

Bundle branch blocks do not cause symptoms. In fact, they *are* a symptom that the conduction system is impaired. The question is, what's causing the BBB? See Table 22-1.

Though RBBB can be seen in normal healthy hearts, LBBB almost always implies extensive cardiac disease. Patients with bundle branch block are at risk for developing severe AV blocks, so it is important to observe their rhythm closely for further signs of conduction disturbance, such as a new first-degree AV block or the development of hemiblocks (see following section). *A new bundle branch block should prompt an immediate assessment of the*

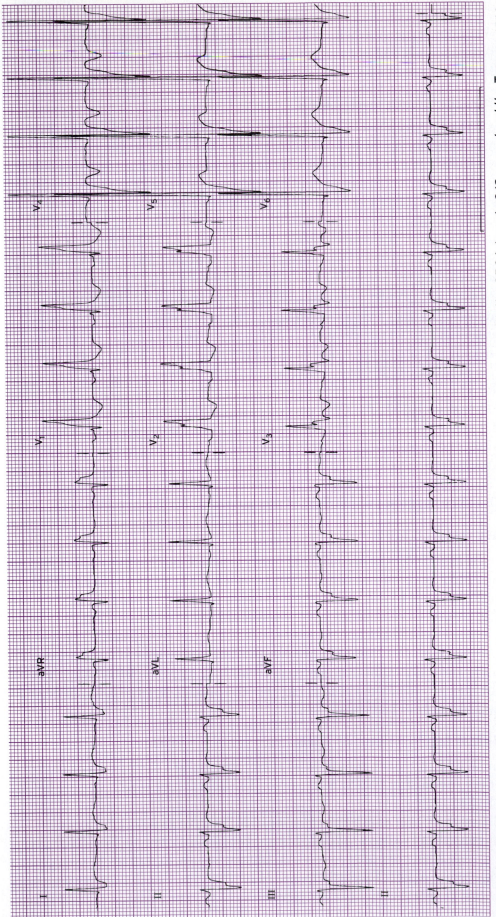

Figure 22-4 Right bundle branch block. Note the RSR' in V₁ and the QRS configuration in V₆, along with the QRS interval ≥0.12 second and the T waves opposite the terminal QRS wave.

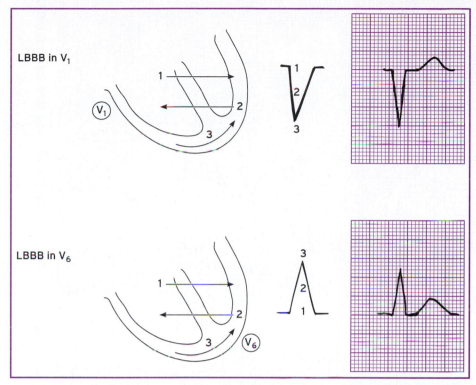

Figure 22-5 LBBB in V₁ and V₆: (1) septal and beginning left ventricular activation, (2) right ventricular activation, (3) final left ventricular activation.

patient. A 12-lead EKG should be done in an effort to determine the cause of the BBB. Remember–the BBB is a symptom of another problem. For example, the BBB might be a result of an MI in progress. Also remember that BBBs cause T wave changes that can be misinterpreted as ischemia. Anterior wall MIs usually cannot be diagnosed in the presence of an LBBB, as the bundle-related changes mask the MI.

Hemiblocks

A hemiblock is a block of one of the fascicles of the left bundle branch. There are two kinds of hemiblocks: **left anterior hemiblock (LAHB),** a block in the left anterior fascicle of the left bundle branch, and **left posterior hemiblock (LPHB),** a block in the posterior fascicle of the left bundle

Table 22-1 Causes of RBBB and LBBB

TYPE OF BBB	CAUSES
RBBB	• Coronary artery disease • Conduction system lesion • Normal variant • Right ventricular hypertrophy • Congenital heart disease • Right ventricular dilatation
LBBB	• Coronary artery disease • Conduction system lesion • Hypertension • Other organic heart disease

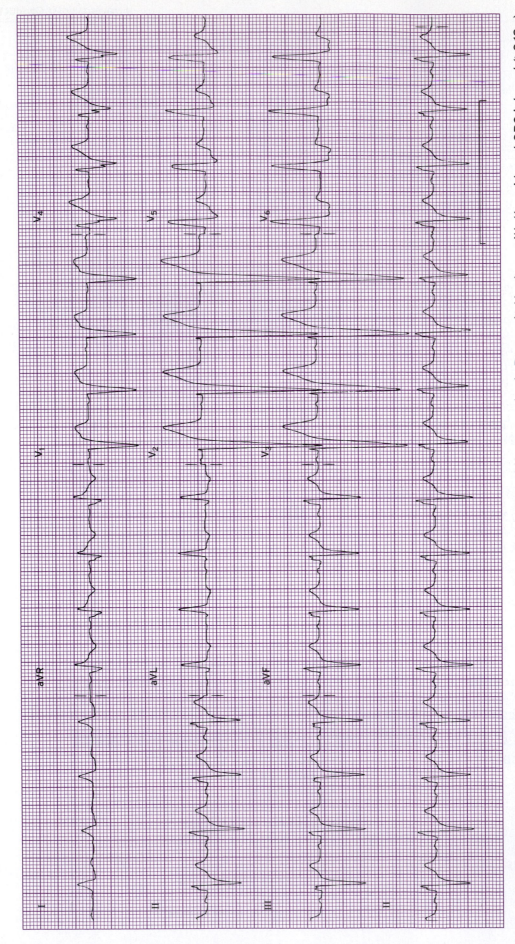

Figure 22-6 Left bundle branch block. Note the RS configuration in V_1 and the monophasic R wave in V_6 along with the widened QRS interval ($\geq$0.12 s) and the T wave opposite the terminal wave of the QRS.

	QRS configuration in V₁	QRS configuration in V₆	QRS interval	T wave
RBBB	RSR′	QRS (wide terminal S)	≥0.12 s	Opposite the terminal QRS
LBBB	QS or RS	Monophasic R	≥0.12 s	Opposite the terminal QRS

Figure 22-7 Summary of criteria for bundle branch blocks.

branch. To find hemiblocks, we look in leads I and III. Let's review the normal QRS configuration in leads I and III. See Figure 22-8.

In Figure 22-8, we see that the QRS complexes in leads I and III are both normally positive, with QRS intervals <0.12 second. In hemiblocks, the QRS interval remains normal, but one of those leads will have negative QRS complexes.

In left anterior hemiblock, lead I has a small Q wave and a taller R wave. Lead III has a small R wave and a deeper S wave. Lead III therefore has a negative QRS deflection in left anterior hemiblock. See Figure 22-9.

In addition to the QRS configuration, there must also be a left axis deviation of at least −30 degrees or more. Without a leftward axis shift, LAHB cannot be diagnosed. LAHB is fairly common and is often seen together with RBBB. In fact, *a left axis deviation in the presence of an RBBB almost always*

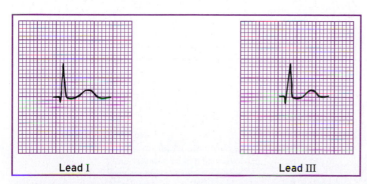

Figure 22-8 Normal QRS configuration in leads I and III.

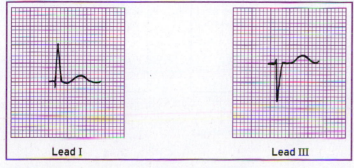

Figure 22-9 QRS configuration in LAHB.

implies a coexisting LAHB. Sometimes the LAHB can distort the shape of a RBBB in V₁ by making the initial R wave very tiny or absent. The left anterior fascicle has a single blood supply—the left anterior descending coronary artery—and is therefore vulnerable in the event of ischemia or infarction. See Figure 22-10 for LAHB on a 12-lead EKG.

Left posterior hemiblock is much less common than LAHB, as the posterior fascicle has a dual blood supply—the circumflex and right coronary arteries. It has a small R and a deeper S in lead I and a small Q and taller R wave in lead III. In LPHB, then, lead I has the negative QRS complex. See Figure 22-11.

LPHB requires a rightward axis shift, often of +120 degrees or more. Sometimes the axis shift of a LPHB is apparent only when comparing the axis of the present EKG to that of previous EKGs done before the LPHB appeared. LPHBs are extremely rare on their own; they are more likely to be seen together with an RBBB. A right axis deviation in the presence of an RBBB indicates an LPHB may be present. Even so, LPHB is not common. See Figure 22-12 for LPHB on a 12-lead EKG.

Causes of hemiblocks are the same as for bundle branch blocks. Let's summarize the criteria for recognition of LAHB and LPHB. See Figure 22-13.

Bundle Branch Block/Hemiblock Algorithm

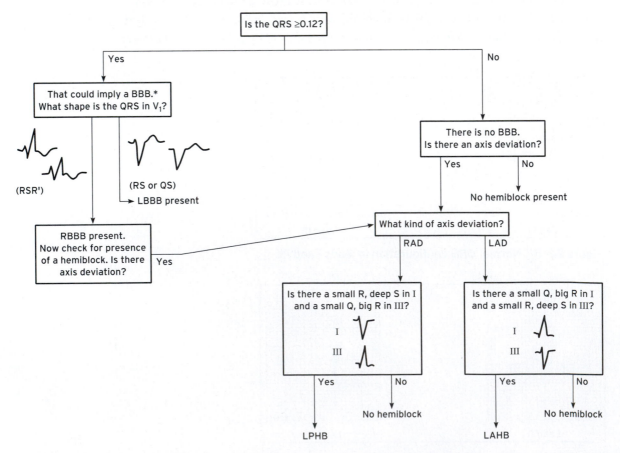

*Wide QRS complexes could be ventricular in origin, rather than a BBB. We'll go over this more in Chapter 23.

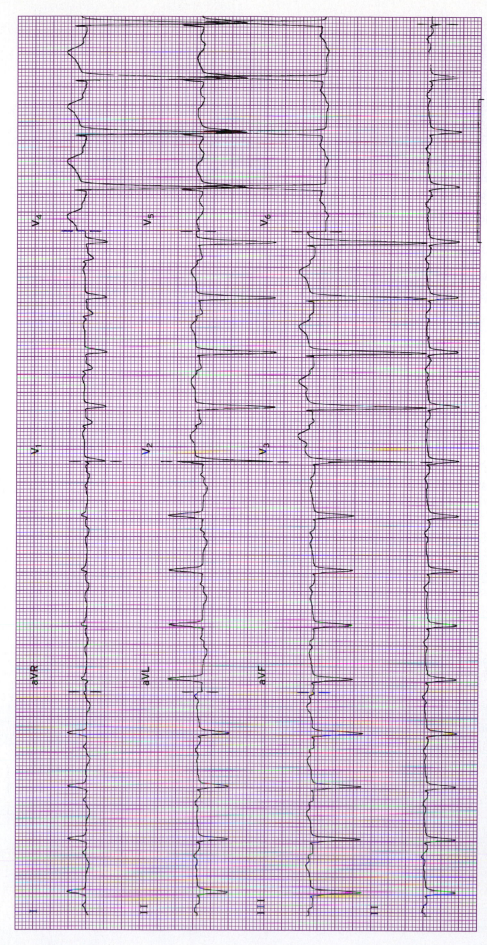

Figure 22-10 Left anterior hemiblock. Note the small Q and taller R in lead I and the small R and deeper S in lead III, along with a left axis deviation of −30°. QRS interval is <0.12 second.

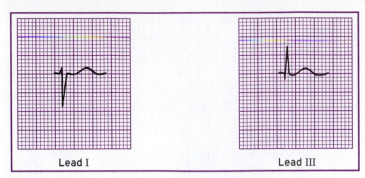

Figure 22-11 QRS configuration in LPHB.

Bifascicular and Trifascicular Blocks

Since the left bundle branch has two fascicles and the right bundle branch provides a third highway for AV conduction, it is common practice clinically to refer to those three highways as three fascicles. If two of those fascicles are blocked, it is called **bifascicular block.** There are several kinds of bifascicular block. See Figure 22-14.

When the term *bifascicular block* is used, most often it refers to RBBB + LAHB. **Trifascicular block** is also possible. There are several possible kinds. See Figure 22-15.

Timely conduction through the AV node is crucial when two of the three bundle branch fascicles are blocked, as the AV node represents the last hope for conduction to reach that one bundle branch fascicle that's still open. First-degree AV block impairs that AV conduction. When the term *trifascicular block* is used, most often it refers to RBBB + LAHB + first-degree AVB.

What are the clinical implications of bifascicular and trifascicular blocks? Having multiple areas of block increases the risk of developing second- or third-degree AV blocks. Let's look at that in more detail.

Bifascicular blocks that intermittently become trifascicular can result in 2:1 AV block or type II second-degree AVB:

- RBBB + LAHB + intermittent LPHB
- RBBB + LPHB + intermittent LAHB
- LBBB + intermittent RBBB
- RBBB + intermittent LBBB

If a fascicle is only intermittently blocked, that means it is open at all other times. Therefore, at least one of the highways to the ventricles is usually open, and conduction can take place then. When that one remaining fascicle becomes intermittently blocked, conduction is not possible, and a dropped QRS occurs. See Figures 22-16 and 22-17.

Certain trifascicular blocks can result in third-degree AVB:

- RBBB + LAHB + LPHB
- RBBB + LBBB

If the fascicles are all permanently blocked, third-degree AV block is the result. There is no conduction possible because all the highways to the ventricles are closed, so an escape pacemaker must take over to depolarize the ventricle and provide the QRS complex. See Figure 22-18.

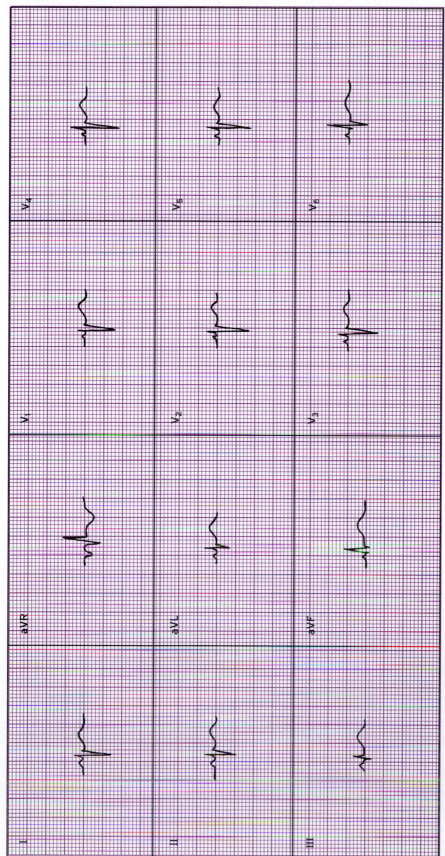

Figure 22-12 Left posterior hemiblock. Note the small R and deeper S in lead I and the small Q and taller R in lead III, along with a right axis deviation.

	Lead I	**Lead III**	**QRS interval**	**Axis**
LAHB	Small Q, taller R	Small R, deeper S	<0.12	Left axis deviation
LPHB	Small R, deeper S	Small Q, taller R	<0.12	Right axis deviation

Figure 22-13   Summary of criteria for hemiblocks.

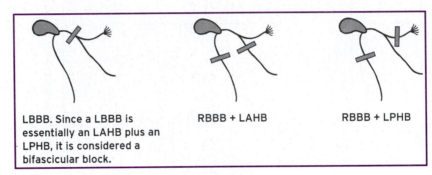

Figure 22-14   Kinds of bifascicular block.

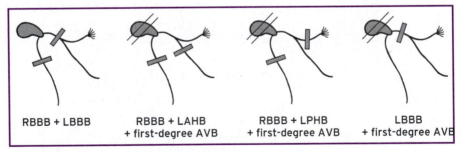

Figure 22-15   Kinds of trifascicular block.

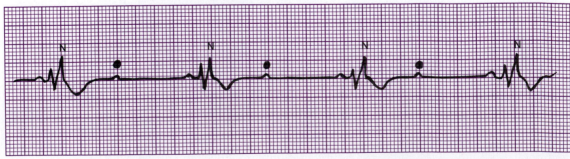

Figure 22-16   2:1 AV block. N = BBB alone or with hemiblock. Conduction is otherwise normal. The dots reveal a sudden block of the other bundle branch or fascicle, causing a dropped QRS.

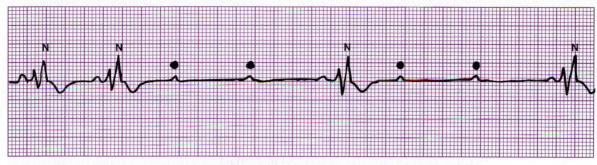

Figure 22-17 Type II second-degree AV block. N = BBB alone or with hemiblock. Conduction is otherwise normal. The dots represent a sudden block of the other bundle branch or fascicle, causing a QRS to be dropped.

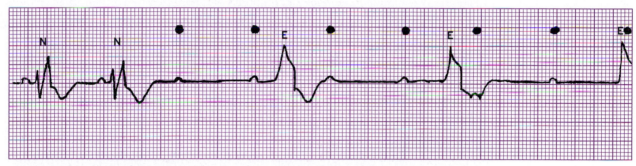

Figure 22-18 Third-degree AV block. N = BBB alone or with hemiblock. The dots represent the block of the other bundle branch. No conduction to the ventricle is possible. E = escape beats that emerge to provide the QRS.

Treatment of Bi- and Trifascicular Blocks

Bifascicular blocks warrant no more than careful monitoring to assess for any deterioration into trifascicular block. In the past, trifascicular blocks were routinely treated with permanent pacemaker insertion. However, because many of the patients with trifascicular block never develop heart block and therefore never benefit from a pacemaker, current thinking suggests it is more prudent to monitor the rhythm closely and insert a pacemaker only if significant AV block develops.

IVCD Practice

1. Type of IVCD (if any): _____

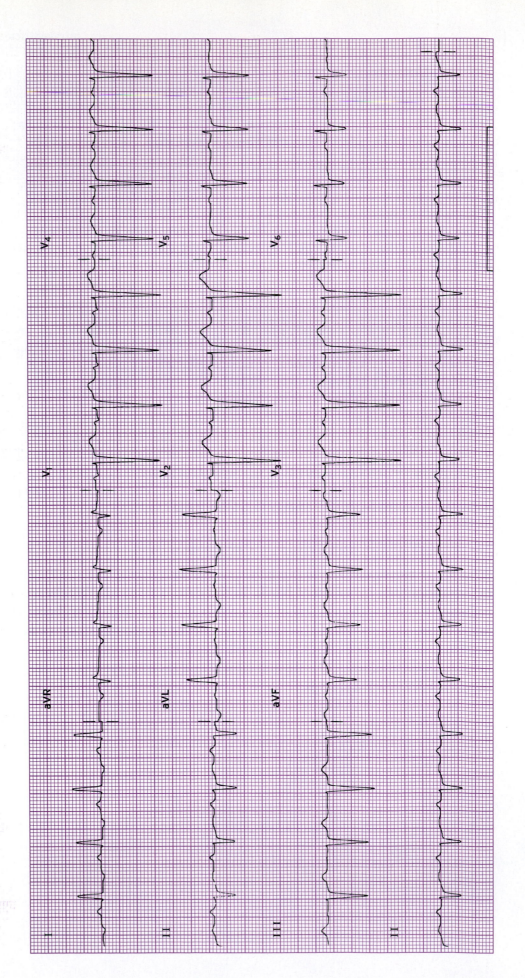

2. Type of IVCD (if any): ______________________

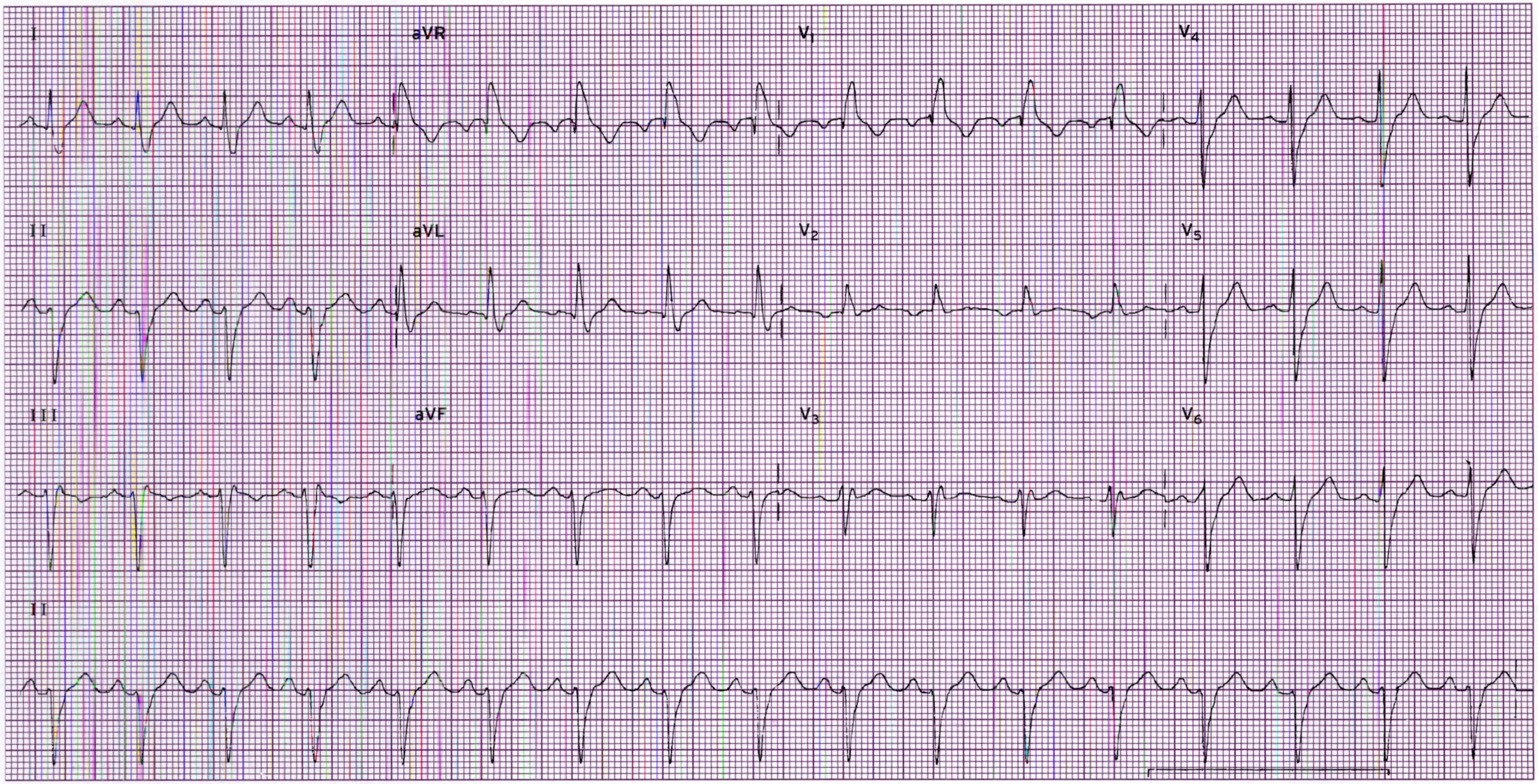

3. Type of IVCD (if any): _____

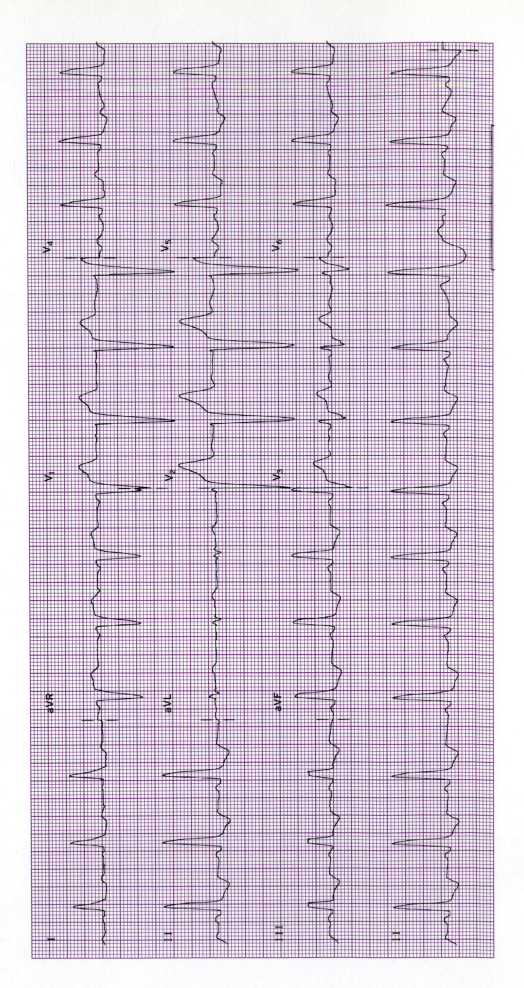

4. Type of IVCD (if any): _____

IVCD Practice (continued)

5. Type of IVCD (if any): _____

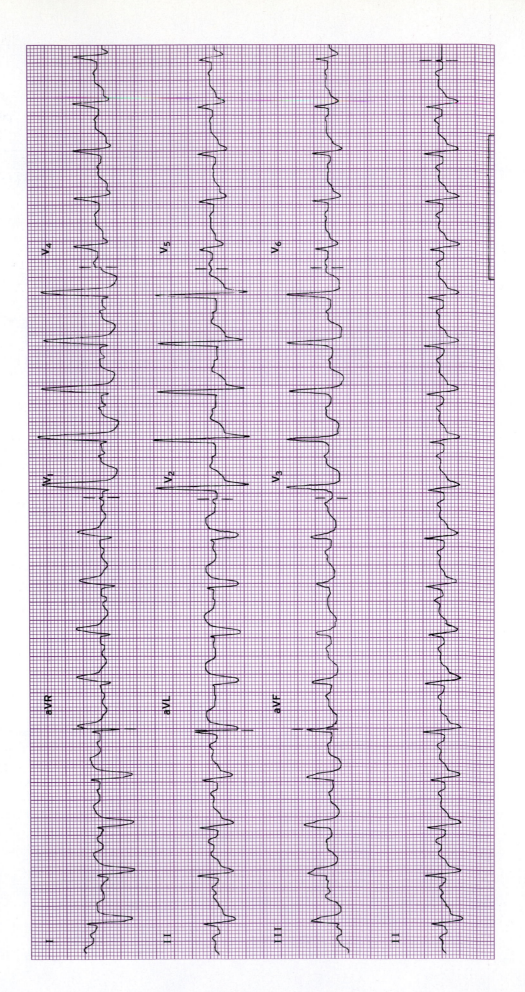

Answers to IVCD Practice

1. **LAHB.** Note the left axis deviation of about −60°. Lead I has a QR configuration and lead III has an RS. The QRS interval is normal (about 0.08 s), so there is no BBB.

2. **RBBB + LAHB.** There is not the typical RSR′ configuration in V_1–the initial R wave is missing–but it is still an RBBB. The QRS is wide (about 0.12 s) and there is a wide terminal S wave in V_6. The T wave slopes off opposite the terminal wave of the QRS complex. There is a left axis deviation of about −90°. You'll recall that a left axis deviation in the presence of an RBBB is almost always indicative of an accompanying LAHB. In fact, the LAHB may be the reason for the loss of the initial R wave in V_1. Or the patient may have had a previous MI that caused a permanent loss of the initial R wave in V_1.

3. **LBBB.** There is a wide QRS (about 0.14 s), a QS complex in V_1, and a monophasic R wave in V_6. The T wave is opposite the terminal part of the QRS.

4. **LBBB.** Again, there is a wide QRS of about 0.13 second, a QS in V_1, and a monophasic R wave in V_6. The T wave is opposite the terminal wave of the QRS complex.

5. **RBBB + possible LPHB.** There is a wide QRS with a QR configuration in V_1 along with a wide terminal S wave in V_6. In addition, there is a right axis deviation of about +150°. This right axis deviation may be caused by an LPHB, but other things can cause this axis shift (we'll get to that in Chapter 24), so the best we can say is that there is a *possible* LPHB. Remember, LPHB is pretty rare. You may see only a few in a lifetime.

Practice Quiz

1. Normal conduction through the bundle branches produces a QRS complex with an interval of what duration? _____

2. A bundle branch block causes the QRS interval to _____

3. In V_1, what is the typical shape of the right bundle branch block? _____

4. In V_1, what is the typical shape of the left bundle branch block? _____

5. Which two coronary arteries supply blood to the left posterior fascicle of the left bundle branch? _____

6. What kind of axis is associated with a left anterior hemiblock? _____

7. What kind of axis is associated with a left posterior hemiblock? _____

8. A bifascicular block is a block of _____ fascicles of the bundle branch system.

9. A permanent trifascicular block can result in what kind of arrhythmia?

10. True or false: First-degree AV block puts conduction to the bundle branches in jeopardy.

Practice Quiz Answers

1. Normal conduction through the bundle branches produces a QRS complex with an interval of **less than 0.12 second.**

2. A bundle branch block causes the QRS interval to **become longer, to ≥0.12 second.**

3. In V_1, the typical shape of a right bundle branch block is **RSR′.**

4. In V_1, the typical shape of a left bundle branch block is **QS** or **RS.**

5. The two coronary arteries that supply blood to the posterior fascicle of the left bundle branch are the **circumflex** and **right coronary arteries.**

6. A **left axis deviation** is associated with a left anterior hemiblock.

7. A **right axis deviation** is associated with a left posterior hemiblock.

8. A bifascicular block is a block of **two** fascicles of the bundle branch system.

9. A permanent trifascicular block can result in **third-degree AV block.**

10. **True.** First-degree AV block puts conduction to the bundle branches in jeopardy.

Aberration versus Ectopy

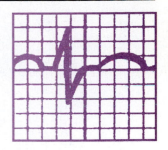

Chapter 23 Objectives

Upon completion of this chapter, the student will be able to:

- Define *aberration*.
- Define *ectopy*.
- List the features favoring aberration.
- List the features favoring ectopy.
- Distinguish between aberration and ectopy on a variety of EKGs and rhythm strips.

Chapter 23 Outline

I. Introduction

II. Features favoring aberration
   A. Triphasic QRS, preceding P waves, same initial deflection, second in a row, same morphology

III. Features favoring ventricular ectopy
   A. Taller left rabbit ear in V_1, indeterminate axis, concordancy in precordial leads, fusion beats, R-on-T phenomenon, absence of atrial activity

IV. Aberration versus ectopy, practice

V. Answers to aberration versus ectopy practice

VI. Practice quiz

VII. Practice quiz answers

Chapter 23 Glossary

Aberration: The temporary abnormality of ventricular conduction that results in an abnormally shaped, and often abnormally widened, QRS complex.

Concordancy: QRS complexes all having either a positive deflection or a negative deflection in the precordial leads.

Ectopy: Beats that arise from a pacemaker other than the sinus node. Understood to mean ventricular beats if the kind of ectopy is not specified.

Triphasic: Having three waves.

Introduction

Aberration is the temporary abnormality of ventricular conduction that results in an abnormally shaped, and often abnormally widened, QRS complex. Aberration occurs when a premature supraventricular impulse arrives at the conduction system while one or more fascicles of the bundle branch system is still refractory from the previous beat. The impulse then is delayed in its travel through the ventricle. Aberration can involve a bundle branch block, a hemiblock, or both.

Ectopy means the beat or rhythm in question originated in a pacemaker other than the sinus node. There can be atrial ectopy in the form of PACs and atrial arrhythmias, junctional ectopy in the form of PJCs and junctional arrhythmias, and ventricular ectopy in the form of PVCs and ventricular arrhythmias. *If the type of ectopy is not specified, it is understood to be ventricular.* For example, saying the patient is "having a lot of ectopy" does not specify what kind of ectopy. It is understood, then, that this implies ventricular ectopy (PVCs). Saying that the patient is having atrial ectopy means PACs. If the patient has an ectopic atrial rhythm, then he or she has an atrial arrhythmia of some sort.

Aberration and ectopy can involve single beats or entire rhythms. Wide QRS complex tachycardias are especially difficult to interpret. Do they represent v-tach (ectopy)? Or are they SVT with a bundle branch block (aberration)? It is an important distinction because treatment is markedly different for the two. Let's look at some features that help in differentiating them.

Features Favoring Aberration

Triphasic QRS

Triphasic contour of the QRS complex (RSR′ in V_1 and/or QRS in V_6) indicates aberration. *Triphasic* means having three waves. This is a right bundle branch block pattern. Ventricular beats almost never have triphasic contours. See Figure 23-1.

Preceding P Waves

P waves preceding ("married to") the wide QRS complexes indicates the rhythm is originating in a pacemaker above the ventricle. A wide QRS in this case would be the result of aberrant conduction through the bundle branch system. See Figure 23-2.

In Figure 23-2, note the premature wide QRS complex (number 4). Also note the abnormal P wave preceding that QRS complex. It's on the downstroke of beat number 3's T wave. See it? This is sinus bradycardia with an

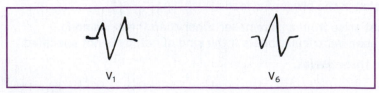

Figure 23-1 Triphasic contours of QRS complexes in V_1 and V_6.

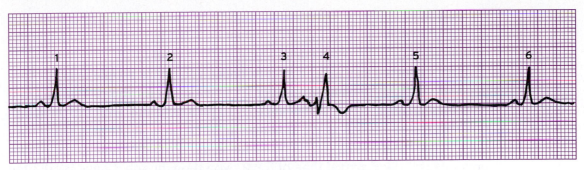

Figure 23-2   Wide QRS beat with preceding P wave.

aberrantly conducted PAC. Reread Chapter 13 (on atrial arrhythmias), particularly the section on PACs, if you've forgotten its criteria.

Same Initial Deflection

Aberration is indicated if the initial deflection of the wide QRS beat or beats is the same as the initial deflection of the surrounding narrow QRS beats. If the initial deflection is the same, then septal and right ventricular depolarization start out the same. This can happen only if the rhythm is originating above the ventricle and heading down the conduction pathway from above, not starting in the bottom (the ventricle) and working its way up. See Figure 23-3.

In Figure 23-3 the third QRS complex is wide. Its initial deflection is the same as the surrounding narrow QRS beats, making it an aberrant beat.

Second-in-a-Row Beat

When the only funny-looking beat is the second beat in a group of rapid beats, aberration is indicated. The second beat in a group of rapid beats is the only one that ends a short R-R cycle preceded by a long R-R cycle. See Figure 23-4. The other beats end a short cycle preceded by a short cycle. The bundle branch refractory period is dependent on the previous R-R cycle length (R-R interval). If there is a long previous R-R cycle, the refractory period is long. If the previous R-R interval is short, the refractory period is short. A long cycle followed by a short cycle results in aberration because

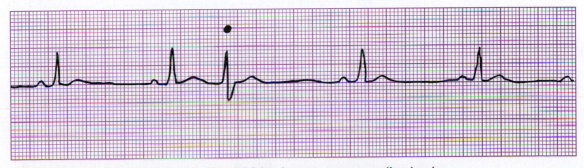

Figure 23-3   Initial deflection of wide QRS beat same as surrounding beats.

the short-cycle impulse arrives at the bundle branches only to find them still partially refractory. This impulse is then delayed in traveling through the ventricles. This delay results in an abnormally shaped QRS.

Here's another way to look at it: Suppose you invite people over for supper and tell them to come whenever it's convenient for them. The first two days they arrive at 5 P.M. The next day you plan your day with the presumption that the guests will arrive at about the same time. What happens if they show up at 3 P.M.? Will you be ready for them? Probably not. Based on the previous two days' arrival time of 5 P.M., you thought you'd have more time to prepare. You have to scramble to prepare everything, and this results in the afternoon going a bit differently than before (aberrant). The next day, you'll be ready at 3 P.M., just in case, won't you? It's the *first* time they arrive early that causes the real problem, and if they come at 3 P.M. thereafter, you're ready. It's the same with the heart's early beats. The first early beat is the one that is "funny-looking." It is so early, it's completely unexpected, and it goes down the pathway in an abnormal (aberrant) manner. The next beat that comes in with the same short R-R cycle can go down the normal way because the conduction system's refractory period has shortened along with the previous R-R interval. This keeps it from getting caught off guard again. See Figure 23-4.

In Figure 23-4, R-R cycles A-B and B-C are relatively long. Beat D comes in early and is wider than the other beats. C-D is a short R-R cycle, as are the other cycles that follow. If you had to draw a circle around the group of rapid beats, you would circle C to K. Because D is the second in this group of rapid beats and is the only one that's "funny-looking," D is aberrant rather than ectopic.

Same Morphology

Aberration is indicated when the wide QRS complex of the beat or rhythm in question has the same morphology as that of a known supraventricular aberrant beat or rhythm. In other words, if the beat or rhythm in question has a wide QRS complex that is the same shape as when the patient was in, say, sinus rhythm with a left bundle branch block, then this wide QRS is also a left bundle branch block. It would be extremely unlikely for an ectopic QRS to have exactly the same morphology as the patient's known supraventricular aberrant QRS. See Figure 23-5.

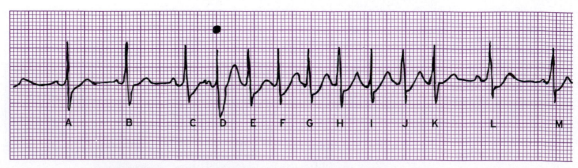

Figure 23-4 Second beat in a group of rapid beats.

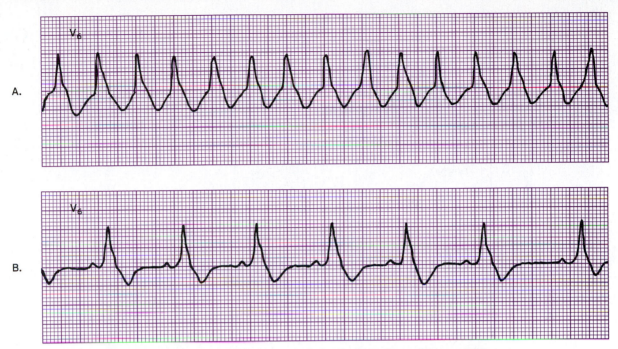

Figure 23-5   (a) The rhythm in question; (b) an obvious sinus rhythm with an LBBB.

In Figure 23-5, both rhythms are from the same patient. In Figure 23-5(a) there is a wide QRS tachycardia. In Figure 23-5(b), we see the same QRS, but this time in an obvious sinus arrhythmia with an LBBB. Thus the wide QRS of the tachycardia is also an LBBB, not ectopic ventricular.

Now let's look at some features that favor ventricular ectopy.

Features Favoring Ventricular Ectopy

Taller Left Rabbit Ear in V₁

It is unusual for an aberrant beat to have this morphology. A taller left rabbit ear is much more suggestive that the beat or rhythm is ventricular in origin (ectopic). See Figure 23-6.

Indeterminate Axis

An axis between −90 and −180 degrees is unusual, though not impossible, for aberrantly conducted supraventricular beats. If it is seen in conjunction with other ectopic-favoring factors (such as absence of atrial activity), however, it is more suggestive of ectopy. See Figure 23-7.

In Figure 23-7, if the QRS in lead I and aVF are both negative, this gives us an axis in the indeterminate quadrant. This likely implies a ventricular ectopic origin for the rhythm in question, but look for other factors as well.

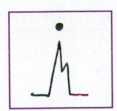

Figure 23-6   Taller left rabbit ear.

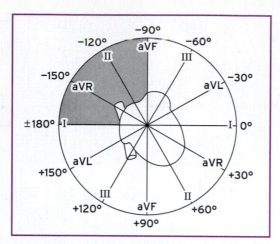

Figure 23-7 Indeterminate axis.

Concordancy in Precordial Leads

This means that precordial leads are either all positive or all negative. Though concordancy favors ectopy, it can be seen at times in aberrant supraventricular rhythms. It is more likely to favor ectopy if there are other ectopy-favoring factors as well. See Figure 23-8.

Note that the precordial leads in Figure 23-8 are all negative. This, combined with the lack of preceding atrial activity, tells us the rhythm is probably ectopic. Here, the rhythm is v-tach.

Presence of Fusion Beats

If fusion beats are present, it implies the ventricle has been firing. Wide QRS beats in the presence of fusion beats are therefore likely to be ectopic. See Figure 23-9.

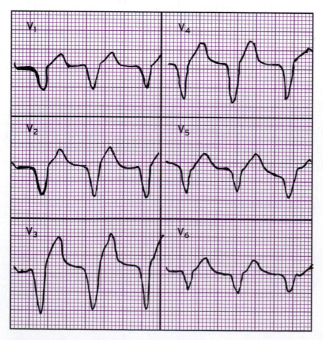

Figure 23-8 Negative concordancy.

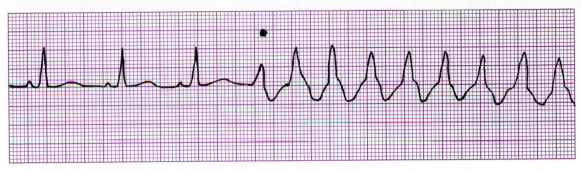

Figure 23-9 Fusion beat preceding a run of v-tach.

On the strip in Figure 23-9, note sinus rhythm, then nine rapid beats with a wide QRS. Note the dot over the fusion beat that starts off the run of v-tach. The fusion beat implies that the wide QRS beats that follow are ventricular (ectopic) rather than aberrant.

R-on-T Phenomenon

A premature wide QRS complex that lands on the T wave of the preceding beat is diagnostic of ectopy rather than aberration. *The P wave of aberrant PACs or PJCs can land on the T wave, but their QRS complexes don't.* If a wide QRS beat lands on the T wave, it's ectopic. See Figure 23-10.

In Figure 23-10, note that the wide QRS beat lands on the T wave of the preceding beat. This is a PVC (ectopic).

Absence of Atrial Activity (or dissociated if present)

Ventricular ectopic beats typically do not have P waves associated with them. Sometimes v-tach will have an occasional dissociated P wave. See Figure 23-11.

In Figure 23-11(a), note the wide QRS and the lack of P waves. This is classic v-tach (ectopy). In Figure 23-11(b), again we have the wide QRS complexes, but now look at the P waves under the dots. They are not in the same place relative to the QRS complexes, and indeed Ps are not even seen on most beats. These Ps are dissociated from the QRS complexes, which indicates that the rhythm is probably ectopic ventricular rather than aberrant. This is v-tach.

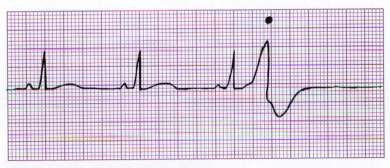

Figure 23-10 R-on-T phenomenon.

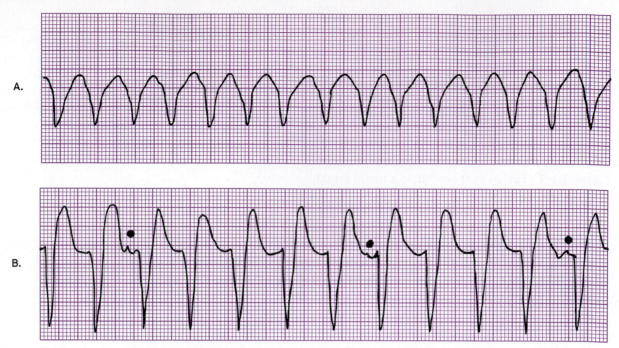

Figure 23-11 (a) Shows no P waves. (b) Shows dissociated P waves. Both have wide QRS complexes.

Now you're ready for some practice.

Aberration versus Ectopy, Practice

1. Aberration or ectopy? _____

If aberration, what kind (RBBB, LBBB, RBBB + LAHB, or RBBB + LPHB? _____

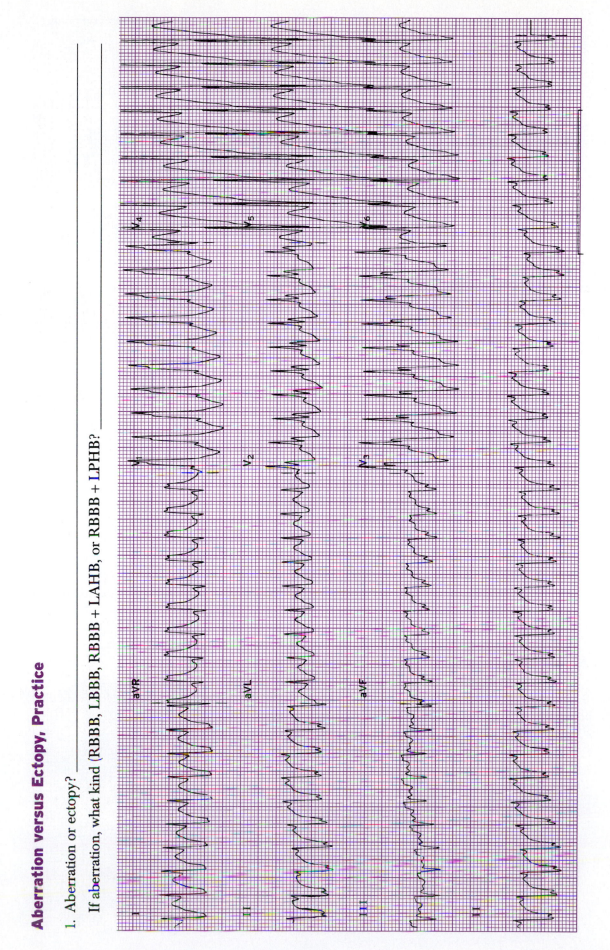

Aberration versus Ectopy, Practice (continued)

2. Aberration or ectopy? _____

   If aberration, what kind? _____

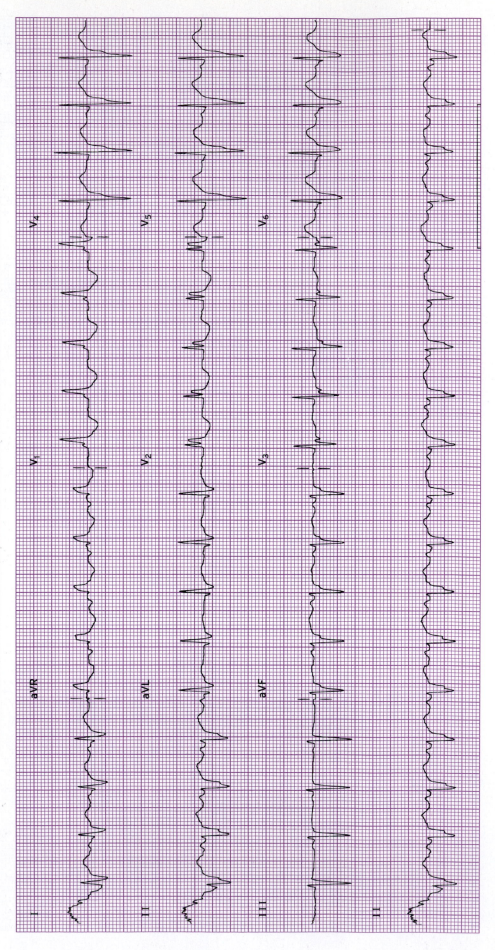

3. Aberration or ectopy? ____________________

If aberration, what kind? ____________________

I
aVR
V1
V4
II
aVL
V2
V5
III
aVF
V3
V6

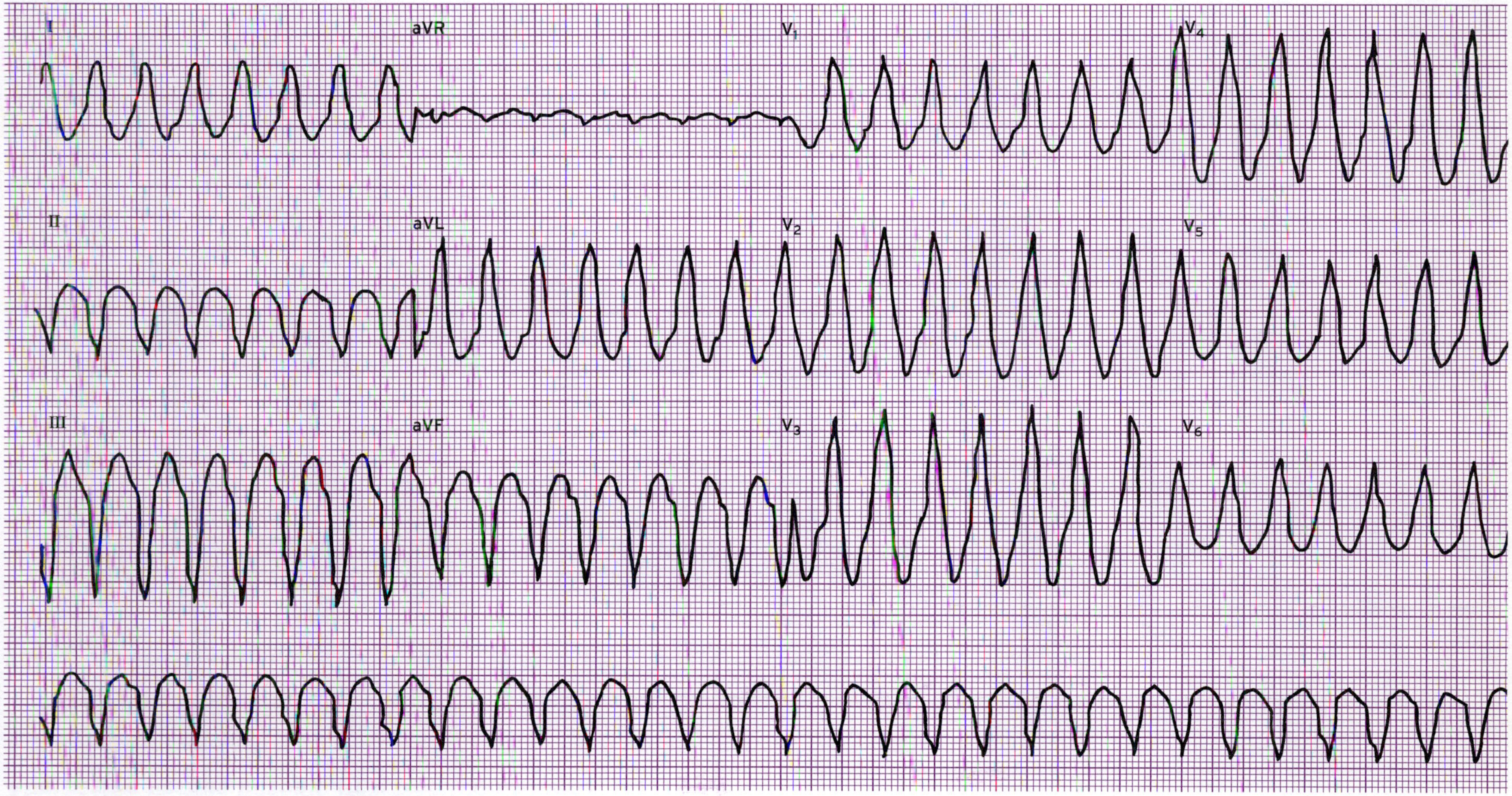

Aberration versus Ectopy, Practice (continued)

4. Aberration or ectopy? _____

   If aberration, what kind? _____

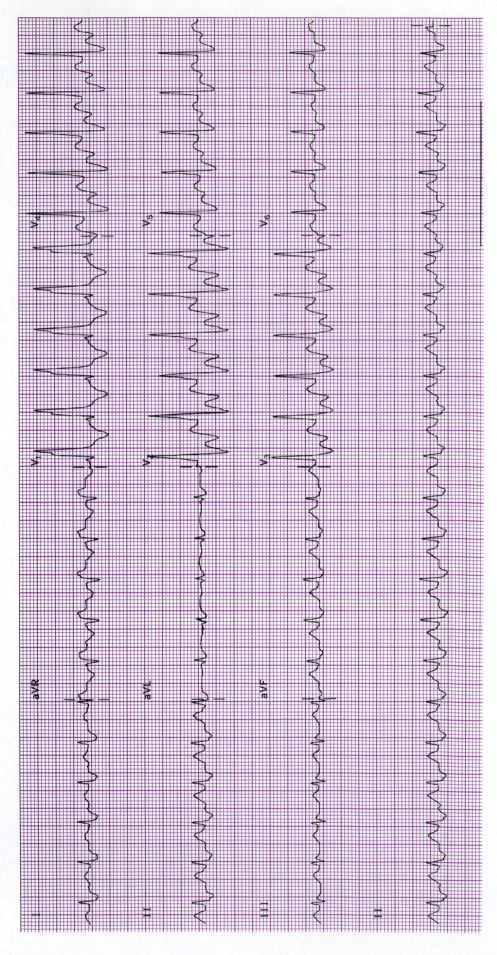

5. Aberration or ectopy? _____

   If aberration, what kind? _____

Aberration versus Ectopy, Practice (continued)

6. This question involves examining two EKGs. The second EKG is actually a manual printout of leads II, aVF, and V₅, done after the patient's heart rate had slowed down. *Compare the two before deciding on your answer.*

Aberration or ectopy? _____

If aberration, what kind? _____

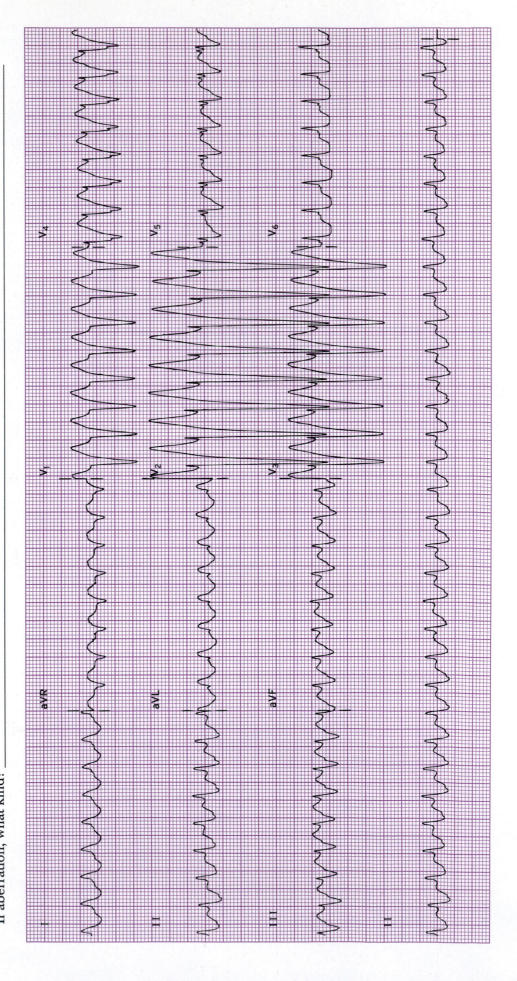

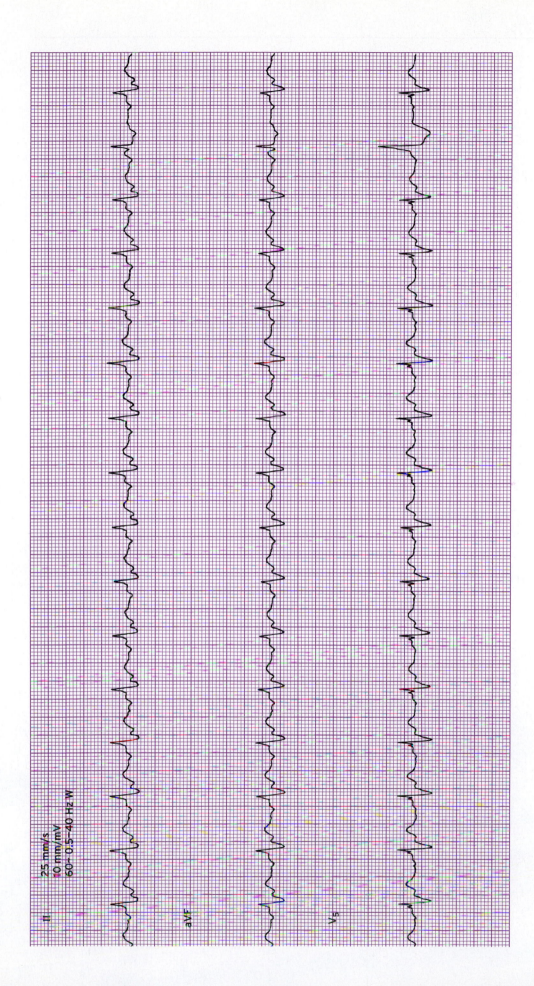

II

aVF

V₅

25 mm/s
10 mm/mV
60~ 0.5~40 Hz W

Answers to Aberration versus Ectopy Practice

1. **Aberration.** Note the RSR′ configuration in V$_1$ (actually seen better in V$_2$). This is SVT with an RBBB and LAHB.

2. **Aberration.** Again, note the RSR′ configuration in V$_1$. Also, there are P waves preceding the QRS complexes. This is sinus tachycardia with an RBBB and LAHB.

3. **Ectopy.** Note the positive concordancy in the precordial leads and the absence of P waves. This is v-tach.

4. **Aberration.** Note the triphasic contour, RSR′, in V$_1$. You'll recall ventricular ectopy rarely has this shape QRS complex. Also note the P waves preceding each QRS. This is sinus tachycardia with a right bundle branch block.

5. **Aberration.** This is 2:1 atrial tachycardia with a left bundle branch block (aberration). Wait a minute, you say, this is clearly a sinus tachycardia! This is a bit subtle, but look in V$_1$. See the two P waves to each QRS? There is a P wave in the ST segment and another just before each QRS. These dual P waves are noticeable only in V$_1$. Can you see how easy it is to miss certain arrhythmias, as some characteristics simply do not show up in certain leads? This shows the true benefit of a 12-lead EKG. It will pick up on things that might otherwise be missed. Even if you saw only one of the P waves per QRS, there is obvious atrial activity, so this would still be aberration.

6. **Aberration.** This is SVT with LBBB. The manual printout of the rhythm after the heart rate slowed down proves the supraventricular origin of this rhythm. Look at leads II and aVF on the manual printout. There are two P waves to each QRS. It is not noticeable as much in V$_5$. Now look at the QRS complexes in the manual printout and the 12-lead EKG. The QRS complexes are the same shape, but the heart rate is much slower. The manual printout is obviously supraventricular, right? It has P waves. Because the tachycardia on the 12-lead EKG has the same shape QRS complexes, it, too, must be supraventricular. It is therefore aberrant. Remember, it is extremely unlikely that an ectopic rhythm or beat would have the exact same configuration as the patient's known aberrant complex.

Practice Quiz

1. Define *aberration*. _____

    _____

2. Define *ectopy*. _____

    _____

3. If the type of ectopy is not specified, it is understood to be _____

4. A QRS complex with a triphasic contour favors _____

5. A QRS complex with a taller left rabbit ear favors _____

6. A tachycardia with an indeterminate axis and no P waves is most likely

_____

7. True or false: Concordancy in the precordial leads is proof that the rhythm is ectopic.

8. True or false: If the second beat in a group of rapid beats is the only "funny-looking" beat, it is likely that these rapid beats are ectopic.

9. A long R-R cycle affects its following refractory period in what way?

_____

10. True or false: Aberrant beats are all supraventricular in origin.

Practice Quiz Answers

1. Aberration is **the temporary abnormality of ventricular conduction that results in an abnormally shaped and often abnormally widened QRS complex.**

2. Ectopy is **the term given to those rhythms or beats that arise from a pacemaker other than the sinus node.**

3. If the type of ectopy is not specified, it is understood to be **ventricular.**

4. A QRS complex with a triphasic contour favors **aberration.**

5. A QRS complex with a taller left rabbit ear favors **ectopy.**

6. A tachycardia with an indeterminate axis and no P waves is most likely **ectopy.**

7. **False.** Concordancy in the precordial leads is suggestive of ectopy, but it is not proof, as some aberrant supraventricular rhythms can have concordancy.

8. **False.** This favors aberration. Remember, the refractory period of the conducting tissues is dependent on the previous R-R cycle length. The second beat in a group of rapid beats is the only one that ended a short cycle preceded by a long cycle. This short-cycle impulse arrives at the bundle branches only to find one still refractory and unable to conduct normally. The beat is then conducted aberrantly.

9. A long R-R cycle **causes the next refractory period to prolong.**

10. **True.** All aberrant beats travel the bundle branches abnormally, so they have to have originated in a pacemaker above the ventricle (supraventricular). Ventricular impulses do not travel through the bundle branches, since they originate below them.

Hypertrophy

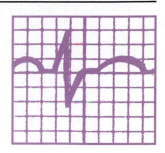

Chapter 24 Objectives

Upon completion of this chapter, the student will be able to:

- Recognize the normal shape of P waves in leads II and V_1.
- Recognize the P wave shapes indicative of right atrial enlargement.
- Recognize the P wave shapes indicative of left atrial enlargement.
- State the causes of right and left atrial enlargement.
- Recognize the normal QRS size and shape in all leads.
- Recognize right ventricular hypertrophy.
- Recognize left ventricular hypertrophy.
- Recognize an EKG with abnormally low voltage.
- State the causes of right and left ventricular hypertrophy.
- State three causes of low-voltage EKGs.
- Use the algorithm to identify atrial enlargement and ventricular hypertrophy.

Chapter 24 Outline

I.   Introduction
II.   Atrial hypertrophy
      A. Right atrial enlargement, left atrial enlargement
III. Ventricular hypertrophy
      A. Right ventricular hypertrophy, left ventricular hypertrophy
IV.   Low-voltage EKGs
V.   Clinical implications of hypertrophy
VI.   Hypertrophy algorithm
VII. Practice quiz
VIII. Practice quiz answers

Chapter 24 Glossary

Dilatation: Stretching of fibers.

Myxedema: A disorder of the thyroid gland that causes low voltage on the EKG.

Pericardial effusion: An excess of pericardial fluid inside the pericardial sac.

Introduction

Hypertrophy refers to excessive growth of tissue. **Atrial hypertrophy** is excessive growth of the atrial muscle. **Ventricular hypertrophy** is an overgrowth of ventricular muscle.

Atrial Hypertrophy

This is often called *atrial enlargement*. To determine the presence of atrial enlargement, we look at P waves. Remember that P waves are normally 1 to 2 mm high, and they should be upright in lead II and upright, biphasic, or inverted in V_1. Atrial enlargement will alter the shape of the P waves. In Figure 24-1, see a normal P wave in leads II and V_1.

Right Atrial Enlargement (RAE)

Most often, right atrial enlargement occurs as a result of chronic lung disease, which causes high pressures in the pulmonary system. These high pulmonary pressures place back pressure on the right ventricle and right atrium, causing them to hypertrophy, or bulk up to do their job of pumping blood into this now-high-pressure lung system. The resultant P waves are tall (≥ 2.5 mm high) and peaked in lead II and/or lead V_1. This tall, peaked P wave is called **P-pulmonale**. RAE is almost always seen accompanying right ventricular hypertrophy. See P waves typical of RAE in Figure 24-2.

Left Atrial Enlargement (LAE)

Left atrial enlargement occurs most often due to mitral valve disease. In mitral stenosis, since the valve opening is abnormally small, the left atrium hypertrophies in its struggle to pump blood through the narrowed valve. In

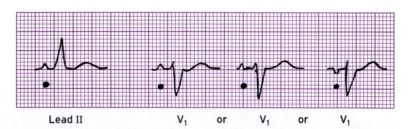

Lead II V_1 or V_1 or V_1

Figure 24-1 Normal P waves in leads II and V_1.

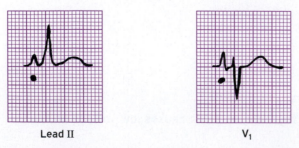

Lead II V_1

Figure 24-2 P waves indicative of right atrial enlargement.

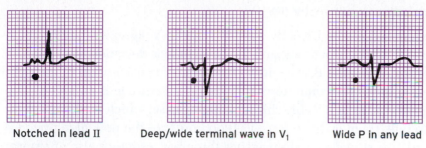

| Notched in lead II | Deep/wide terminal wave in V₁ | Wide P in any lead |

Figure 24-3   P waves indicative of left atrial enlargement.

mitral regurgitation, the valve is floppy, resulting in back flow of blood from left ventricle to left atrium. The left atrium then dilates to accommodate the extra fluid volume. In LAE, the resultant P waves can be any of the following:

- Notched with 0.04 second between notch peaks (called **P-mitrale**) in lead II or

- Biphasic in V_1, with the terminal negative deflection ≥1 mm deep and ≥1 mm wide or

- ≥0.11 second wide in any lead

See P waves indicative of left atrial enlargement in Figure 24-3.

Ventricular Hypertrophy

To determine if ventricular hypertrophy exists, we look for greater-than-normal amplitude (voltage) of the QRS complexes in the leads over the hypertrophied ventricle. Let's look at an example of normal QRS amplitude. See Figure 24-4.

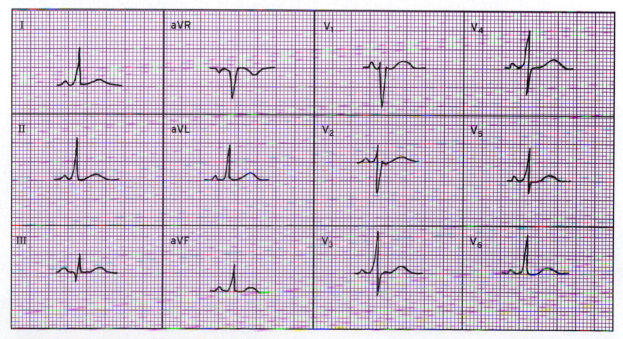

Figure 24-4   Normal QRS amplitude (voltage).

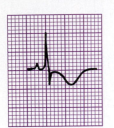

Figure 24-5 QRST configuration typical of RVH in V_1.

Right Ventricular Hypertrophy (RVH)

RVH is evidenced on the EKG by a tall R wave in V_1 (greater than or equal to the size of the S wave), accompanied by a right axis deviation and, often, T wave inversion. Since the R wave in V_1 represents depolarization of the right ventricle, it will be taller than normal if the right ventricle is enlarged. The most common cause of RVH is chronic lung disease, which forces the right ventricle to bulk up in order to force its blood out into the now-high-pressure lung system. This struggle to pump against this great resistance also often produces a **strain pattern.** A right ventricular strain pattern is evidenced by ST depression and T wave inversion in the right-sided leads, such as V_1 and V_2. RVH is almost always accompanied by RAE. See Figure 24-5 for an example of the typical QRST configuration in right ventricular hypertrophy in V_1.

Now let's see what RVH looks like on a 12-lead EKG. See Figure 24-6.

Left Ventricular Hypertrophy (LVH)

LVH is most commonly caused by hypertension, which causes the left ventricle to bulk up in order to expel its blood against the great resistance of the abnormally high blood pressure. LVH has several possible criteria:

- The R wave in V_5 or V_6 (whichever is taller) + the S wave in $V_1 \geq 35$ mm or
- The R wave in aVL ≥ 11 mm or
- The R wave in V_5 or $V_6 > 27$ mm.

Leads I, aVL, and V_5 and V_6 will have taller-than-normal R waves as the current travels toward their positive electrodes; leads V_1 and V_2 will have

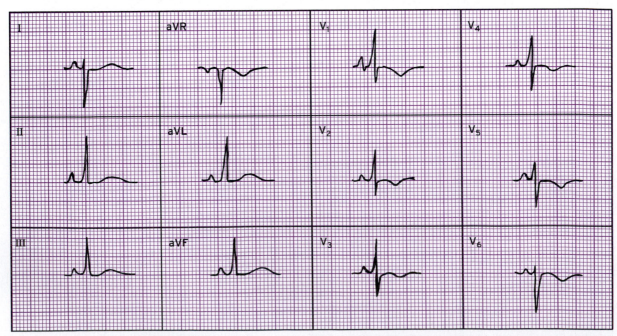

Figure 24-6 Right ventricular hypertrophy. Note that the R wave in V_1 is taller than the S wave is deep; there is right axis deviation and T wave inversion.

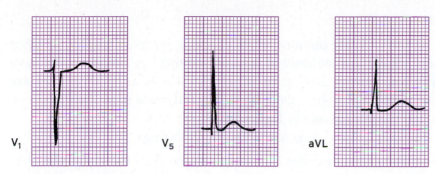

Figure 24-7 LVH by voltage criteria.

deeper-than-normal S waves as the current travels away from their positive electrode. See Figure 24-7. Add the height of the R wave in V_5 to the depth of the S wave in V_1. The result is ≥35 mm. This is LVH as evidenced by adding the voltages.

LVH, like RVH, often has an associated strain pattern. For LVH, that would involve ST depression and T wave inversion in the left-sided leads I, aVL, and V_5 and V_6. In addition, LAE often accompanies LVH. See Figure 24-8 for a 12-lead EKG example of LVH.

Ventricular hypertrophy does not usually prolong the QRS interval beyond normal limits. When you're evaluating 12-lead EKGs, always check the P waves for atrial enlargement and the QRS complexes for ventricular hypertrophy.

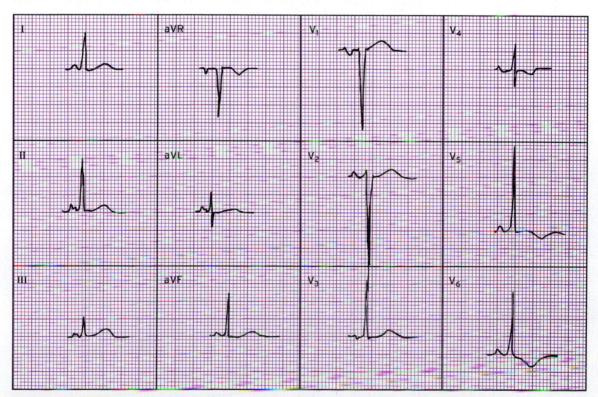

Figure 24-8 Left ventricular hypertrophy. Note the S wave in V_1 is 22 mm deep, and the R wave in V_5 is 24 mm tall, for a total voltage of 46 mm. This meets and exceeds the criteria for LVH.

Low-Voltage EKGs

It should be immediately obvious, when checking for hypertrophy, whether there is abnormally **low voltage** of the QRS complexes. Some people have abnormally low-voltage EKGs, in which the waves and complexes are shorter than usual. See Figure 24-9. Note the difference in voltage between this EKG and the normal one in Figure 24-4.

Some causes of a low-voltage EKG are the following:

- *Obesity.* Fatty tissue muffles the cardiac impulse on its way to the electrodes on the skin.

- *Emphysema.* Air trapping in the lungs muffles the impulse.

- *Myxedema.* The thyroid gland function is abnormally low, causing decreased voltage.

- *Pericardial effusion.* In this condition, excessive fluid inside the pericardial sac surrounding the heart muffles the impulse on its way to the skin.

Clinical Implications of Hypertrophy

Hypertrophy is the heart's way of attempting to meet a contractile demand that cannot be met by normal-size heart muscle, whether that be atrial or ventricular muscle. Unfortunately, hypertrophy also places increased demands on the coronary circulation to feed that extra muscle bulk. When that increased blood and oxygen demand cannot be adequately met, ischemia results. Hypertrophy increases the likelihood of ischemia and infarction simply by increasing the amount of muscle to be nourished by the coronary arteries.

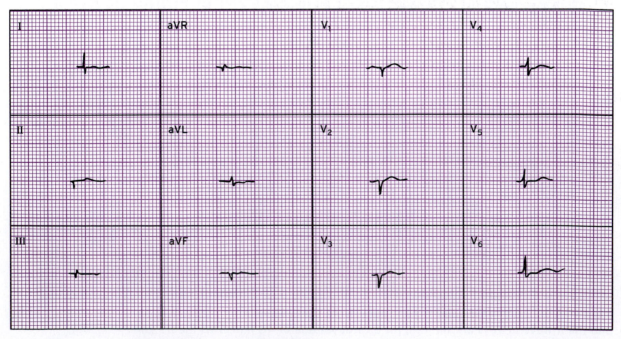

Figure 24-9 Low voltage EKG.

Ventricular dilatation, a stretching of the myocardial fibers that results from overfilling of the ventricles or inadequate pumping of blood out of the ventricles, can also result in a hypertrophy pattern on the EKG. Remember Starling's law? If the heart's fibers are overstretched, the tissue becomes floppy and incapable of adequate contraction.

Low-voltage EKGs, contrary to what may seem logical, do not imply that the heart is smaller than normal, or that it is generating less current than normal. It is usually caused by an outside influence that affects the heart's current on its way to the electrodes on the skin.

Hypertrophy Algorithm

This algorithm will point out atrial and ventricular hypertrophy. Just answer the questions and follow the arrows. *If none of the criteria are met, there is no hypertrophy.*

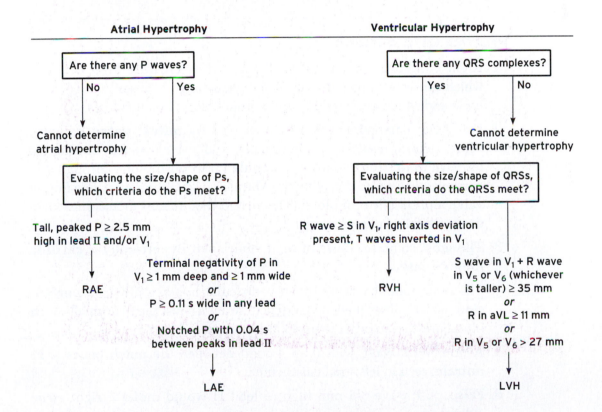

Practice Quiz

1. Right atrial enlargement is usually caused by _____

2. Left atrial enlargement is usually caused by _____

3. The most common cause of right ventricular hypertrophy is _____

4. The most common cause of left ventricular hypertrophy is_____

   _____

5. A notched P wave with 0.04 second between the notch peaks is_____

   _____

6. True or false: A P wave 3.5 mm high in lead II would indicate that the atria are normal size.

7. True or false: Right ventricular hypertrophy is noted by the presence of a tall R wave in V_1 along with an inverted T wave and a right axis deviation.

8. True or false: If the S wave in V_1 is 8 mm deep and the R wave in V_5 is 16 mm tall, the criteria for left ventricular hypertrophy has been met.

9. Define *hypertrophy*. _____

10. In what way does mitral regurgitation result in left atrial enlargement?

    _____

Practice Quiz Answers

1. Right atrial enlargement is usually caused by **chronic lung disease,** which causes high pressures in the lung system and causes the right ventricle and right atrium to bulk up to propel blood into the lungs.

2. Left atrial enlargement is usually caused by **mitral valve disease.** Mitral stenosis results in an abnormally small valve opening, causing the left atrium to struggle harder and bulk up to push blood through this narrowed valve into the ventricle. Mitral regurgitation results in a floppy valve and backflow of blood. The atrium then dilates to accommodate this extra fluid volume.

3. The most common cause of right ventricular hypertrophy is **chronic lung disease.**

4. The most common cause of left ventricular hypertrophy is **hypertension,** which causes the left ventricle to strain against the abnormally high blood pressure in order to expel its blood.

5. A notched P wave with 0.04 second between the notch peaks is **P-mitrale,** seen in left atrial enlargement.

6. **False.** A P wave 3.5 mm high in lead II would indicate right atrial enlargement.

7. **True.** Right ventricular hypertrophy is noted by the presence of a tall R wave in V_1 along with an inverted T wave and a right axis deviation.

8. **False.** If the S wave in V_1 is 8 mm deep and the R wave in V_5 is 16 mm tall, the sum is 24 mm, which does not meet the criteria for left ventricular hypertrophy. The sum must meet or exceed 35 mm to be LVH.

9. Hypertrophy is **excessive growth of tissue.**

10. **Mitral regurgitation is a backflow of blood from the left ventricle into the left atrium. This causes the left atrium to dilate to accommodate this extra fluid volume.**

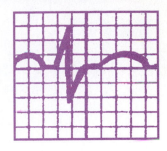

Myocardial Infarction (MI)

Chapter 25 Objectives

Upon completion of this chapter, the student will be able to:

- Describe the difference between Q wave MI and non-Q wave MI.
- Describe the three Is of infarction.
- Describe what EKG changes are associated with ischemia, injury, and infarction.
- Draw the different kinds of ST segment abnormalities and explain what each implies.
- Draw the different T wave abnormalities and explain what each implies.
- Describe how a significant Q wave differs from a normal Q wave.
- Describe normal R wave progression.
- Identify the transition zone in a variety of EKGs.
- Describe where the transition zone is for clockwise and counterclockwise rotation.
- Describe the EKG changes associated with MI evolution and give the timeline associated with each change.
- Explain how to determine the age of an MI.
- Name the four walls of the left ventricle.
- Name the leads that look at each of the four walls of the left ventricle.
- Describe an easy way to find posterior MIs.
- Name the coronary artery that feeds each of the four walls of the left ventricle.
- Describe how to determine if a right ventricular infarction is present.
- Describe precordial lead placement for a right-sided EKG.
- Describe how pericarditis and early repolarization mimic an MI.

Chapter 25 Outline

Chapter 25 Glossary

Acute: Within a day or two.

Indicative changes: EKG changes (ST elevation, significant Q wave, T wave inversion) that indicate where the MI is.

Necrosis: Death of tissue.

Non–Q wave MI: An MI that does not cause the development of significant Q waves. May include subendocardial MI.

Occlusion: Blockage.

Pericarditis: An inflammation of the pericardium and the myocardium just beneath it.

Q wave MI: An MI that results in development of significant Q waves on the EKG.

Reciprocal changes: Those EKG changes (ST depression) seen in the area electrically opposite the damaged area.

Subendocardial: Referring to the innermost layer of the myocardium just beneath the endocardium.

Transmural: Through the full thickness of the wall at that location.

Introduction

Myocardial infarctions involve death of myocardial tissue in an area deprived of blood flow by an **occlusion** (blockage) of a coronary artery. Actual death of tissue is the end of a process that begins with ischemia and injury.

There are two types of myocardial infarctions: **Q wave MIs** and **non–Q wave MIs.**

- Q wave MIs tend to be **transmural** (i.e., they usually, though not always, damage the entire thickness of the myocardium in a certain area of the heart). Q wave MIs result in ST segment elevation, T wave inversion, and significant Q waves, along with the usual symptoms of an MI.

- The non–Q wave MI tends to be **subendocardial** or **incomplete,** damaging only the innermost layer of the myocardium just beneath the endocardium. This kind of MI typically does less damage than a Q wave MI and does not result in the typical EKG changes associated with Q wave MIs. Non–Q wave MIs can be difficult to diagnose. They sometimes present with widespread ST segment depression and T wave inversion. At other times the MI is diagnosed only by patient history, ST segment changes, and elevated lab values that indicate myocardial damage. With non–Q wave MIs, the patient will have the usual symptoms of an MI, and will typically go on to have a Q wave MI within a few months if treatment for the coronary artery blockage is not rendered. Non–Q wave MIs are less common than Q wave MIs. See Figure 25-1.

Three I's of Infarction

The sequence of events that occurs when a coronary artery becomes occluded is known as the *three I's of infarction.*

- **Ischemia.** Experiments on dogs have shown that almost immediately after a coronary artery becomes occluded, the *T wave inverts* in the EKG leads overlooking the occluded area. This indicates that myocardial tissue is ischemic, starving for blood and oxygen due to the lack of blood flow. Myocardial tissue becomes pale and whitish in appearance.

- **Injury.** Soon, as the coronary occlusion continues, the once-ischemic tissue becomes injured by the continued lack of perfusion. The tissue becomes bluish in appearance. The *ST segment rises,* indicating a current of injury and the beginning of an acute MI.

- **Infarction.** If occlusion persists, the jeopardized myocardial tissue **necroses** (dies) and turns black. *Significant Q waves develop* (in Q wave MIs) on the EKG. In time, the dead tissue will become scar tissue.

Ischemia and injury to myocardial tissue cause repolarization changes, so the ST segments and the T waves will be abnormal. Infarction causes depolarization changes, so the QRS complex on the EKG will show telltale signs of permanent damage. See Figure 25-2.

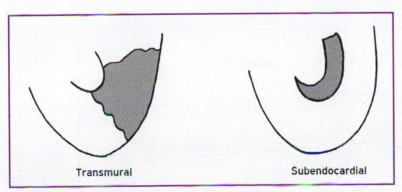

Transmural   Subendocardial

Figure 25-1 Transmural and subendocardial MIs.

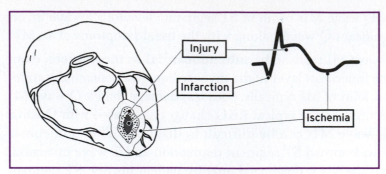

Figure 25-2 The three I's of infarction.

In Figure 25-2, an occlusion in a coronary artery is blocking the blood flow to the portion of myocardium fed by that artery. This creates three distinct zones. The innermost zone is the infarcted zone. It is the area that has been deprived of oxygen the longest, as it's the deepest layer and thus farthest away from the blood supply. Immediately surrounding that area is the injured zone, and surrounding that is the ischemic zone.

Ischemia and injury are reversible if circulation is restored. Once the tissue has infarcted, however, the tissue is permanently dead. Myocardial cells do not regenerate.

To determine if an MI is present, we look at the ST segments, the T waves, and the QRS complexes. Let's look at each of those separately.

ST Segment

The normal ST segment should be on the baseline at the same level as the PR segment. (Think of the PR segment as the baseline for ST segment evaluation purposes.) Abnormal ST segments can be elevated or depressed. To see if the ST segment is elevated or depressed, draw a straight line extending from the PR segment out past the QRS. An elevated ST segment is one that is above this line. A depressed ST segment is one that is below this line. *ST segment elevation implies myocardial injury.* ST elevation can be either concave or convex. Convex ST segment elevation (also called a **coved ST segment**) is most often associated with an MI in progress. Concave ST elevation is often associated with **pericarditis,** an inflammation of the pericardium and the myocardium immediately beneath it, but it can also be seen in MIs. *ST depression implies ischemia or reciprocal changes opposite the area of infarct.* See Figure 25-3.

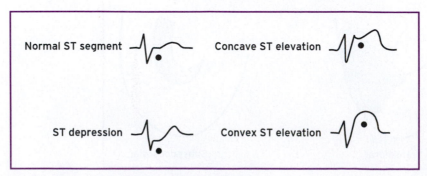

Figure 25-3 ST segment abnormalities.

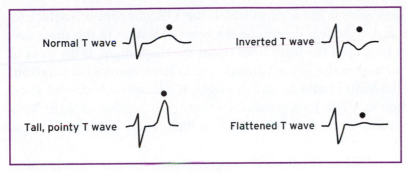

Figure 25-4   T wave abnormalities.

In Figure 25-3, note how the ST segment is right on line with the PR segment in the normal ST example.

T Wave

The normal T wave should be rounded with an amplitude less than or equal to 5 mm in the frontal leads and should be upright in all leads except aVR and V_1. aVR's T wave should be negative. V_1's T wave can be flat, inverted, or upright. See Figure 25-4.

All the abnormal T waves in Figure 25-4 can imply myocardial ischemia. The tall, pointy T can also signal hyperkalemia or **hyperacute** changes of an MI in progress. Hyperacute changes are those that accompany an MI in its earliest stages.

QRS Complexes

We look for significant Q waves and poor R wave progression as clues to an MI. Normal Q waves imply septal and right ventricular depolarization. A significant (i.e., pathological) Q wave implies myocardial necrosis. For a Q wave to be significant, it must be *either* 0.04 second (one small block) wide *or* at least one-fourth the size of the R wave. In Figure 25-5, see the difference between a normal Q and a significant Q.

R Wave Progression and Transition

In the precordial leads, you'll recall that the QRS starts out primarily negative in V_1 and goes through a transition around V_3 or V_4, where the QRS is isoelectric. The QRS then ends up primarily positive by V_6. This means that, accordingly, the R waves progress from very small in V_1 to very large in V_6. If the R waves do not get progressively larger in the precordial leads, as they should, this can imply myocardial infarction. Sometimes, poor R wave progression is the only electrocardiographic evidence of an MI.

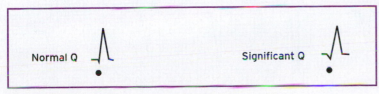

Figure 25-5   Normal versus significant Q waves.

The transition zone is the lead in which the QRS becomes isoelectric. This transition zone can help determine the heart's rotation in the chest cavity. Imagine looking up at the heart from under the diaphragm. If the front of the heart rotates toward the left, it's considered to have **clockwise rotation.** If the front of the heart rotates toward the right, it's **counterclockwise rotation.** A transition in V_1 or V_2 is counterclockwise; a transition in V_5 or V_6 is clockwise. Rotation in the precordial leads is like axis in the frontal leads. See Figure 25-6.

In Figure 25-6, look at the R wave progression in the normal transition example. The R waves grow progressively taller across the precordium, and the transition zone is in V_4. See how V_4's QRS complex is mostly isoelectric? Here, V_1 through V_3 are mostly negative, V_5 and V_6 are positive, and V_4 is where the transition from negative to positive occurs.

In the counterclockwise example, the transition zone is between V_1 and V_2. There is no real isoelectric complex. V_1 is negative and V_2 is already positive, so the transition zone would have to be between the two. The R wave progression is also abnormal. The R waves progress from very small in V_1 to unusually large in V_2.

In the clockwise example, the transition zone is between V_5 and V_6. R wave progression is abnormal–the R wave is small in V_5 and very tall in V_6.

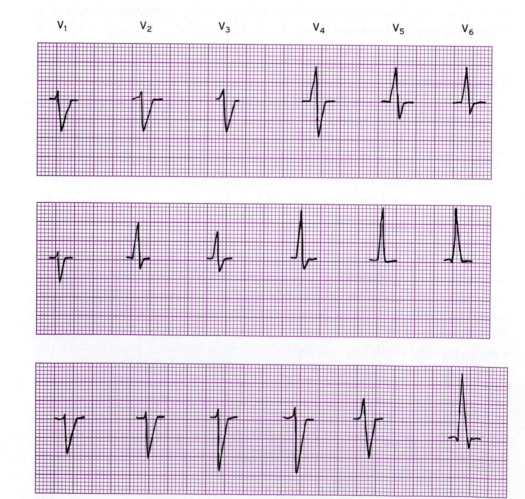

Normal transition

Counterclockwise rotation

Clockwise rotation

Figure 25-6 R wave progression and transition zones in the precordial leads.

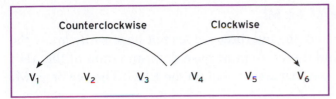

Figure 25-7 Clockwise versus counterclockwise rotation.

Here's a quick way to determine the heart's rotation: Imagine leads V_3 and V_4 as the hub of a clock's hand. Between V_3 and V_4 is the normal transition zone. If the transition is in V_1 or V_2, draw a rounded arrow from V_3 and V_4 to V_1 and V_2. The arrow is going counterclockwise. If the transition is in V_5 or V_6 draw a rounded arrow from V_3 and V_4 to V_5 and V_6. This arrow is going clockwise. See Figure 25-7.

Evolution of an MI

MIs occur over a period of time. The EKG changes over the course of an MI are its **evolution.** See Figure 25-8.

TIMELINE	AGE OF MI	EKG CHANGE	IMPLICATION
Immediately before the actual MI starts		T wave inversion	Cardiac tissue is ischemic, as evidenced by the newly inverted T waves.
Within hours after the MIs start	Acute	Marked ST elevation + upright T wave	Acute MI has begun, starting with myocardial injury.
Hours later	Acute	Significant Q + ST elevation + upright T	Some of the injured myocardial tissue has died, while other tissue remains injured.
Hours to a day or two later	Acute	Significant Q + less ST elevation + marked T inversion	Infarction is almost complete. Some injury and ischemia persist at the infarct edges.
Days to weeks later (in some cases this stage may last up to a year)	Age indeterminate	Significant Q + T wave inversion	Infarction is complete. Though there is no more ischemic tissue (it has either recovered or died), the T wave inversion persists.
Weeks, months, years later	Old	Significant Q only	The significant Q wave persists, signifying permanent tissue death.

Figure 25-8   Evolution of an MI.

Determining the Age of an MI

When an EKG is interpreted, the interpreter does not necessarily know the patient's clinical status and therefore must base determination of the MI's age on the indicative changes that are present on the EKG. The age of an MI is determined as follows:

- An MI that has ST segment elevation is **acute** (one to two days old or less).

- An MI with significant Q waves, baseline (or almost back to baseline) ST segments, and inverted T waves is of **age indeterminate** (several days old, up to a year in some cases). Some authorities call this a **recent MI.**

- The MI with significant Q waves, baseline ST segments, and upright T waves is **old** (weeks to years old).

Walls of the Left Ventricle

Though it is possible to have an infarction of the right ventricle, infarctions occur mostly in the left ventricle, since it has the greatest oxygen demand and thus is impacted more adversely by poor coronary artery flow. MIs can affect any of the four walls of the left ventricle (see Figure 25-9):

- **Anterior wall.** The front wall–fed by the left anterior descending coronary artery.

- **Inferior wall.** The bottom wall–fed by the right coronary artery.

- **Lateral wall.** The left side wall of the heart–fed by the circumflex coronary artery.

- **Posterior wall.** The back wall–fed by the right coronary artery.

Each of these left ventricular walls can be "seen" by our EKG electrodes. You'll recall that the positive pole of leads II, III, and aVF sit on the left foot. They look at the heart from the bottom. Which wall of the heart would they see? Good for you if you said the inferior wall.

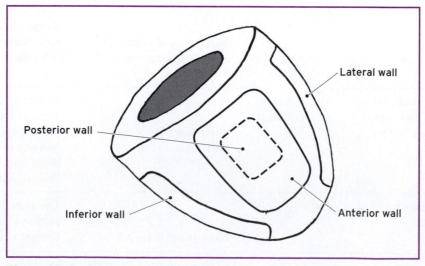

Figure 25-9   Walls of the left ventricle.

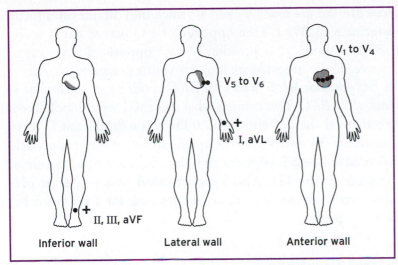

Figure 25-10 Leads looking at the anterior, inferior, and lateral walls of the left ventricle.

What about leads I, aVL, and V_5 and V_6? They sit pretty much on the heart's left side, so they look at the lateral wall.

Leads V_1 through V_4 sit right in the front of the heart, looking at the anterior wall. See Figure 25-10.

What about the posterior wall? Unlike the other infarct locations, there are no leads looking directly at the posterior wall because we do not put EKG electrodes on the patient's back for a routine 12-lead EKG. Therefore, the only way to look at the posterior wall is to look *through* the anterior wall. See Figure 25-11.

The ventricles depolarize from endocardium to epicardium (from inside to outside). You'll note on Figure 25-11 that the vectors representing depolarization of the anterior and posterior walls are opposite each other. Therefore, *the only way to diagnose a posterior MI is to look for changes opposite those that would be*

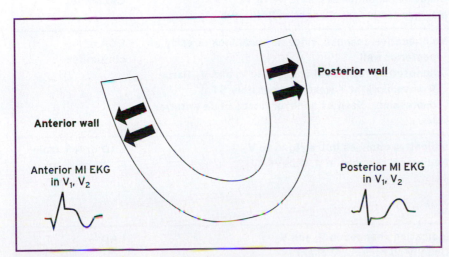

Figure 25-11 Posterior wall MI changes.

seen with an anterior MI. We use leads V_1 and V_2 since they sit almost directly opposite the posterior wall. What's the opposite of a Q wave? An R wave. What's opposite ST elevation? ST depression. What's opposite T wave inversion? Upright T wave. Those are what we look for with a posterior infarct.

An easy way to find posterior MIs is to turn the EKG upside down and look at V_1 and V_2 from the back of the EKG. This mimics what the EKG would look like if we had leads directly over the posterior wall. If there is a significant Q wave and T wave inversion in V_1 and V_2 in this upside-down reverse approach, there is a posterior MI. The ST segment may be elevated or at baseline, depending on the age of the MI. Also keep in mind that posterior MIs almost always accompany an inferior MI, so always look for a posterior MI when an inferior MI is present.

Myocardial Infarct Locations

A Q wave MI is diagnosed on the EKG by **indicative changes** (i.e., ST elevation, T wave inversion, and significant Q waves) in the leads for that area. Depending on the age of the infarct, not all of those indicative changes will be present.

In the area electrically opposite the infarct area are **reciprocal changes** (i.e., ST depression). Reciprocal ST depression is seen only when there is ST elevation in the indicative leads.

Table 25-1 Infarct Locations

LOCATION OF MI	EKG CHANGES	CORONARY ARTERY
Anterior	Indicative changes in V_1 to V_4 Reciprocal changes in II, III, aVF	Left anterior descending (LAD)
Inferior	Indicative changes in II, III, aVF Reciprocal changes in I, aVL, and V leads	Right coronary artery (RCA)
Lateral	Indicative changes in I, aVL, V_5 to V_6 May see reciprocal changes in II, III, aVF	Circumflex
Posterior	No indicative changes, since no leads look directly at posterior wall Diagnosed by reciprocal changes in V_1 and V_2 (large R wave, upright T wave, and possibly ST depression). Seen as a mirror image of an anterior MI.	RCA or circumflex
Extensive anterior (sometimes called *extensive anterior-lateral*)	Indicative changes in I, aVL, V_1 to V_6 Reciprocal changes in II, III, aVF	LAD or left main
Anteroseptal	Indicative changes in V_1 and V_2 Usually no reciprocal changes	LAD

Let's look at the EKG changes associated with the different infarct locations. It is not necessary to have every single change listed in order to determine the kind of infarct, but most of the criteria should be met. Note the coronary artery involved. See Table 25-1.

The MIs in Table 25-1 involve only one wall of the left ventricle. MIs can extend across into other walls as well. For example, a patient might have an inferior-lateral MI, which would involve the inferior leads as well as the lateral leads. Combination MIs such as this do not always involve every one of the usual leads. For example, an inferior-lateral MI might involve the inferior leads and only a few lateral leads. An anterior-lateral MI might include the anterior leads and only a few lateral leads.

On the next several pages you will find helpful ways of determining the kind of MI you're seeing. First you will find infarction squares, then a pictorial of the different MI types, and finally an MI algorithm. Let's take a look.

Infarction Squares

In Table 25-2, each lead square is labeled with the wall of the heart at which it looks. When you analyze an EKG, note which leads have ST elevation and/or significant Q waves. Then use the infarction squares to determine the type of infarction. For example, if there were ST elevation in leads II, III, aVF, and V_5 and V_6, you would note that the MI involves inferior and lateral leads. The MI would be inferior-lateral.

Next let's look at some MI pictorials. Ignore the QRS width in these pictorials—the drawings are just to illustrate what these types of MIs look like.

Table 25-2   Infarction Squares

I	aVR	V_1	V_4
Lateral	Ignore this lead when looking for MIs	Anterior (posterior if mirror image)	Anterior
II	aVL	V_2	V_5
Inferior	Lateral	Anterior (posterior if mirror image)	Lateral
III	aVF	V_3	V_6
Inferior	Inferior	Anterior	Lateral

MI Pictorials

Anterior MI

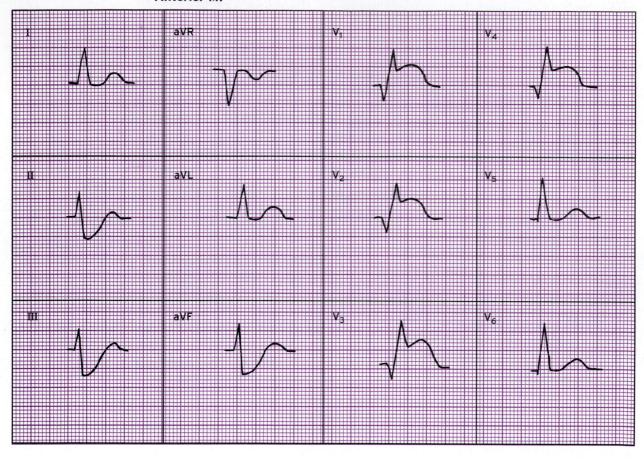

This is an **acute anterior MI,** as evidenced by the ST elevation in V_1 to V_4. Also note the reciprocal ST depression in leads II, III, and aVF.

If this MI were **age indeterminate,** it would have more normal ST segments, significant Q waves, and T wave inversions in V_1 to V_4.

If this MI were **old,** it would have only the significant Q wave remaining. The ST segment would be back at baseline and the T wave would be upright.

Inferior MI

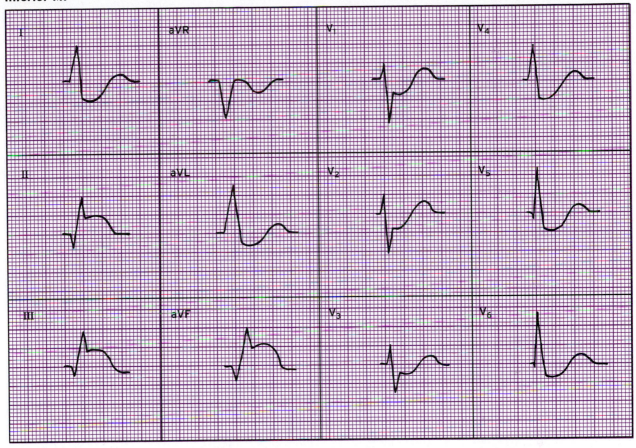

This is an **acute inferior MI.** Note the ST elevation in leads II, III, and aVF. Note also the reciprocal ST segment depression in leads I, aVL, and V_1 to V_6.

The **age indeterminate inferior MI** would have more normal ST segments along with significant Q waves and inverted T waves in leads II, III, and aVF.

The **old inferior MI** would have only significant Q waves in II, III, and aVF. The ST segments would be at baseline and T waves would be upright.

Lateral Wall MI

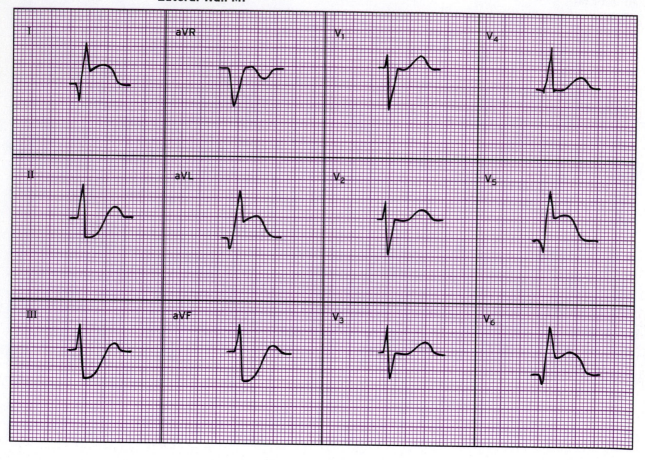

This is an **acute lateral wall MI,** as evidenced by the ST elevation in leads I, aVL, and V$_5$ to V$_6$. Note also the reciprocal ST depression in leads II, III, and aVF.

If this were an **age indeterminate lateral MI,** there would be more normal ST segments along with significant Q waves and inverted T waves in I, aVL, and V$_5$ to V$_6$.

An **old lateral wall MI** would have baseline ST segments, significant Q waves, and upright T waves in I, aVL, and V$_5$ to V$_6$.

Posterior MI

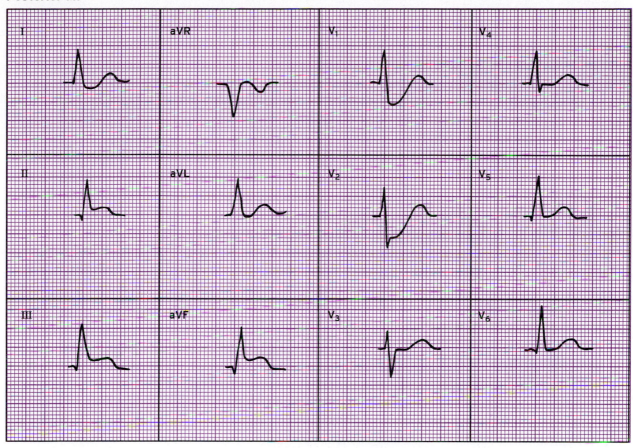

This is an **acute posterior wall MI.** Note the tall R wave in V_1 to V_2 along with ST segment depression and an upright T wave. Remember, a posterior MI is diagnosed by a mirror image of the normal indicative changes of an MI in V_1 to V_2. Note that there is an acute inferior MI as well.

An **age indeterminate posterior MI** would have more normal ST segments, a tall R wave, and an upright T wave.

The **old posterior MI** would have only the tall R wave remaining. The ST segments would be at baseline and the T wave would be inverted.

Extensive Anterior MI

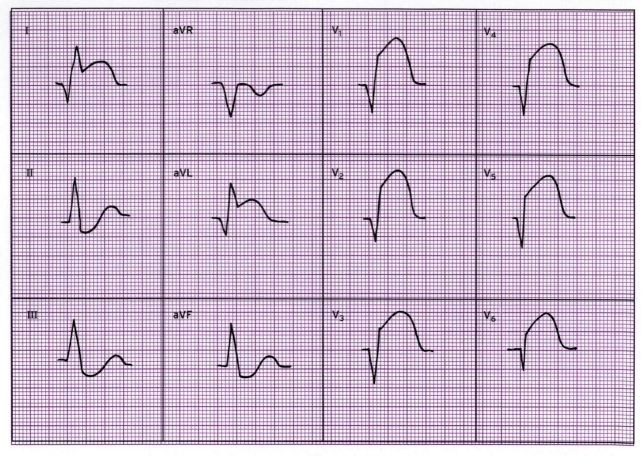

Here we have a huge MI, the **acute extensive anterior MI.** Note the significant Q waves and ST elevation in I, aVL, and V_1 to V_6 and the reciprocal ST depression in II, III, and aVF.

The **age indeterminate extensive anterior MI** would have more normal ST segments along with significant Q waves and T wave inversion.

The **old extensive anterior MI** would have baseline ST segments, significant Q waves, and upright T waves in I, aVL, and V_1 to V_6.

Anteroseptal MI

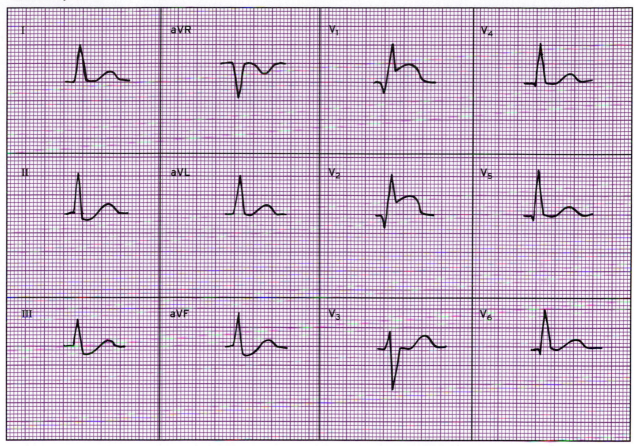

This is an **acute anteroseptal MI.** Note the ST elevation in leads V_1 to V_2.

An **age indeterminate anteroseptal MI** would have more normal ST segments, significant Q waves, and inverted T waves in V_1 to V_2.

The **old anteroseptal MI** would have only significant Q waves remaining in V_1 to V_2. The ST segments would be at baseline and the T waves would be upright.

Subendocardial MI

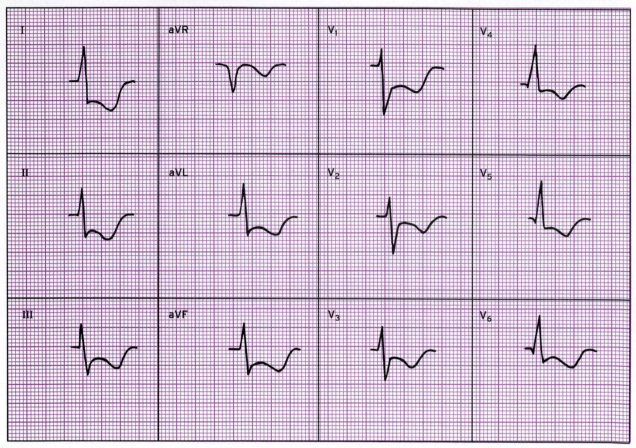

This is an **acute subendocardial MI.** It is one kind of non–Q wave MI. It is characterized by widespread ST depression and T wave inversions. Subendocardial infarctions are diagnosed only in the acute phase, as they do not cause significant Q waves, and their T waves are already inverted.

Myocardial Infarction Algorithm

This algorithm is designed to point out the myocardial infarction area. Just answer the questions and follow the arrows.

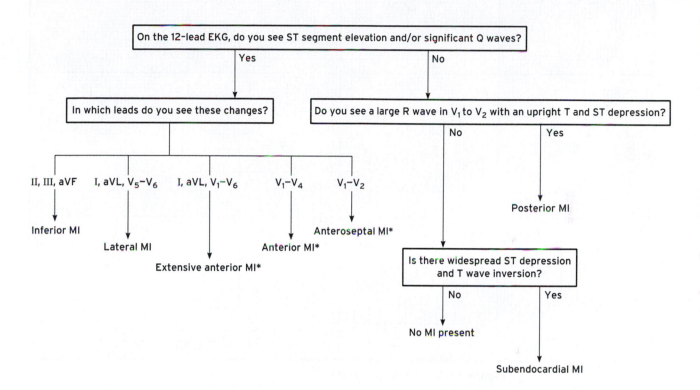

*If LBBB is present, these types of MIs cannot be diagnosed. The high take-off to the T wave of LBBB mimics the ST elevation of these kinds of MI.

How to Use the MI Algorithm

Refer to the EKG in Figure 25-12. Do you see any ST segment elevation or significant Q waves? Yes, there are significant Q waves and also there is ST elevation.

In which leads do you see these changes? These are noted in V_1 to V_4. The arrow points to anterior MI.

Right Ventricular Infarction

On occasion, an inferior MI will be accompanied by a right ventricular (RV) infarction. RV infarctions occur when the blockage to the right coronary artery system is so extensive that damage extends into the right ventricle. RV infarctions are not detectable by the routine 12-lead EKG, which looks at the left ventricle. To diagnose an RV infarction, two conditions must be met: First, there must be electrocardiographic evidence of an inferior wall MI on a standard 12-lead EKG. Second, a right-sided EKG must reveal ST

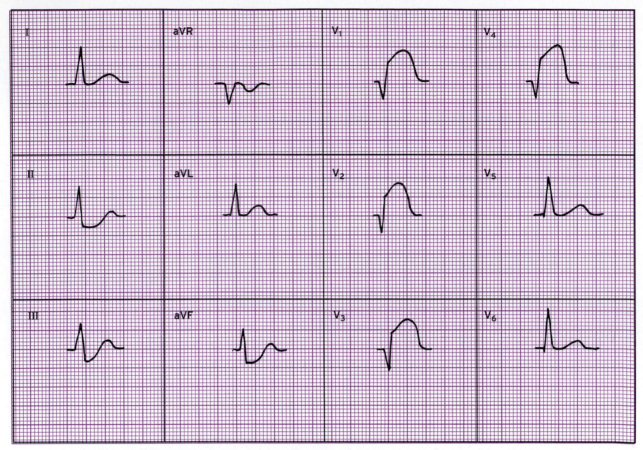

Figure 25-12 MI for algorithm.

elevation in V$_3$R and/or V$_4$R. This right-sided EKG is done only if an RV infarction is suspected (i.e., the patient exhibits symptoms, particularly hypotension, beyond what is expected with just an inferior MI).

A right-sided EKG is done with the limb leads in their normal places, but with the precordial leads placed on the right side of the chest instead of the left. See Figure 25-13.

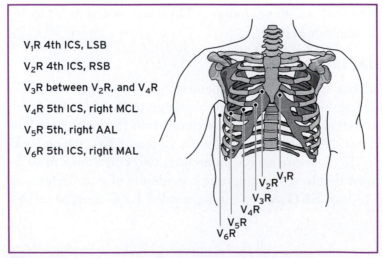

V$_1$R 4th ICS, LSB
V$_2$R 4th ICS, RSB
V$_3$R between V$_2$R, and V$_4$R
V$_4$R 5th ICS, right MCL
V$_5$R 5th, right AAL
V$_6$R 5th ICS, right MAL

Figure 25-13 Lead placement for a right-sided EKG.

Right Ventricular Infarction (Right-Sided EKG)

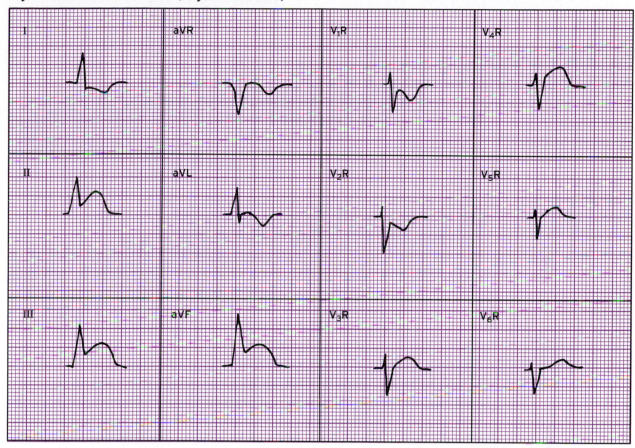

On this right-sided EKG, note the ST elevation in leads V_3R to V_4R. This proves there is an RV infarction. You'll note also that there is ST elevation in leads II, III, and aVF that indicate an inferior MI. Remember, the right-sided EKG leaves the limb leads in their normal place, but moves the precordial leads to the right side of the chest. So the inferior MI will still be obvious on the right-sided EKG.

Conditions That Can Mimic an MI

Now that you have a feel for the different kinds of MIs, let's look at some conditions that can cause EKG changes that look just like an MI. In most cases, the only difference is in the patient's medical symptoms and history.

Acute Pericarditis

Though ST segment elevation is most often associated with an MI in progress, there are times when it may instead imply an inflammation of the pericardium, called **pericarditis.** In acute pericarditis, the pericardium and the myocardium just beneath it are inflamed, causing repolarization abnormalities that present as concave ST segment elevation. Since pericarditis does not involve coronary artery blockage, the ST elevation will not be limited to leads overlying areas fed by a certain coronary artery—it will be widespread throughout many leads.

The ST elevation of pericarditis differs from that of an MI in that an MI usually produces *convex* ST elevation, whereas pericarditis produces *concave*

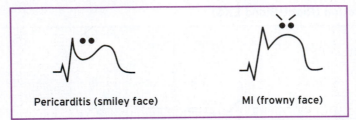

Pericarditis (smiley face)   MI (frowny face)

Figure 25-14 Smiley-face (concave) and frowny face (convex) ST elevations.

elevation. These are often referred to as the *smiley-face* and *frowny-face* ST segments. The smiley face is concave ST elevation. The frowny face is convex. See Figure 25-14.

Like an MI, pericarditis also causes chest pain, and it is crucial to differentiate between the two, as treatment differs greatly. See Figure 25-15.

In Figure 25-15, note the widespread concave ST elevation in leads I, II, III, aVL, aVF, and V_1 to V_6. This is *not* typical of an MI because it is so widespread. Is it possible this is a huge MI instead of pericarditis? Sure. But based on the concave ST elevation scattered across many leads, it's more likely that it's pericarditis. Only by examining the patient would we know for sure.

Early Repolarization

A normal variant sometimes seen in young people, especially young black males, early repolarization results in ST elevation that may be convex or concave. Repolarization begins so early in this condition that the ST seg-

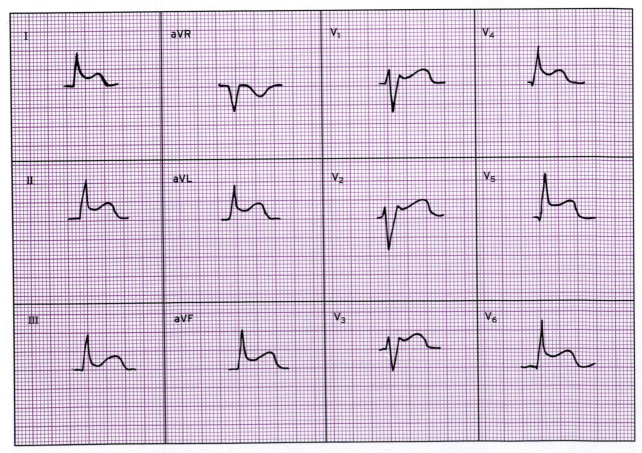

Figure 25-15 Pericarditis.

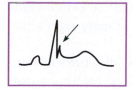

Figure 25-16   Fishhook of early repolarization.

ment appears to start even before the QRS complex has finished, thus making it appear that the ST segment is mildly elevated. Often there is a "fishhook" at the end of some of the QRS complexes that makes recognition of early repolarization easier. Note the ST elevation and the fishhook (see arrow) in Figure 25-16.

It is not always possible to distinguish early repolarization from an MI based on only a single EKG. A series of EKGs would reveal the typical evolutionary changes if an MI is present, and they would remain unchanged if early repolarization is present. The ST segment elevations of early repolarization are most often evident in leads V_2 to V_4, though they may be more widespread. Of great help in differentiating early repolarization from an MI is the age and presentation of the patient. A 20-year-old black male with no cardiac complaints who has mild ST elevations probably has early repolarization. A 65-year-old male with chest pain and ST elevation is more likely to have an MI in progress. Only by examining the patient can the definitive diagnosis of early repolarization versus MI be made. But the EKG will give hints. See Figure 25-17.

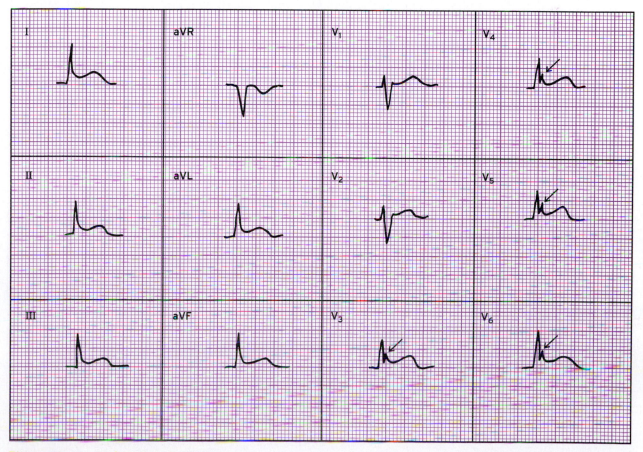

Figure 25-17   Early repolarization.

In Figure 25-17, note the mild ST segment elevation in almost all leads and the fishhook in V_3 to V_6 (see arrows). This is typical of early repolarization.

Now it's time for some practice. The EKGs that follow all represent standard left-sided EKGs. The first five EKGs are like the MI pictorials, consisting of only one beat in each lead box. The last five are genuine 12-lead EKGs. Use the infarction squares and/or the MI algorithm if you need help.

MI Practice

Tell which wall of the heart is affected and how old the MI is (if there is indeed an MI).

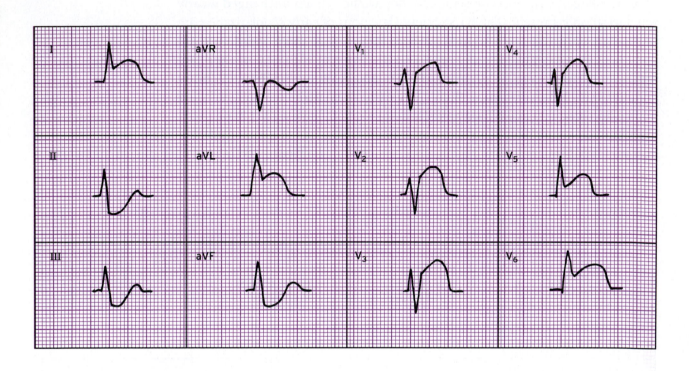

1. _____

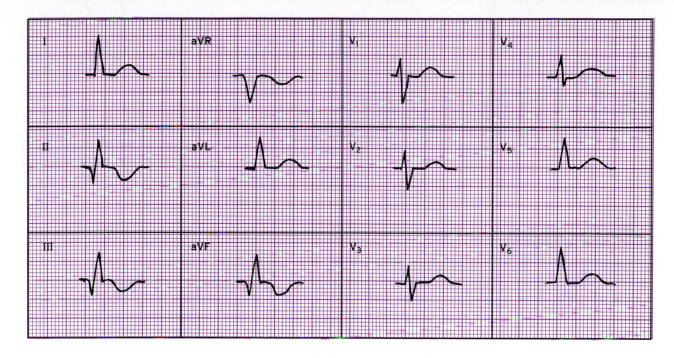

2. _____

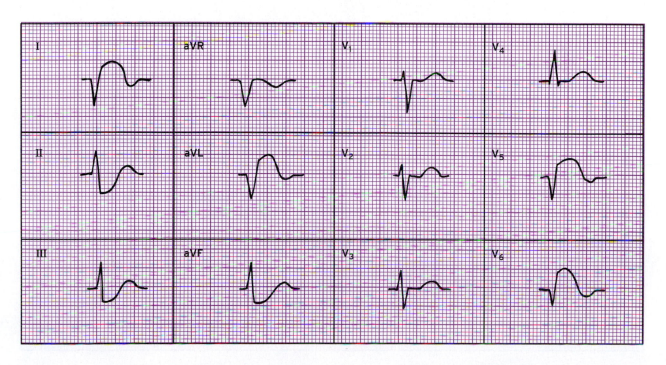

3. _____

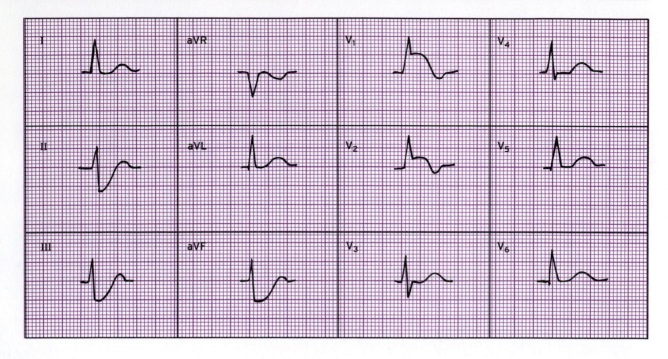

4. _____

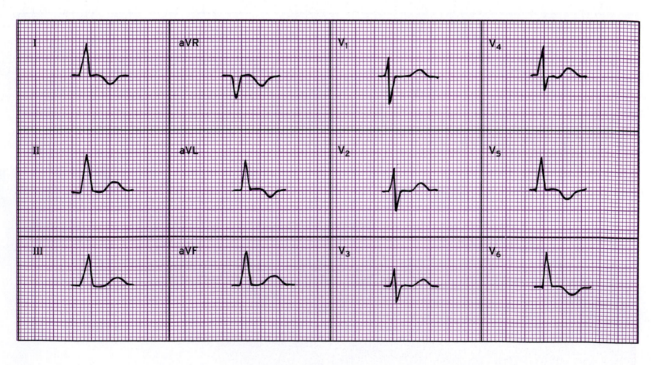

5. _____

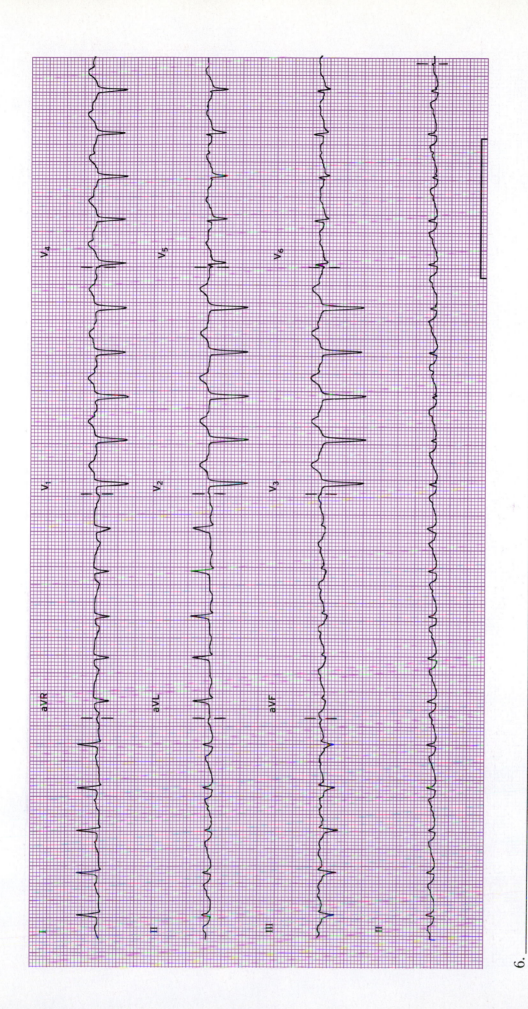

6.

459

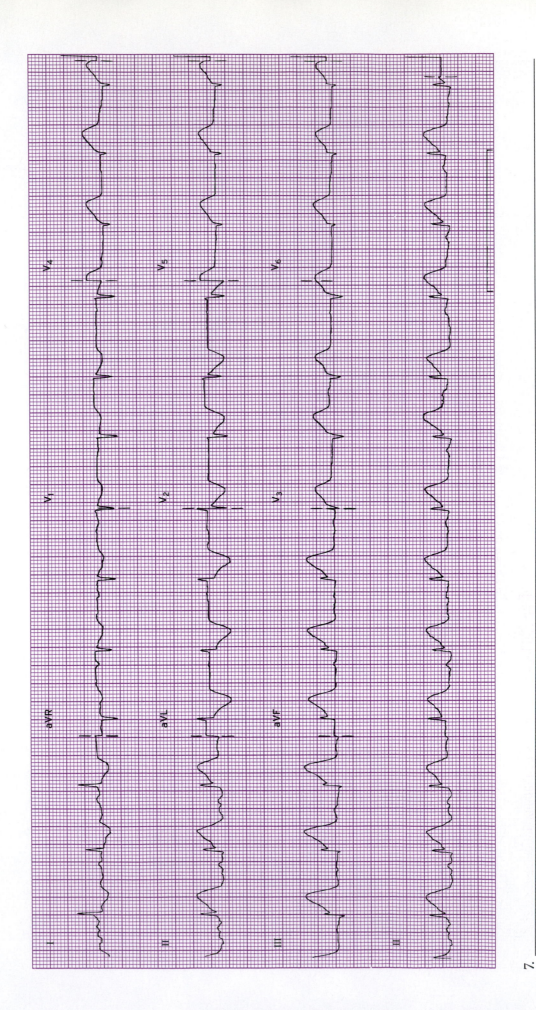

7.

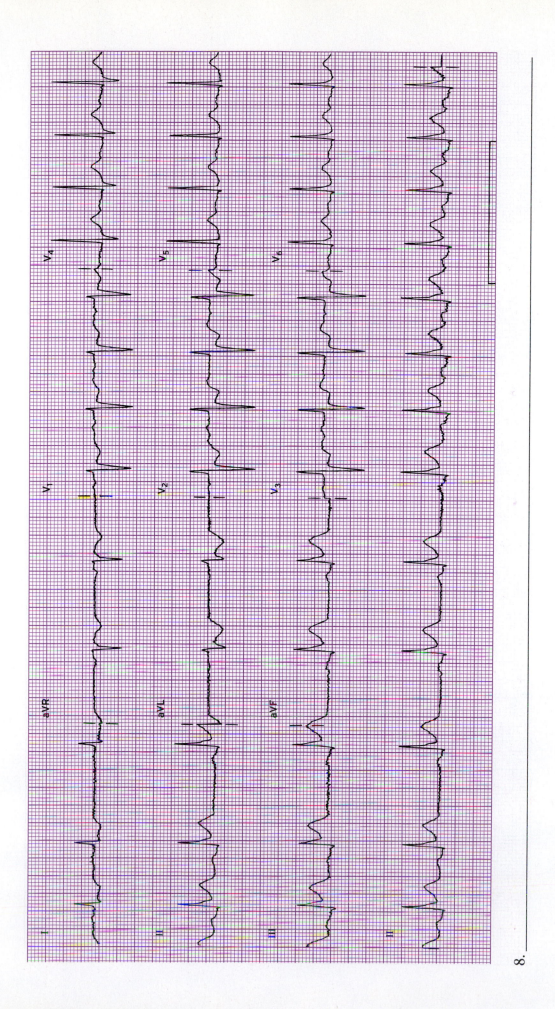

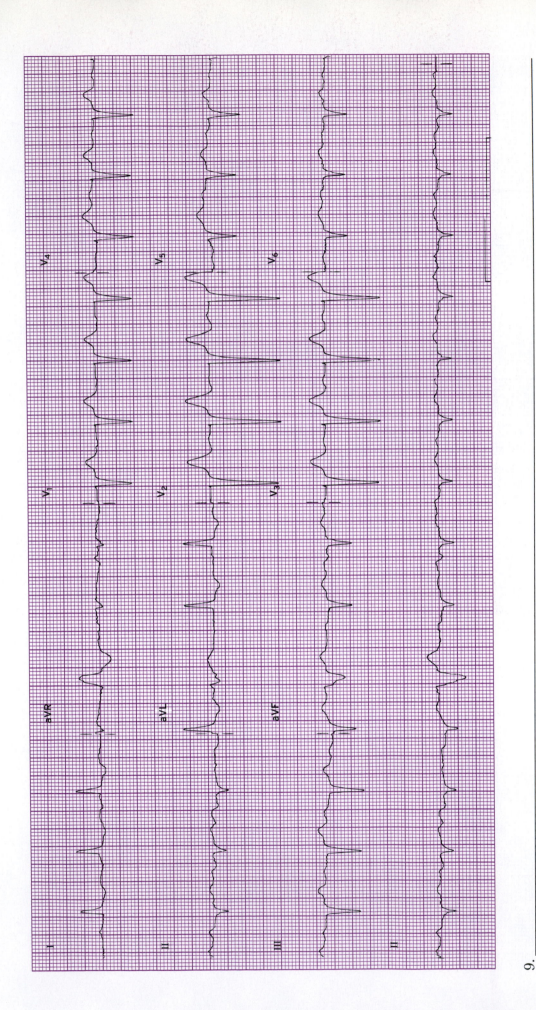

9.

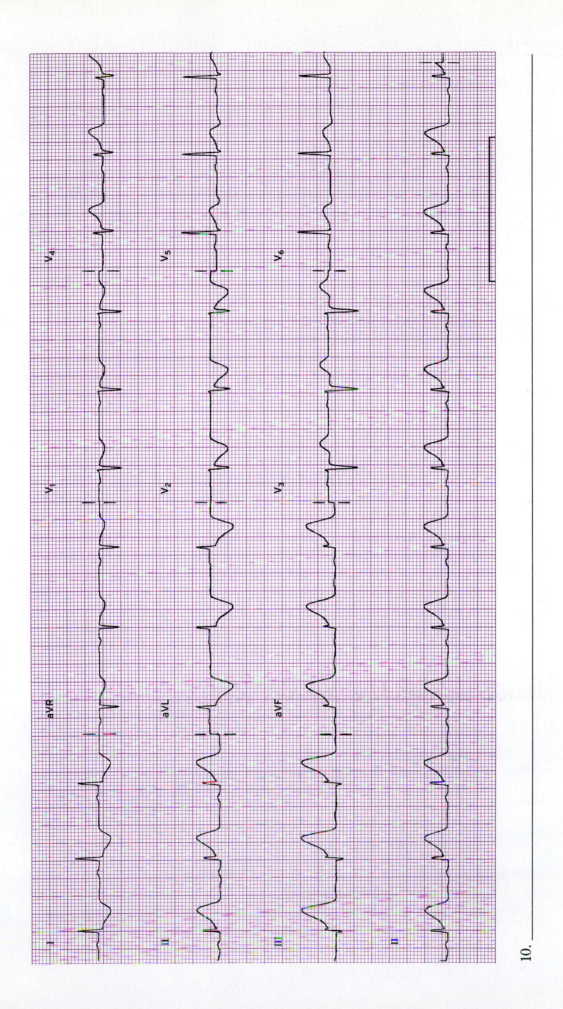

10.

Answers to MI Practice

1. **Extensive anterior MI, acute.** Note the ST segment elevation in leads I, aVL, V_1 to V_6, along with reciprocal ST depression in II, III, and aVF. The T waves are upright.

2. **Inferior MI, age indeterminate.** Note the significant Q waves in II, III, and aVF, along with inverted T waves. The ST segment is at baseline.

3. **Lateral wall MI, acute.** Note the ST elevation, significant Q waves, and inverted T waves in I, aVL, and V_5 to V_6, along with reciprocal ST depression in II, III, and aVF.

4. **Anteroseptal MI, acute.** Note the ST elevation and inverted T in V_1 to V_2, along with reciprocal ST depression in II, III, and aVF.

5. **No MI. Lateral wall ischemia present.** Note the T wave inversion in I, aVL, and V_5 to V_6. Remember that T wave inversion represents ischemia. There is no ST elevation or depression and no significant Q waves.

6. **Anterior and inferior MI, both old.** Note the significant Q waves in V_1 to V_4 (anterior leads), along with essentially normal ST segments. The ST does slope upward a bit in V_1 to V_4, but it is not frankly elevated. There is also an old inferior MI. There are significant Q waves in III and aVF, but not in II. aVF is tiny, but you can see a Q wave there. That Q wave in aVF is significant because it is about half the size of the R wave—more than deep enough to meet the criteria. The T waves in the inferior leads are not inverted.

7. **Inferior and anterior-lateral MI, acute.** There is ST elevation in II, III, and aVF (inferior leads) and ST elevation and QS complexes in V_3 to V_6 (anterior and lateral leads). Leads V_1 and V_2 both have tiny R waves—those are not QS complexes there. It appears this patient started off with an anterior-lateral MI, which then extended into the inferior wall. The Q waves in V_3 to V_6 indicate that that infarct area is older than that in the inferior leads, where there are no significant Q waves.

8. **Inferior MI, acute.** There is ST elevation in II, III, and aVF, along with upright T waves and no significant Q waves as yet. Also note the reciprocal ST depression in I, aVL, and V_1 to V_3.

9. **Inferior-lateral MI, old.** There are significant Q waves in II, III, aVF (inferior leads), and V_6 (lateral lead) with upright T waves and baseline ST segments. Lead V_5 looks like it has a tiny R wave, not a Q wave. Also note the essentially nonexistent R wave progression in the precordial leads. This could imply an additional old anterior MI, or it could be caused by other factors.

10. **Inferior MI, acute.** Note the ST elevation in II, III, and aVF with reciprocal ST depression in I, aVL, and V_1 to V_3. There is a significant Q in III, but not yet in II or aVF.

Practice Quiz

1. List the three Is of infarction. _____

_____

_____

2. State the differences between a Q wave MI and a non–Q wave MI.

_____

3. Which coronary artery's occlusion results in an anterior wall MI?

_____

4. Name the three normal indicative changes of an MI.

_____

5. Reciprocal changes are seen in which area of the heart?

_____

6. If there is ST elevation in leads II, III, and aVF, how old is the MI and in which wall of the heart? _____

_____

7. If there is a significant Q wave in V_1 to V_2 with baseline ST segments and upright T waves, how old is the MI and in which wall of the heart?

_____

8. If the transition zone of the precordial leads is in V_1 to V_2, what kind of rotation is the heart said to have? _____

9. The kind of MI that can be diagnosed by inverting the EKG and looking at leads V_1 and V_2 from behind is the_____

10. Which coronary artery supplies the lateral wall of the left ventricle?

_____

Practice Quiz Answers

1. The three Is of infarction are **ischemia, injury,** and **infarction.**

2. **A Q wave MI causes ST elevation, T wave inversion, and significant Q waves to develop on the EKG. The non–Q wave MI does not cause development of significant Q waves.**

3. Occlusion of the **left anterior descending coronary artery** causes anterior MI.

4. The normal indicative changes of an MI are **ST elevation, significant Q waves,** and **T wave inversions.**

5. Reciprocal changes are seen **in the area electrically opposite the damaged area.**

6. If there is ST elevation in II, III, and aVF, **the MI is acute inferior.**

7. If there is a significant Q wave in V_1 to V_2 with baseline ST segments and upright T waves, **the MI is an old anteroseptal MI.**

8. If the transition zone is in V_1 to V_2, **there is counterclockwise rotation of the heart.**

9. The kind of MI that can be diagnosed by inverting (turning over) the EKG and looking at leads V_1 and V_2 from behind is the **posterior MI.**

10. The **circumflex coronary artery** supplies the lateral wall of the left ventricle.

Miscellaneous EKG Effects

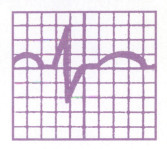

Chapter 26 Objectives

Upon completion of this chapter, the student will be able to:

- Describe the digitalis effect on the EKG.
- Describe the quinidine effect on the EKG.
- Describe the effect of hypo- and hyperkalemia on the EKG.
- Describe the effect of hypo- and hypercalcemia on the EKG.

Chapter 26 Outline

Chapter 26 Glossary

Hypercalcemia: Elevated blood calcium level.

Hyperkalemia: Elevated blood potassium level.

Hypocalcemia: Low blood calcium level.

Hypokalemia: Low blood potassium level.

Introduction

Electrolyte abnormalities and certain medications can affect the EKG. Let's look at some of these effects.

Medication Effects

Digitalis

Digitalis preparations are notorious for causing sagging ST segment depression (also called a **scooping** ST segment) that is easily misinterpreted as ischemia. The cause of this ST segment change is still not understood. Digi-

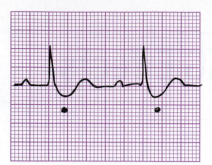

Figure 26-1 Digitalis effect.

talis also prolongs the PR interval because it slows conduction through the AV node. These effects are not necessarily indicative of digitalis toxicity, as they also occur at normal therapeutic levels. See Figure 26-1.

See the sagging ST segments and prolonged PR interval in figure 26-1? This is typical of the digitalis effect.

Quinidine

Quinidine causes a widened T wave and prolongs the QT interval to such a degree that arrhythmias such as torsades de pointes can occur. These effects are due to quinidine's prolonging effect on repolarization. See Figure 26-2.

Note the incredibly wide T wave and the prolonged QT interval. With quinidine effect, the prolonged QT is caused by the widened T wave.

Electrolyte Abnormalities

Hyperkalemia

A high potassium level in the bloodstream has two main EKG effects. First, at potassium levels of about 6, it causes tall, pointy, narrow T waves. You'll recall that normal blood potassium level is 3.5 to 5. As the potassium level continues to rise to around 8, the tall T wave is replaced by a very widened QRS complex. This widened QRS is a sign that cardiac arrest may be imminent if the potassium level is not lowered quickly. These EKG effects are due to potassium's effect on depolarization and repolarization, and will return to normal once the potassium level is normalized. One way to remember potassium's effect on the T wave is to think of the T wave as a tent contain-

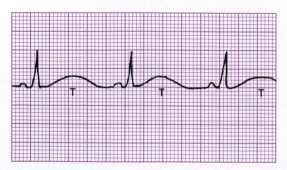

Figure 26-2 Quinidine effect.

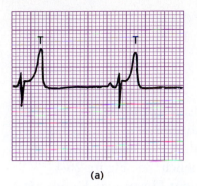

Figure 26-3 Hyperkalemia.

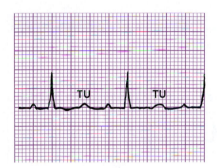

Figure 26-4 Hypokalemia.

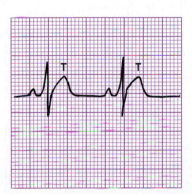

Figure 26-5 Hypercalcemia.

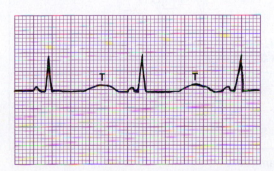

Figure 26-6 Hypocalcemia.

ing potassium. The more potassium, the taller the tent. See Figure 26-3. In Figure 26-3(a), note the tall, pointy T waves. In Figure 26-3(b), note the widened QRS complex.

Hypokalemia

A low potassium level in the bloodstream results in a prominent U wave and flattened T waves. The potassium tent is almost empty, so it flattens out. These effects are due to the fact that repolarization, especially phase 3 of the action potential, is disturbed by the potassium deficit. See Figure 26-4.

Note the flattened T wave and the prominent U wave in Figure 26-4. Recall the U wave is not usually seen on the EKG, but if it is present it follows the T wave. T waves always follow QRS complexes. *If there are no obvious T waves on the strip, be sure the QRS complexes are really QRS complexes and*

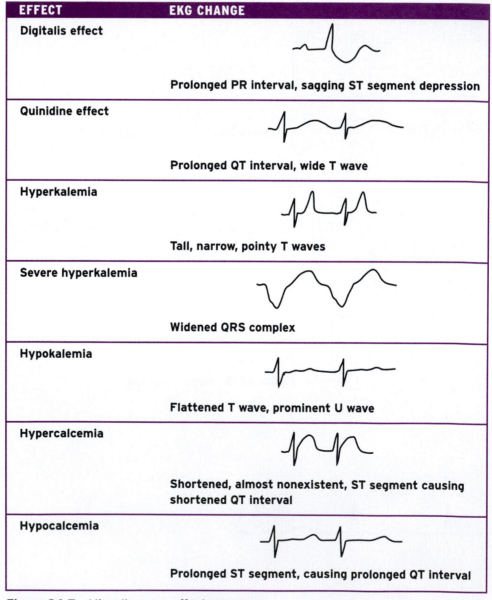

EFFECT	EKG CHANGE
Digitalis effect	Prolonged PR interval, sagging ST segment depression
Quinidine effect	Prolonged QT interval, wide T wave
Hyperkalemia	Tall, narrow, pointy T waves
Severe hyperkalemia	Widened QRS complex
Hypokalemia	Flattened T wave, prominent U wave
Hypercalcemia	Shortened, almost nonexistent, ST segment causing shortened QT interval
Hypocalcemia	Prolonged ST segment, causing prolonged QT interval

Figure 26-7 Miscellaneous effects summary.

not artifact. Then, if you still can't really see T waves following those QRS complexes, you can be reasonably sure the potassium level is quite low, usually around 2.0. T waves will improve after supplemental potassium is given.

Hypercalcemia

An elevated blood calcium level causes the ST segment to shorten to such an extent that the T wave seems to be almost on top of the QRS. This effect occurs because the elevated calcium level shortens the repolarization phase of the action potential. See Figure 26-5.

In Figure 26-5, note the extremely short ST segment, which in turn causes a very short QT interval. The ST segment and QT interval will return to normal once the calcium level is normalized.

Hypocalcemia

Low calcium levels in the bloodstream prolong repolarization and cause a very prolonged ST segment, thus prolonging the QT interval. See Figure 26-6.

In Figure 26-6, note how far the T wave is from the QRS complex. This demonstrates a very prolonged ST segment and QT interval.

Summary of Miscellaneous Effects

See Figure 26-7 for a summary of miscellaneous effects.

Practice Quiz

1. What effect does digitalis have on the EKG? _____

   _____

   _____

2. Prolonged QT interval can be caused by what two factors? _____

   _____

3. A prolonged QT interval caused by prolonging of the ST segment is caused by _____

   _____

4. Tall, narrow, pointy T waves are a sign of _____

5. A very short ST segment is typical of _____

Practice Quiz Answers

1. Digitalis causes **sagging ST segment depression and prolonged PR intervals.**

2. Prolonged QT interval can be caused by **quinidine** and **hypocalcemia.** Quinidine lengthens the QT by widening the T wave. Hypocalcemia lengthens the QT by prolonging the ST segment.

3. A prolonged QT interval caused by prolonging of the ST segment is caused by **hypocalcemia.**

4. Tall, narrow, pointy T waves are a sign of **hyperkalemia.**

5. A very short ST segment is typical of **hypercalcemia.**

12-Lead EKG Practice

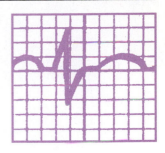

Chapter 27 Objectives

Upon completion of this chapter, the student will be able to:

- Practice the six steps in analyzing EKGs.
- Using this method, correctly interpret a variety of 12-lead EKGs.

Chapter 27 Outline

I.   Introduction

II.   12-lead EKG interpretation in a nutshell

III. 12-lead EKG interpretation checklist

IV. Practice EKGs

V.   Answers to practice EKGs

Chapter 27 Glossary

There are no new terms introduced in this chapter.

Introduction

This chapter will pull together everything you've learned so far about rhythm and 12-lead EKG interpretation. First you will find a summary of what to look for on every EKG, then a checklist. Refer to these when evaluating the 12-lead EKGs that follow.

There are 10 EKGs to interpret in this chapter. Take your time and be methodical. Don't hesitate to go back and review portions of this text if you find that you're a little rusty in certain areas. Practice does indeed make perfect.

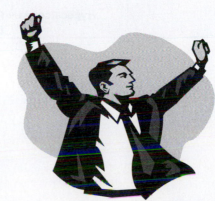

Now let's get down to work.

Think positively. You know this stuff . . .

12-Lead EKG Interpretation in a Nutshell

You've now seen all the criteria for 12-lead EKG interpretation. Let's put it all in condensed form. Look for the following on every 12-lead EKG:

The Basics	Rhythm, Rate, Intervals (PR, QRS, QT)
Axis	Don't forget to put the + or − signs on the degree marking.
IVCDs	RBBB = RSR′ in V_1, QRS ≥ 0.12 s LBBB = QS or RS in V_1, monophasic R in V_6, QRS ≥ 0.12 s LAHB = Small Q in I, small R in III, left axis deviation LPHB = Small R in I, small Q in III, right axis deviation
Hypertrophy	RAE = Tall peaked P ≥ 2.5 mm in II or V_1 LAE = Notched P in II with 0.04 s between notches *or* P in any lead ≥ 0.11 s wide *or* biphasic P with terminal negative portion 1 mm wide and/or 1 mm deep. RVH = R ≥ S in V_1, inverted T, RAD LVH = S in V_1 + R in V_5 or V_6 ≥ 35 *or* R in aVL ≥ 11 mm *or* R in V_5 or V_6 > 27 mm
Infarction	Anterior MI = ST elevation and/or significant Q in V_1 to V_4 Inferior MI = ST elevation and/or significant Q in II, III, aVF Lateral MI = ST elevation and/or significant Q in I, aVL, V_5 to V_6 Anteroseptal MI = ST elevation and/or significant Q in V_1 to V_2 Extensive anterior (extensive anterior-lateral) = ST elevation and/or significant Q in I, aVL, V_1 to V_6 Posterior MI = Large R + upright T in V_1 to V_2; may also have ST depression. Subendocardial = Widespread ST depression and T wave inversion in many leads Ischemia = Inverted T waves in any lead, as long as not BBB-related
Miscellaneous effects	Digitalis effect = Sagging ST segments, prolonged PR interval Quinidine effect = Wide T waves causing prolonged QT interval Hyperkalemia = Tall, pointy, narrow T waves Severe hyperkalemia = Wide QRS complex Hypokalemia = Prominent U waves, flattened T waves Hypercalcemia = Shortened ST segment causing short QT interval Hypocalcemia = Prolonged ST segment causing prolonged QT interval

12-Lead EKG Interpretation Checklist

The Basics

- Rhythm _____
- Rate _____
- Intervals   PR _____   QRS _____   QT _____

Axis

- Degree marking _____

Intraventricular Conduction Defects (IVCDs)

Circle if present:

- RBBB
- LBBB
- LAHB
- LPHB

Hypertrophy

Circle if present:

- RAE
- LAE
- RVH
- LVH

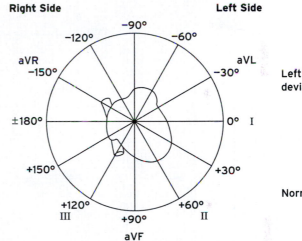

Infarction

Circle if present:

- Anterior MI
- Inferior MI
- Lateral MI
- Posterior MI
- Anteroseptal MI
- Extensive anterior (anterior-lateral) MI
- Subendocardial MI
- Ischemia

Miscellaneous Effects

Circle if present:

- Hyperkalemia
- Severe hyperkalemia
- Hypokalemia
- Hypercalcemia
- Hypocalcemia
- Digitalis effect
- Quinidine effect

Practice EKGs

1. Rhythm and rate _____ PR _____ QRS _____ QT _____

Axis _____ IVCDs _____

Hypertrophy _____

Infarction _____

Miscellaneous effects _____

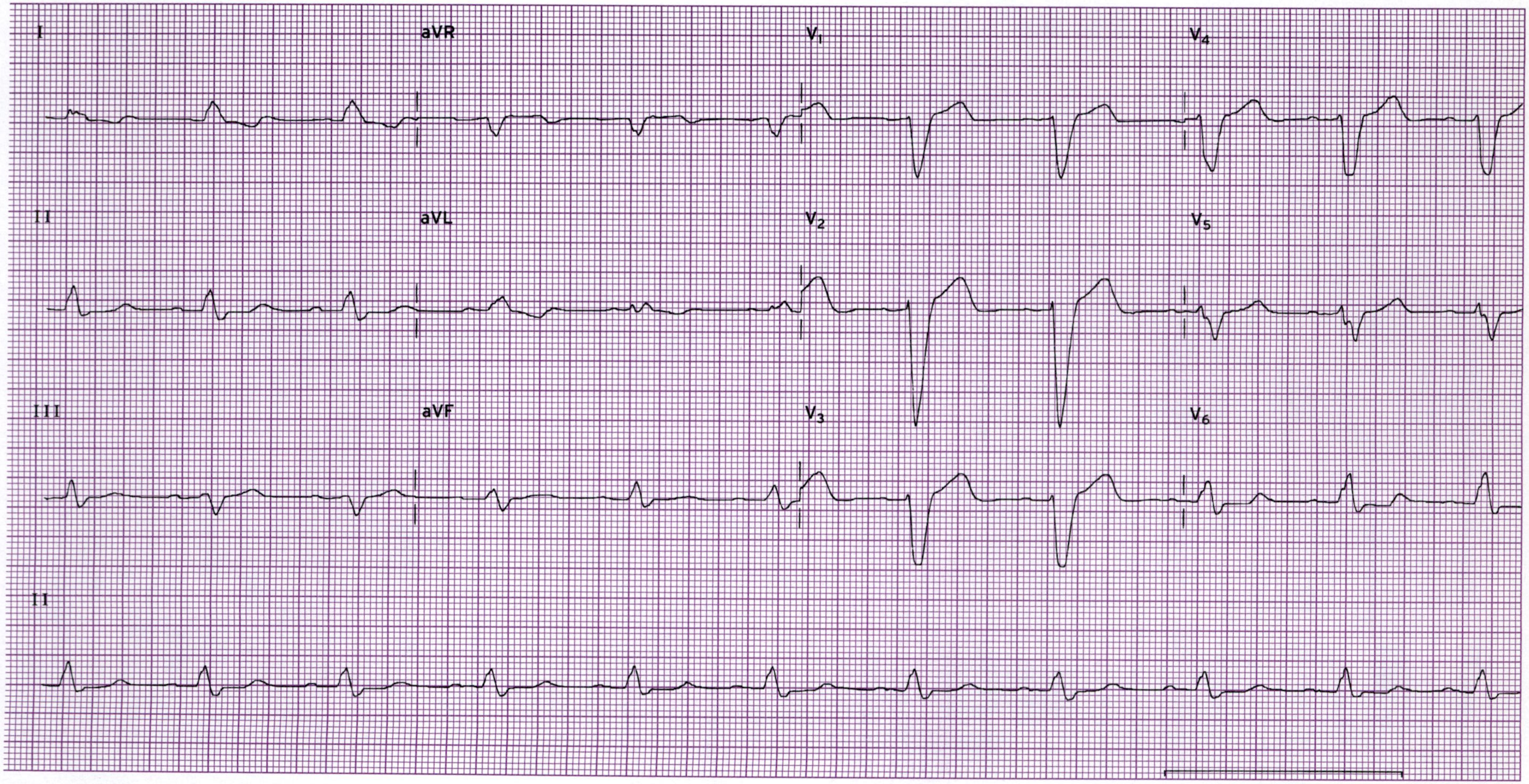

2. Rhythm and rate _____ PR _____ QT _____

Axis _____ IVCDs _____

Hypertrophy _____

Infarction _____

Miscellaneous effects _____

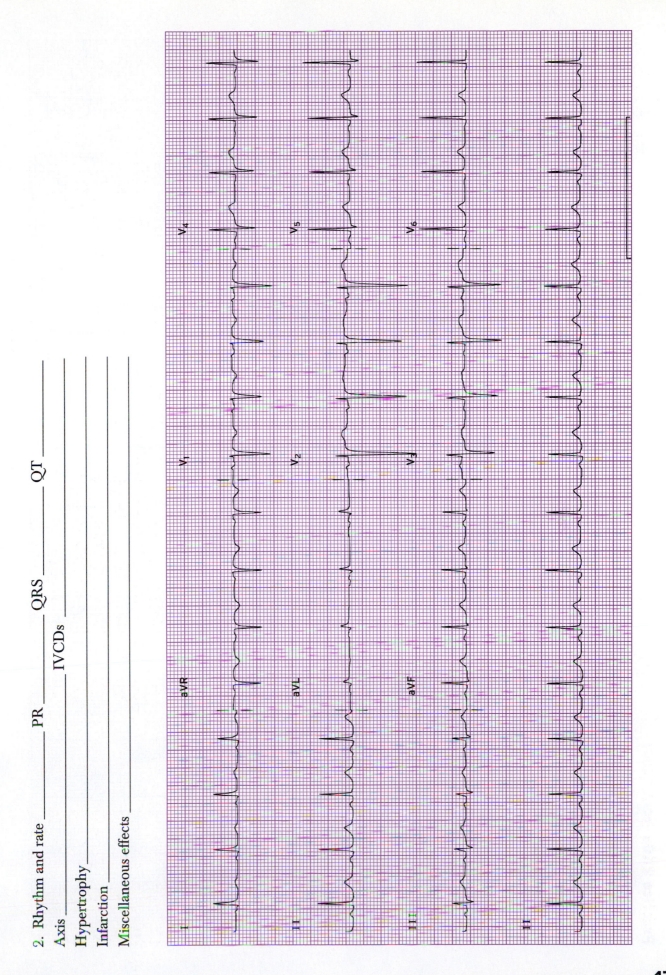

477

Practice EKGs (continued)

3. Rhythm and rate _____ PR _____ QRS _____ QT _____

Axis _____ IVCDs _____

Hypertrophy _____

Infarction _____

Miscellaneous effects _____

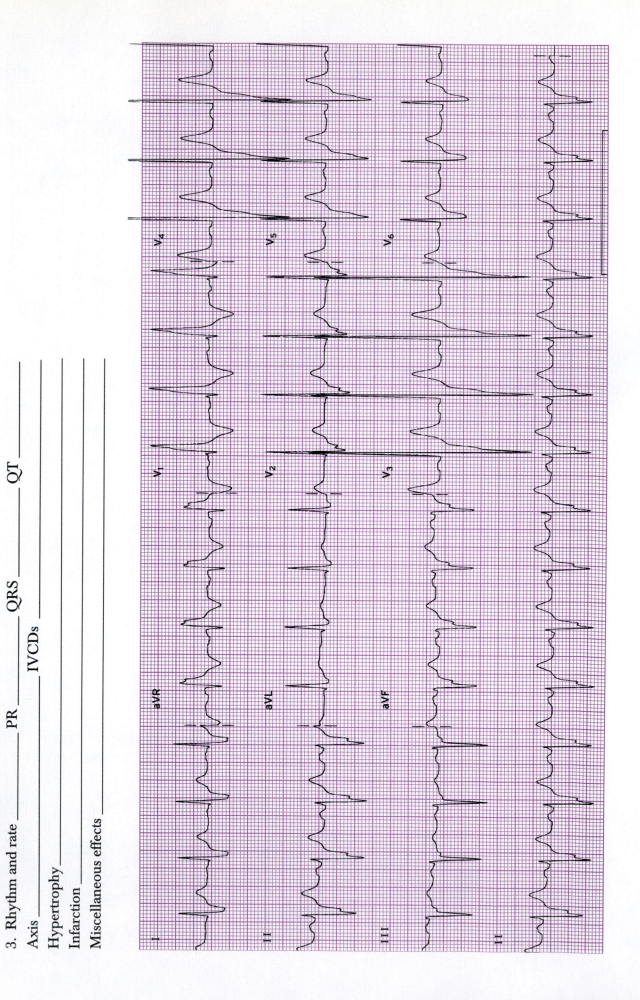

4. Rhythm and rate _____ PR _____ QRS _____ QT _____

Axis _____ IVCDs _____

Hypertrophy _____

Infarction _____

Miscellaneous effects _____

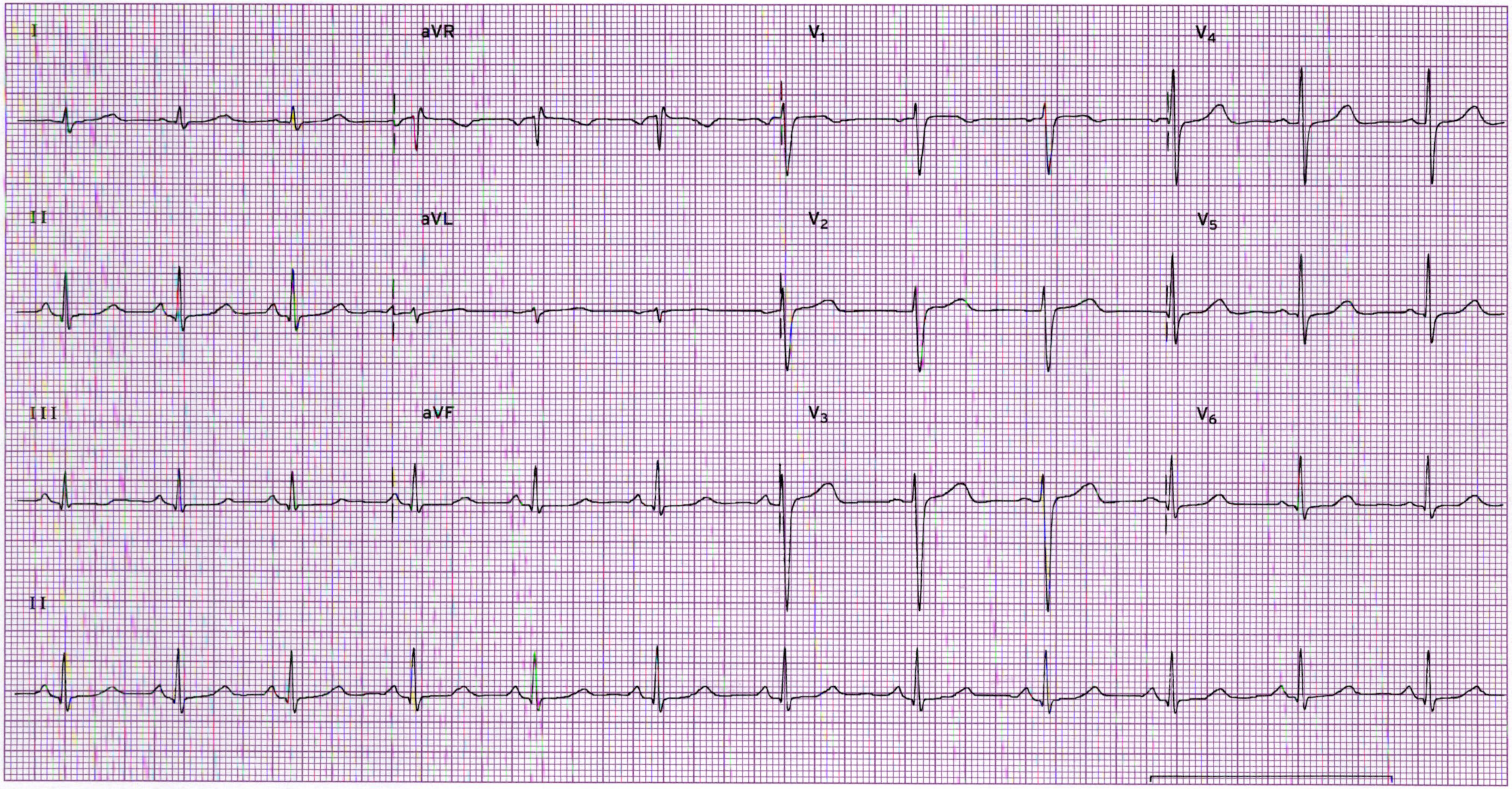

5. Rhythm and rate _____ PR _____ QRS _____ QT _____

Axis _____ IVCDs _____

Hypertrophy _____

Infarction _____

Miscellaneous effects _____

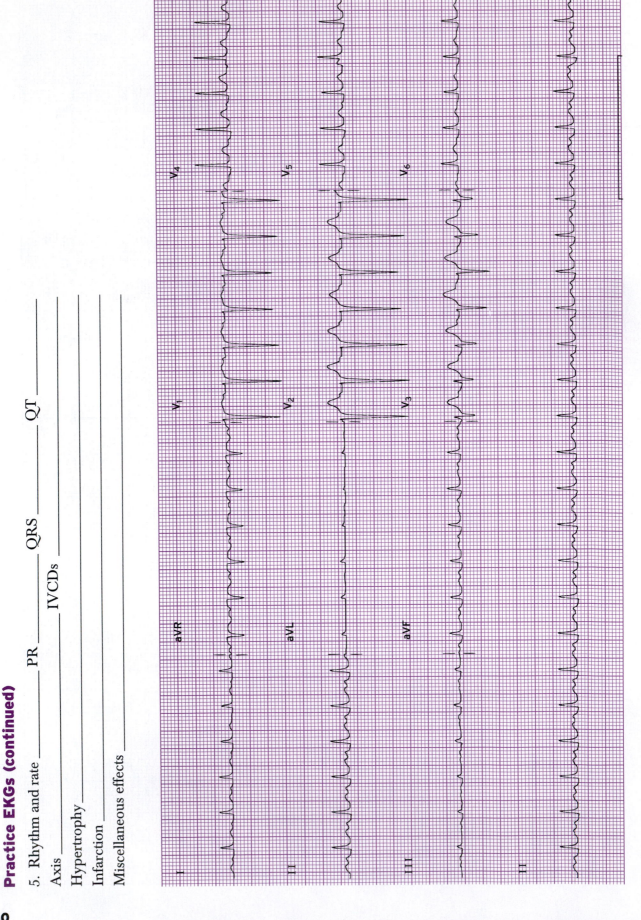

6. Rhythm and rate _____ PR _____ QRS _____ QT _____

Axis _____ IVCDs _____

Hypertrophy _____

Infarction _____

Miscellaneous effects _____

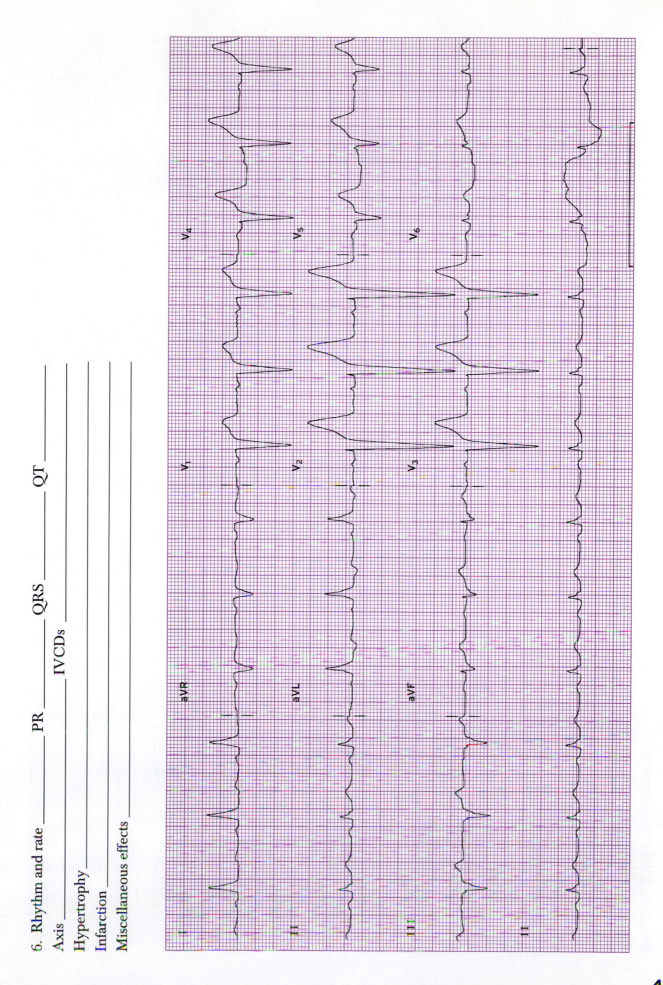

Practice EKGs (continued)

7. Rhythm and rate _____ PR _____ QRS _____ QT _____

Axis _____ IVCDs _____

Hypertrophy _____

Infarction _____

Miscellaneous effects _____

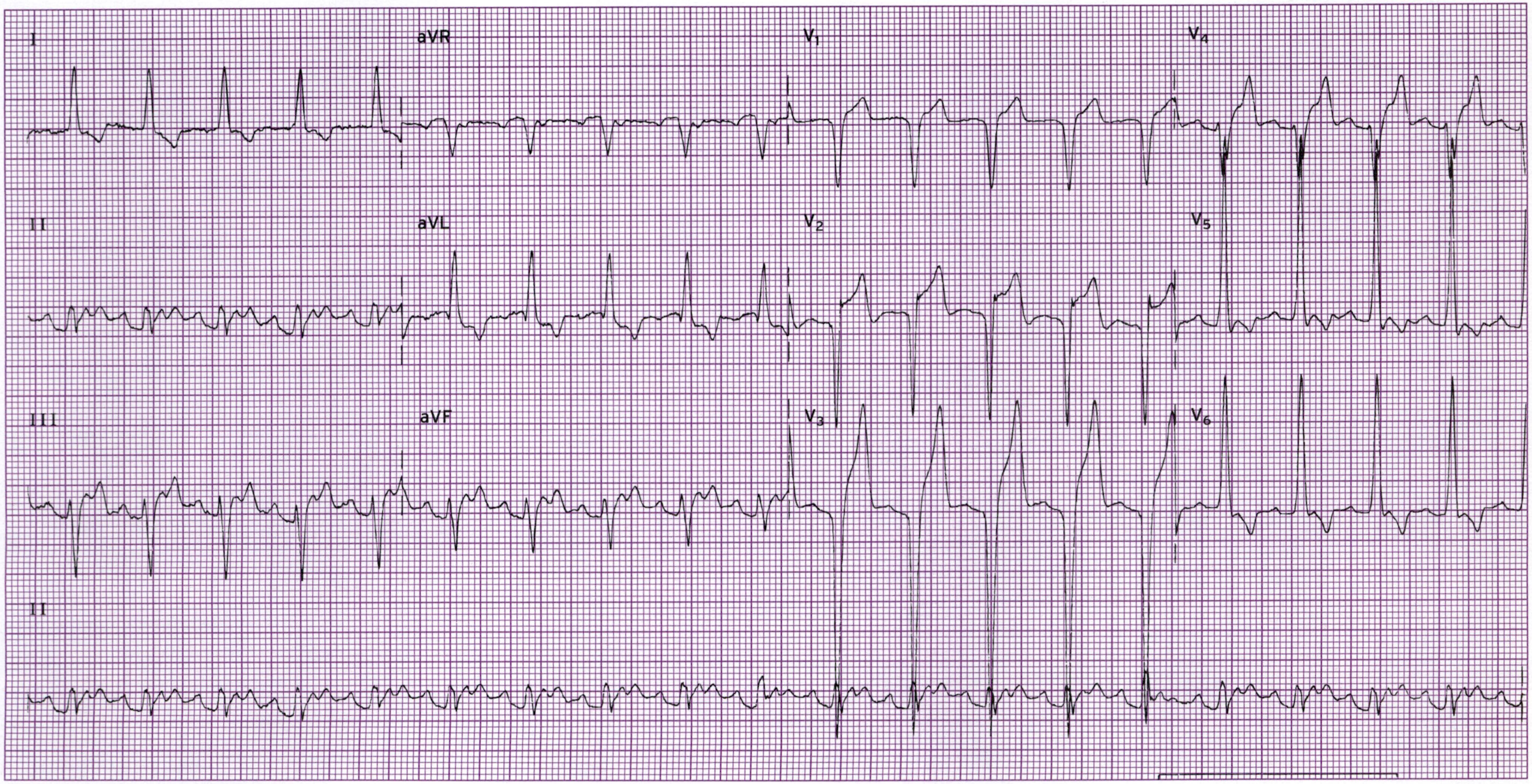

8. Rhythm and rate _____ PR _____ QRS _____ QT _____

Axis _____ IVCDs _____

Hypertrophy _____

Infarction _____

Miscellaneous effects _____

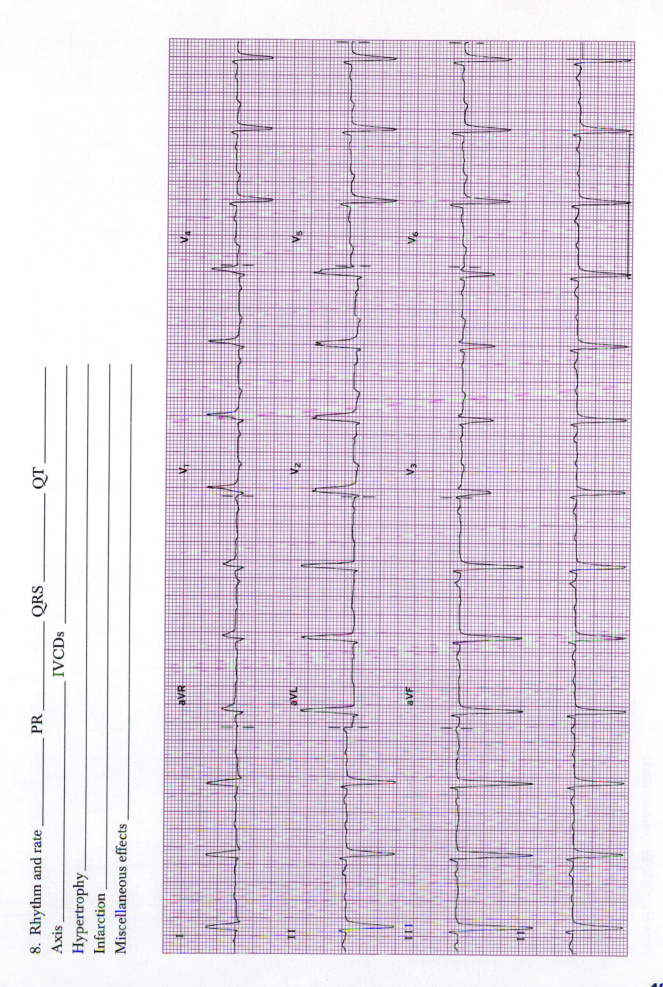

Practice EKGs (continued)

9. Rhythm and rate _____ PR _____ QRS _____ QT _____

Axis _____ IVCDs _____

Hypertrophy _____

Infarction _____

Miscellaneous effects _____

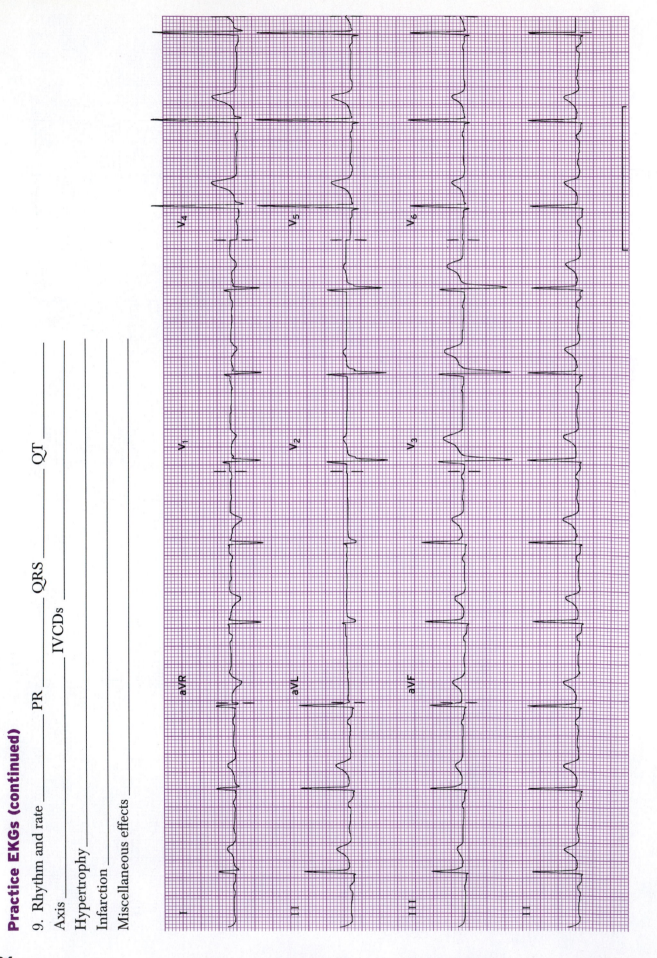

10. **R**hythm and rate _____ PR _____ QRS _____ QT _____

Axis _____ IVCDs _____

Hypertrophy _____

Infarction _____

Miscellaneous effects _____

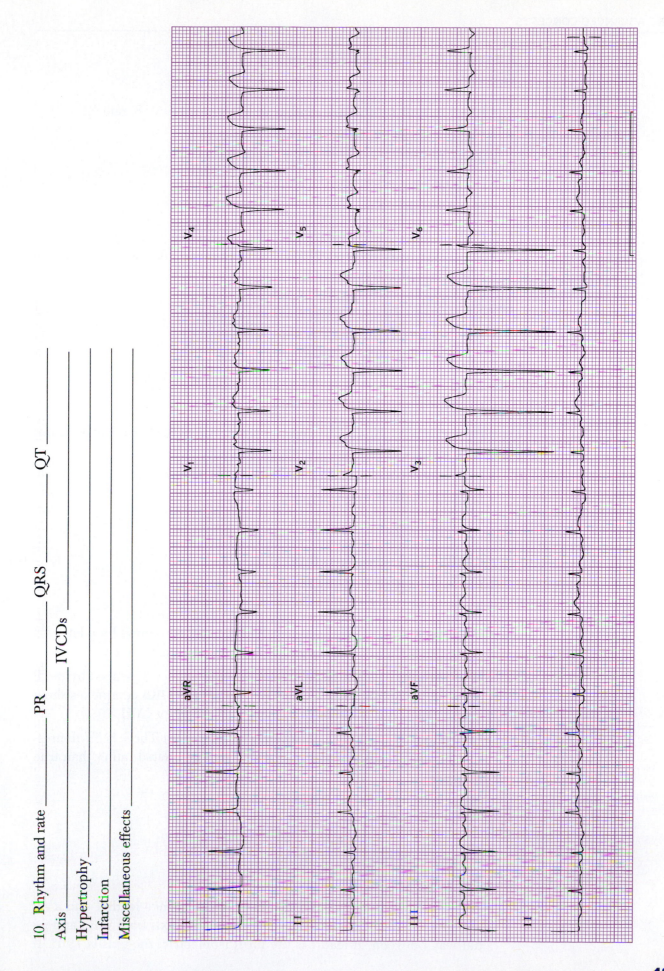

Answers to 12-Lead EKG Practice

EKG 1

- **Rhythm and rate:** Sinus rhythm with first-degree AVB, rate 62.
- **PR:** 0.20–0.24   **QRS:** 0.16   **QT:** 0.44–0.48
- **Axis:** 0°
- **IVCDs:** Left bundle branch block.
- **Hypertrophy:** None.
- **Infarction:** No evidence of ischemia or infarction.
- **Miscellaneous effects:** None. The widened QRS here is from the LBBB, not from hyperkalemia.

EKG 2

- **Rhythm and rate:** Sinus rhythm, rate 94.
- **PR:** 0.12   **QRS:** 0.06   **QT:** 0.34
- **Axis:** +30°
- **IVCDs:** None.
- **Hypertrophy:** None. The negative deflection of the P wave in V_1 is not deep enough to be LAE.
- **Infarction:** No evidence of ischemia or infarction.
- **Miscellaneous effects:** None.

EKG 3

- **Rhythm and rate:** Sinus rhythm, rate 94.
- **PR:** 0.16   **QRS:** 0.14   **QT:** 0.40
- **Axis:** −60°
- **IVCDs:** RBBB + LAHB. (When RBBB is accompanied by a left axis deviation, it almost always signifies an accompanying LAHB.)
- **Hypertrophy:** Left atrial enlargement is present, as evidenced by the P wave of 0.12 second wide in lead II. Though the QRS complexes show great voltage, it is not enough to meet the criteria for LVH.
- **Infarction:** No evidence of ischemia or infarction. There is ST depression in many leads, but this is probably bundle-related rather than true ischemia.
- **Miscellaneous effects:** None.

EKG 4

- **Rhythm and rate:** Sinus rhythm, rate 68.
- **PR:** 0.16   **QRS:** 0.08   **QT:** 0.40
- **Axis:** +75°. Where did *that* axis come from? Since leads I and aVL are almost equally isoelectric, we figure out the axis both ways and go halfway between. If lead I is the most isoelectric, the axis is +90°. If

it's aVL, the axis is +60°. So we fudge halfway between and call it +75°. Only do this if you can't decide which lead is the most iso-electric. If you said +60 or +90, that's fine. Consider it correct.

- **IVCDs:** None.
- **Hypertrophy:** None.
- **Infarction:** No evidence of ischemia or infarction.
- **Miscellaneous effects:** None.

EKG 5

- **Rhythm and rate:** Sinus tachycardia, rate 150.
- **PR:** 0.14   **QRS:** 0.06   **QT:** 0.24
- **Axis:** +60°. aVL looks slightly more isoelectric than lead III.
- **IVCDs:** None.
- **Hypertrophy:** None. In fact, the voltage is pretty low throughout.
- **Infarction:** No evidence of ischemia or infarction. Those are not Q waves in V_1 to V_2, in case you thought it was an anteroseptal MI. There's a small R wave there.
- **Miscellaneous effects:** None.

EKG 6

- **Rhythm and rate:** Sinus rhythm, rate 71.
- **PR:** 0.20   **QRS:** 0.12   **QT:** 0.40
- **Axis:** 0°
- **IVCDs:** LBBB
- **Hypertrophy:** LAE is probably present, as evidenced by the wide P waves of 0.12 second and the terminal negativity of the biphasic P in V_1 being ≥1 mm deep/wide.
- **Infarction:** No evidence of ischemia or infarction.
- **Miscellaneous effects:** None.

EKG 7

- **Rhythm and rate:** Atrial tachycardia with 2:1 block versus atrial flutter with 2:1 conduction. Atrial rate 250, ventricular rate 115.
- **PR:** 0.16   **QRS:** 0.10   **QT:** 0.28
- **Axis:** −30°
- **IVCDs:** LAHB.
- **Hypertrophy:** LVH by voltage criteria.
- **Infarction:** Anterior and inferior wall MI. Note the ST segment elevation in II, III, aVF, and V_1 to V_4. There are already significant Q waves in V_1 to V_3. This is a massive MI.
- **Miscellaneous effects:** No miscellaneous effects. The incredibly tall, pointy T wave in V_3 is related to the huge QRS voltage in that lead.

EKG 8

- **Rhythm and rate:** Sinus rhythm, rate 75.
- **PR:** 0.18   **QRS:** 0.13   **QT:** 0.42
- **Axis:** −60°
- **IVCDs:** RBBB + LAHB.
- **Hypertrophy:** LVH. See how tall the R wave is in aVL? It's taller than 11 mm, so it meets the criteria for LVH. Also note the left ventricular strain pattern in V_4 to V_6. There is also LAE, as evidenced by the widened P waves. Also note the notching of the P waves in lead II.
- **Infarction:** Probable old anteroseptal MI, as there is a loss of the normal small R wave in V_1 to V_2.
- **Miscellaneous effects:** None.

EKG 9

- **Rhythm and rate:** Sinus rhythm, rate 65.
- **PR:** 0.18   **QRS:** 0.06   **QT:** 0.36
- **Axis:** +60°
- **IVCDs:** None.
- **Hypertrophy:** None, but very close to meeting voltage criteria for LVH.
- **Infarction:** Probable early repolarization. Note the very slight concave ST elevation in II, III, aVF, and V_3 to V_5. It would help to know the age of this patient and the symptoms (if any) to identify this with a higher probability of accuracy.
- **Miscellaneous effects:** None.

EKG 10

- **Rhythm and rate:** Atrial flutter with 2:1 conduction. No way, you say? Look at V_1. See the spike in the ST segment? That's a flutter wave. There's another one before the QRS. Atrial rate is about 250, ventricular rate is 125.
- **PR:** Not applicable   **QRS:** 0.06   **QT:** 0.24
- **Axis:** 0° (aVF is the most isoelectric).
- **IVCDs:** None. The axis is still normal. There is no LAHB.
- **Hypertrophy:** None. In fact, the voltage is rather low in the frontal leads.
- **Infarction:** Acute anterior-lateral MI. Note the ST elevation in V_1 to V_6. There are significant Q waves in V_1 to V_5. There is also *very slight* ST coving in III and aVF, so there may also be an inferior MI.
- **Miscellaneous effects:** None.

Cardiac Medications

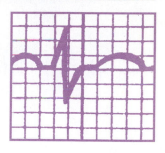

Chapter 28 Objectives

Upon completion of this chapter, the student will be able to:

- Describe the effect of each class of antiarrhythmic medication on the action potential.
- Give examples of each class of antiarrhythmic medication.
- Describe the effects of digitalis and adenosine on the heart rate.
- Name the emergency medications and describe the mode of action of each.
- Describe the danger of giving supplemental oxygen to patients with chronic lung disease.

Chapter 28 Outline

I.   Introduction
II. Antiarrhythmics
     A. Class I, class II, class III, class IV
III. Emergency cardiac medications
     A. Atropine, epinephrine, lidocaine, verapamil, sodium bicarbonate, isoproterenol, oxygen
IV. Practice quiz
V.   Practice quiz answers

Chapter 28 Glossary

Antiarrhythmic: A class of medications that treats or prevents arrhythmias.
Bronchi: The large airways leading from the trachea to the lungs.
Endotracheal: Into the trachea.
Intramuscular: Into a muscle.
Intravenous: Through a vein.
Oral: By mouth.
Sublingual: Under the tongue.
Tachyarrhythmias: Rapid arrhythmias.
Trachea: Windpipe.
Transdermal: Through the skin.

Vasoconstriction: Clamping down of the arterial wall tight against the blood inside. Causes the artery opening to become smaller.

Vasodilation: Loosening of the arterial wall, causing the artery to open up wider.

Introduction

Cardiac medications are used to treat arrhythmias or abnormalities in cardiac function. We will look at various classifications of medications.

Antiarrhythmics

These medications are used to treat and/or prevent arrhythmias. They all affect the action potential. See Figure 28-1 for the effects of each class on the action potential. There are four classes of antiarrhythmic medications. Let's look at the four classes.

Class I: Sodium Channel Blockers

Class I medications block the influx of sodium ions into the cardiac cell during depolarization. This results in decreased excitability of the cardiac cell and decreased myocardial contractility. Class I antiarrhythmic medications affect phase 0 of the action potential. There are three categories of class I antiarrhythmics:

- *Class Ia.* These medications include *quinidine* and *procainamide,* and they cause prolonged QT interval as well as decreased cardiac contractility. They can also cause hypotension. Quinidine is especially notorious for causing wide T waves. Most class Ia antiarrhythmics can be used to treat supraventricular as well as ventricular arrhythmias. Quinidine is

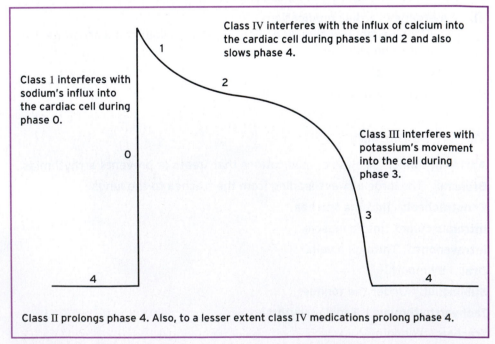

Class IV interferes with the influx of calcium into the cardiac cell during phases 1 and 2 and also slows phase 4.

Class 1 interferes with sodium's influx into the cardiac cell during phase 0.

Class III interferes with potassium's movement into the cell during phase 3.

Class II prolongs phase 4. Also, to a lesser extent class IV medications prolong phase 4.

Figure 28-1 Effects of each class of antiarrhythmic medications on the action potential.

usually given orally. In rare instances it may be given intravenously. Procainamide can be given orally or intravenously.

- *Class Ib.* These medications include *lidocaine* and *tocainide,* both of which have a local anesthetic effect. They are used for treatment of ventricular arrhythmias only. They suppress the ventricles' irritability and raise the fibrillatory threshold, making it less likely the ventricles will fibrillate. Class Ib medications have minimal, if any, effect on conductivity. Lidocaine is given intravenously. Tocainide is given orally.

- *Class Ic.* These medications slow impulse conduction and are useful in treating SVT and ventricular arrhythmias. Unfortunately, they are also very prone to causing arrhythmias and are therefore used only in life-threatening situations. These medications include *flecainide* and *propafenone,* both of which are given orally.

Class II: Beta-Blockers

Beta-blockers slow the heart rate by blocking the sympathetic nervous system's beta receptors. There are two kinds of beta receptors: *Beta-1 receptors* increase heart rate, conductivity, and contractility. *Beta-2 receptors* relax smooth muscle in arteries and bronchi. Blocking these receptors decreases or blocks these actions. Beta-blockers decrease the automaticity of the sinus node, slow AV conduction, and slow the process of depolarization. They are used to treat supraventricular tachyarrhythmias. They depress phase 4 of the action potential. Beta-blockers include medications such as *propranolol* and *atenolol.* Propranolol can be given orally or intravenously. Atenolol is given orally. Beta-blockers should be used with caution in patients with asthma or heart failure, as the effects could be life-threatening.

Class III: Potassium Channel Blockers

These medications interfere with the movement of potassium ions into the cardiac cell during phase 3 of the action potential. They therefore can prolong the PR, QRS, and QT intervals. Class III medications can be used to treat supraventricular and/or ventricular arrhythmias. Medications include *amiodarone* and *bretylium,* which are used to treat ventricular arrhythmias, and *ibutilide,* used for supraventricular tachyarrhythmias. Amiodarone can be given orally or intravenously. Bretylium and ibutilide are given intravenously.

Class IV: Calcium Channel Blockers

These medications interfere with the influx of calcium into the cardiac cell during phases 1 and 2 of the action potential and also slow phase 4 of the action potential. Thus, AV conduction is prolonged and contractility decreased. The PR interval will prolong and the heart rate will slow. Calcium blockers are used for supraventricular arrhythmias. Medications include *verapamil* and *diltiazem,* both of which can be given orally or intravenously.

There are other antiarrhythmic medications that do not fall into any of the four classes. These include but are not limited to *adenosine,* which is used to treat SVT, and *digitalis,* classified as a cardiac glycoside, which is used to treat heart failure and supraventricular arrhythmias.

Let's summarize the antiarrhythmic medications. See Table 28-1.

Table 28-1 Antiarrhythmic Medications Summary

CLASS	KNOWN AS	MODE OF ACTION	EXAMPLES	KIND OF ARRHYTHMIAS TREATED
I	Sodium channel blockers	Block sodium's influx into the cardiac cell, decrease myocardial excitability and contractility	*Ia.* Quinidine, procainamide *Ib.* Lidocaine, tocainide *Ic.* Flecainide, propafenone	*Ia.* Supraventricular and ventricular *Ib.* Ventricular only *Ic.* Supraventricular and ventricular
II	Beta-blockers	Block the sympathetic nervous system's beta receptors, slow the heart rate	Propranolol, atenolol	Supraventricular
III	Potassium channel blockers	Decrease potassium's movement into the cardiac cell, prolong PR, QRS, and QT intervals	Amiodarone, bretylium, ibutilide	Ventricular *or* supraventricular
IV	Calcium channel blockers	Decrease calcium's influx into the cardiac cell, slow AV conduction, decrease contractility	Verapamil, diltiazem	Supraventricular

Emergency Cardiac Medications

These medications are used during cardiac arrest or in situations in which the patient's condition is rapidly deteriorating because of an arrhythmia.

- *Atropine.* Atropine is used to increase the heart rate during asystole or bradycardias. It nullifies any vagal influence. It is usually given intravenously, but in situations in which there is no IV line in place, it can be given via the **endotracheal tube,** a breathing tube inserted into the trachea by way of the nose or mouth.

- *Epinephrine.* This medication became famous for saving the unfortunate Uma Thurman's character's life in the movie *Pulp Fiction.* Epinephrine is a catecholamine that causes vasoconstriction, thus increasing the blood pressure, and beta receptor stimulation, thus restoring the heartbeat in cardiac arrest. It is given intravenously (or endotracheally if an IV line is not in place). In very rare instances, it may be given **intracardiac**—injected directly into the heart through the chest wall.

- *Lidocaine.* A class Ib antiarrhythmic, Lidocaine is useful in abolishing ventricular arrhythmias such as ventricular tachycardia or ventricular fibrillation. It is given intravenously (or endotracheally if no IV line is in place).

- *Verapamil.* A calcium channel blocker, verapamil is used in emergency situations to convert supraventricular tachycardias back to sinus, or at least to slow the heart rate to a more tolerable level. It is given intravenously in emergency situations. Verapamil cannot be given endotracheally.

- *Sodium bicarbonate.* This medication combats the acidity of the blood caused by lactic acid buildup in a cardiac arrest situation. Remember lactic acid builds up in an anaerobic environment. Cardiac arrest produces such an environment. Combating this acidity can help convert arrhythmias back to normal in a cardiac arrest.

- *Isoproterenol (Isuprel).* Isuprel was once a first-line drug used to treat cardiac arrest and bradycardias. It has fallen out of favor in recent years because it causes a monumental increase in the heart's oxygen consumption and can extend the size of an MI. Nowadays, it is used only as a last resort to treat symptomatic bradycardias that are resistant to atropine and epinephrine. It is turned off once a pacemaker can be utilized. Isuprel is given by continuous intravenous infusion. It cannot be given endotracheally.

- *Oxygen.* Though most people do not think of oxygen as a medication, when it is used to treat disease or a medical condition it is indeed a medication. And, like any medication, oxygen has its benefits and its risks. Oxygen is used in emergency situations to provide the tissues with the oxygen they are lacking. This alone can help convert arrhythmias back to normal. Overzealous use of oxygen in nonemergency situations, however, can have disastrous results for people with chronic lung disease, as it can deprive them of their **hypoxic drive** (i.e., stimulus to breathe based on their blood oxygen level being lower than normal) and cause them to stop breathing. The average person breathes because carbon dioxide levels in the body become high, and this stimulates breathing in order to blow off this carbon dioxide. People with chronic lung disease, however, typically live with a higher-than-normal carbon dioxide level. Thus their stimulus to breathe is a not a high carbon dioxide level but rather a *low oxygen level.* When their blood oxygen level is low enough, they breathe in order to take in more oxygen. Giving these patients too much oxygen makes their blood oxygen level climb so high that they lose the stimulus to breathe. So they stop. It is therefore very important to monitor just how much oxygen the person receives. Oxygen can be given by mask, nasal cannula (small prongs in the nose), endotracheal tube, and **tracheostomy** (surgically inserting a tube through the neck into the trachea).

Let's summarize the emergency medications. See Table 28-2.

Table 28-2 Emergency Medications Summary

MEDICATION	MODE OF ACTION	INDICATION
Atropine	Increases heart rate	Bradycardias, asystole
Epinephrine	Stimulates contractility, increases heart rate and BP	Cardiac arrest, bradycardias
Lidocaine	Decreases ventricular irritability	Rapid ventricular arrhythmias, PVCs
Verapamil	Decreases heart rate	Rapid supraventricular arrhythmias
Sodium bicarbonate	Decreases blood's acidity	Cardiac arrest with acidosis
Isoproterenol	Increases heart rate	Bradycardias resistant to atropine and epinephrine
Oxygen	Increases tissue oxygenation	Symptomatic arrhythmias, cardiac arrest

Practice Quiz

1. Digitalis is classified as what kind of medication? _____

2. Class I antiarrhythmic medications have what effect on the action potential? _____
_____

3. What effect does atropine have on the heart rate? _____

4. What effect does vasoconstriction have on the blood pressure? _____
_____

5. True or false: Beta-blockers cause the heart rate to increase.

6. What effect do class III antiarrhythmic medications have on the action potential? _____
_____

7. True or false: Giving oxygen cannot be hazardous to the patient.

8. True or false: Epinephrine is classified as a cardiac glycoside.

9. In what ways may lidocaine be given to the patient? _____
_____

10. Isoproterenol is used nowadays in treating what problem? _____
_____

Practice Quiz Answers

1. Digitalis is classified as a **cardiac glycoside.**

2. Class I antiarrhythmic medications **affect phase 0 of the action potential by blocking the influx of sodium into the cardiac cell.**

3. Atropine **increases the heart rate.**

4. Vasoconstriction **causes the blood pressure to increase.**

5. **False.** Beta-blockers cause the heart rate to decrease.

6. Class III antiarrhythmic medications **affect phase 3 of the action potential. They interfere with the movement of potassium into the cardiac cell during repolarization.**

7. **False.** Giving oxygen can indeed be hazardous to the patient. It can cause certain patients to stop breathing.

8. **False.** Epinephrine is not a cardiac glycoside. It is an unclassified antiarrhythmic medication.

9. Lidocaine may be given **intravenously or endotracheally.**

10. Isoproterenol is used nowadays to **treat symptomatic bradycardias unresponsive to atropine and epinephrine.**

Diagnostic Electrocardiography

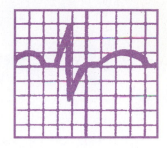

Chapter 29 Objectives

Upon completion of this chapter, the student will be able to:

- Define *stress testing.*
- State the goal of stress testing.
- Define *MET.*
- Describe the indications for stress testing.
- Describe the relative and absolute contraindications to stress testing.
- State how to calculate target heart rate.
- Describe how a stress test is done.
- Describe how a pharmacologic stress test is done.
- Name the three most commonly used protocols for treadmill exercise testing.
- Describe the reasons to terminate the test.
- Describe normal signs and symptoms during the stress test.
- Describe the normal EKG changes that occur during stress testing.
- Describe the EKG changes that indicate a positive stress test.
- Explain Bayes' theorem as it relates to the reliability of stress testing.
- Define *specificity* and *sensitivity.*
- Describe the indications for Holter monitoring.
- State the contraindications to Holter monitoring.
- Describe the artifact associated with Holter monitoring.
- Explain why an event monitor might be superior to a Holter monitor for some patients.
- State what a positive Holter or event monitor is.

Chapter 29 Outline

I.   Introduction
II. Stress testing
    A. Goal
    B. Indications
    C. Absolute contraindications
    D. Relative contraindications
    E. Preparation techniques

Chapter 29 Glossary

Bayes' theorem: The theorem that states that the predictive value of a test is based not only on the accuracy of the test itself but also on the patient's probability of disease, as determined by a risk assessment done prior to testing.

Chronotropic: Affecting the heart rate.

Hyperventilate: To breathe very rapidly.

Inotropic: Affecting contactility.

MET: Metabolic equivalent, a measurement of oxygen consumption.

Patency: Openness.

Sensitivity: The ability of a test to pick out the people who are truly diseased.

Specificity: The ability of a test to exclude people who are not diseased.

Introduction

Diagnostic electrocardiography involves an EKG done to rule out disease. It can involve a resting EKG, a stress test, or ambulatory monitoring such as Holter monitoring. We've talked about resting EKGs in depth. Let's look at the other two now.

Stress Testing

Stress testing is a diagnostic procedure done to determine the likelihood of coronary artery disease (CAD). The heart is stressed by physical exertion, usually on a bicycle or a treadmill, or by administration of medication that causes increased heart rate and thus stresses the heart. The patient's symptoms and EKG during the stress test give vital information regarding the **patency** (openness) of his or her coronary arteries.

Goal of Stress Testing

The goal of stress testing, whether exercise or pharmacologic, is to increase the heart rate to a maximal level that increases myocardial oxygen demand and to evaluate the EKG and subjective responses of the patient. Decreased flow through narrowed coronary arteries will usually become evident as the test progresses. In other words, are there EKG changes that signal ischemia or infarction? Does the patient experience chest pain or arrhythmias with this stress? The test is concluded when the patient's symptoms (chest pain, fatigue, or ST segment changes) preclude continuing, or, for submaximal tests, when a target heart rate is reached.

Indications for Stress Testing

Stress testing is usually done to search for coronary artery disease in a patient having suspicious symptoms. But there are other indications as well. Here are a few:

- *Post-CABG or postangioplasty evaluation.* The patient has had bypass surgery or a balloon procedure to open up blocked coronary arteries. The stress test is a way to determine if those procedures have improved coronary flow.

- *Diagnosis or treatment of exercise-induced arrhythmias.* Some patients have arrhythmias only on exertion. The stress test is a safe way to induce those arrhythmias in a controlled environment so they can be identified and treated.

- *Follow-up to cardiac rehab.* The post-MI patient has gradually worked up to more normal exercise levels. The stress test helps determine if his or her heart is tolerating this increased exertion.

- *Family history of heart disease.* The individual with a family history of heart disease and two or more of the recognized heart disease risk factors is advised to have a stress test at age 40 and periodically thereafter. If coronary artery disease is detected, treatment can begin early.

Absolute Contraindications

Who is *not* a candidate for stress testing under any circumstances? For people with the following conditions, the risks of the test greatly outweigh the potential benefits. Testing these people could have serious or fatal consequences.

- *Acute MI.* The heart is too unstable to tolerate exertion. Stress testing could cause the infarct area to extend.

- *Unstable angina or angina at rest.* Patients who have angina at rest will not tolerate stress. It could cause them to infarct.

- *Uncontrolled ventricular rhythms.* They could deteriorate to v-fib.

- *Severe aortic stenosis.* Due to a very narrowed aortic valve opening, cardiac output is low, and stressing these patients could cause them to pass out or suffer cardiac arrest.

- *Dissecting aneurysm.* This is a ballooning out of the wall of an artery. Stress causes an increase in blood pressure, which could cause the aneurysm to blow.

- *Heart block greater than first degree.* These patients cannot get their heart rate up to the target level, and they may already have decreased cardiac output that exertion would worsen.

Relative Contraindications

Some individuals can have a stress test *only* if the benefits outweigh the risks. In other words, it must be determined that the information to be gained from the stress test is so valuable that it outweighs the risks involved to individuals with the following conditions:

- *Uncontrolled rapid supraventricular rhythms.* With the heart rate already fast prior to the stress test, it won't take much to make the cardiac output fall.

- *Frequent PVCs.* It's possible that ventricular tachycardia or fibrillation could result, so it's important to determine if the information the stress test will provide is worth the risk.

- *Uncontrolled hypertension.* The person with this condition has either not received treatment for hypertension or has not taken the prescribed medication, and his or her BP is extremely high. Stress testing this person could result in stroke.

- *Mild or moderate aortic stenosis.* The cardiac output could drop.

Preparation Techniques

The single most important piece of equipment in performing a stress test is a 12-lead EKG machine that has the capability to run continuously for a period of time. The electrode patches should adhere securely to the skin, and they may be taped if necessary. Female patients are advised to wear a bra in order to decrease artifact. To prevent nausea, patients are advised not to eat a large meal for at least four hours prior to the test. They should wear comfortable, loose clothing and walking shoes or other appropriate footwear. They should take their routine medications as usual unless specifically instructed not to by the physician. Certain medications, such as beta-blockers and calcium channel blockers, may be held for a period of time before the test, as they prevent the heart rate from reaching target levels. Also, nitrates might be held, as they could prevent symptoms of coronary artery disease, such as chest pain, and could thus result in a false-negative test.

How Is It Done?

Before all stress tests, a resting EKG is done. A history is obtained, with special emphasis on a description of any symptoms the patient has been having that prompted the test (chest pain, shortness of breath, etc.). Baseline vital signs (heart rate, blood pressure, respiratory rate) are checked with the patient lying down and standing. An EKG will be done with the patient standing up **hyperventilating** (breathing very rapidly). ST segment and T wave changes can be caused by hyperventilation, and during the stress test it's important to know if any ST-T changes are from ischemia or simply from hyperventilating.

For the **exercise test,** the patient then exercises on a treadmill or bicycle, or uses a special arm bicycle called an *arm ergometer,* while a continuous EKG is run. A nurse or technician checks the patient's blood pressure at frequent intervals and inquires about any symptoms the patient may be developing. The stress test is continued until at least 85% of the target heart rate is achieved or the patient develops EKG changes or symptoms that require termination of the test. *The target heart rate is 220 minus the patient's age.* A sixty-year-old patient would thus have a target heart rate of $220 - 60 = 160$. For the test to be valid for interpretation, a heart rate of 85% of 160, or 136, would be required. For a submaximal test following an MI, the test is concluded when 70% of the target heart rate is achieved, assuming the patient is asymptomatic. If myocardial perfusion is to be studied, radioisotopes such as thallium-201 can be injected during the last minute of exercise and then special x-rays done. Thallium follows potassium ions into the heart and diffuses into the tissues. Poor myocardial uptake of the thallium produces a "cold spot" on the x-ray (compared to the "hot spots" from adequate thallium uptake) and indicates impaired myocardial blood flow in the artery supplying that area. Multiple gated acquisition (MUGA) scans can also be done after the exercise test to check myocardial perfusion. MUGA scans are nuclear scans that use an injected radioisotope to point out areas of poor myocardial blood flow.

The **pharmacologic stress test** does not involve exercise. This kind of testing is appropriate for individuals with physical limitations that preclude exercise, such as amputations, or for the elderly who could not do enough exercise to reach the target heart rate. For this test, an IV line is started and the patient is given an intravenous dose of medication that causes the heart rate to climb to the target level. This increased heart rate stresses the heart and should provide the same symptoms and EKG changes as an exercise test. As with the exercise test, a continuous EKG is run, vital signs are checked, and symptoms are assessed. After at least 85% of the target heart rate is achieved, the test is concluded. The most common medications used in pharmacologic stress tests are *cardiolyte, dobutamine, dipyridamole,* and *adenosine.*

Exercise Protocols

There are three main protocols used in treadmill exercise stress tests. Speed and incline of the treadmill, as well as the frequency of the changes in the protocol's stages, are determined by the protocol used. The intensity of exercise is measured in metabolic equivalents (**METs**), which are reflections of oxygen consumption. One MET is the oxygen consumption of a person sitting down resting. Most average adults can reach a MET level of 13 with exertion. Those with CAD may have symptoms of ischemia at very low MET levels, such as 4 METs. Sometimes a **double product** is calculated in order to determine the level of exercise achieved. Double product is calculated as the heart rate times the systolic blood pressure ($HR \times SBP = DP$). A double product greater than 25,000 indicates that an acceptable level of exercise has been achieved during stress testing. Let's look at the different protocols.

- **Bruce.** This is the most commonly used protocol, used for maximal testing. The treadmill's speed and incline are increased every 3 minutes up to a total of 21 minutes. Let's look at the stages of the Bruce protocol. See Table 29-1.

Table 29-1 Bruce Protocol Stages

STAGE	SPEED	INCLINE
I	1.7 mph	10°
II	2.5 mph	12°
III	3.4 mph	14°
IV	4.2 mph	16°
V	5.0 mph	18°
VI	5.5 mph	20°
VII	6.0 mph	22°

As you can see in Table 29-1, the speed starts out at a comfortable walking pace at a low incline, then every 3 minutes accelerates until by stage VII the patient is running uphill at a 22° incline. An advantage of the Bruce protocol is the relatively short duration needed to produce maximal effort in the patient. On the downside, this protocol can be very demanding and may be too ambitious for the sedentary individual.

- **Modified Bruce.** Many institutions have modified the Bruce protocol so that the initial work is less strenuous, and the stages change in smaller increments. This is appropriate for patients who might not tolerate the standard Bruce protocol.

- **Naughton.** This is a slower-moving submaximal test in which the settings are changed every two minutes. Though the settings change more quickly than in the Bruce protocol, they are more gradual and allow the individual to adjust more easily. The Naughton protocol is used most often for testing post-MI patients just before or shortly after hospital discharge.

Termination of the Test

The stress test should be immediately stopped if any of the following occur:

- *ST segment elevation.* This indicates severe transmural myocardial ischemia and injury. The sudden development of ST segment elevation is an ominous sign. Continuing the test could result in irreversible cardiac damage.

- *Ventricular tachycardia.* Cardiac arrest could result if the test is not stopped.

- *Chest pain, especially if accompanied by ST segment depression or elevation.* Mild chest pain unaccompanied by ST segment changes may not be indicative of significant coronary artery disease. More severe chest pain, especially that accompanied by ST segment changes, is more reflective of significant disease.

- *Drop in blood pressure or failure of the BP to rise with exercise.* The blood pressure usually rises in response to exercise. Failure of the blood pressure to rise with exercise indicates poor cardiac reserve. A drop in BP can indicate pump failure.

- *Bradycardia, especially the development of AV blocks.* The heart rate should increase with exertion. If it slows down, it is a sign of poor cardiac reserve. The development of AV blocks, especially type II second-degree AV block and third-degree AV block, could signal ischemia to the AV node or bundle branches, which are supplied by the right coronary artery and the LAD, respectively. Continuing the test could prove dangerous to the patient.

- *Patient indicates inability to continue due to fatigue, shortness of breath, or dizziness.* Trust the patient who says he or she feels too bad to continue.

- *Patient requests to stop.* Again, listen to the patient. But inquire about the symptoms that prompt the patient to want to stop the test. There may be an occasional unmotivated patient who requests to stop the test before achieving target levels. In this case the physician might gently encourage the patient to continue, since the test that is stopped at too early a stage will be inadequate at ruling out CAD.

- *ST depression greater than 3 mm.* This is a strongly positive stress test. Continuing the test could cause the patient to infarct.

- *Elevation of the systolic blood pressure above 240 mmHg or the diastolic blood pressure above 120 mmHg.* This is controversial. Though some experts say that blood pressure that rises too high during exercise puts the patient at risk for stroke, others downplay this risk.

- *Patient becomes very pale and diaphoretic (cold and clammy).* These are signs of decreased cardiac output. The patient is not tolerating the test.

Test Interpretation

The following EKG changes are normal on the stress test:

- *Shortened PR interval.* AV conduction and heart rate usually accelerate with exertion.

- *Tall P waves.* This is often a result of increased lung capacity.

- *Lower-voltage QRS complexes.* This may be due to increased volume of air in the lungs muffling the cardiac impulse as it heads toward the skin.

- *Increased heart rate (shorter R-R intervals).* The ability of the heart rate to increase with exercise is known as the **chronotropic reserve.** Heart rate that does not increase with stress is **chronotropic incompetence.**

Normal Signs and Symptoms

The following patient signs and symptoms are normal during a stress test:

- *Decreased systemic vascular resistance due to vasodilation.* Exercise causes blood vessels to dilate, lowering the resistance to the outflow of blood from the heart and increasing cardiac output.

- *Increased respiratory rate.* Exercise causes increased oxygen demand, so the respiratory rate increases to allow more oxygen intake.

- *Sweating.*

- *Fatigue.*

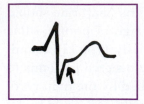

Figure 29-1 J point depression.

- *Muscle cramping in calves or sides.* This is a common phenomenon in exercise and does not imply poor myocardial function.

- *Increased blood pressure.* The ability of the blood pressure to rise with exercise is known as **inotropic reserve.** Blood pressure that does not rise with exercise can imply **inotropic incompetence.**

- *J point depression.* The J point is the point at which the QRS joins the ST segment. J point depression means the ST segment takes off before the QRS complex has gotten back up to the baseline. Note the J point in Figure 29-1. It is below the baseline. This is J point depression.

Positive Stress Test

The following indicate a positive (abnormal) stress test:

- *ST segment depression greater than or equal to 1.0 to 1.5 mm that does not return to the baseline within 0.08 s (two little blocks) after the J point.* ST depression can be of three different types: upsloping, horizontal, and downsloping. In terms of cardiac implications, upsloping is the least indicative of coronary artery disease, horizontal is intermediate, and downsloping is the most indicative of CAD. See Figure 29-2.

Let's compare ST segments on a preexercise resting EKG and a stress test EKG. See Figures 29-3 and 29-4. Ignore the QRS width on these examples. In Figure 29-3, note the normal ST segments and the relatively slow heart rate. Now see Figure 29-4 for the stress test EKG. Note the normal increase in heart rate along with significant downsloping ST segment depressions in leads II, III, and aVF. This is a positive stress test.

- *U wave inversion or new appearance of U waves.* Though a much less common phenomenon than ST segment changes, U wave inversion—or indeed the sudden appearance of U waves during the exercise test—is indicative of coronary ischemia. See Figure 29-5, and note the inverted U waves following the upright T waves.

- *ST segment elevation.* Elevation of the ST segment is an indication of considerable transmural myocardial ischemia progressing to the injury

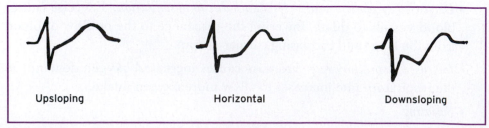

Upsloping   Horizontal   Downsloping

Figure 29-2 Types of ST segment depression.

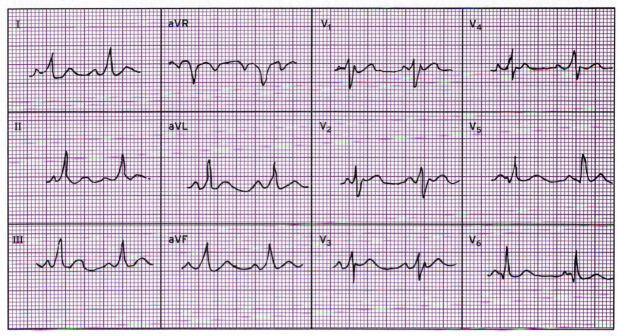

Figure 29-3   Preexercise resting EKG.

phase. The stress test should be stopped immediately to prevent permanent tissue damage.

Reliability of Stress Tests

How reliable are stress tests in diagnosing coronary artery disease? Like any medical testing, the stress test is not infallible. There can be false-positives and false-negatives. The validity of stress test results can be absolutely determined only by angiogram, a procedure in which dye is injected into the

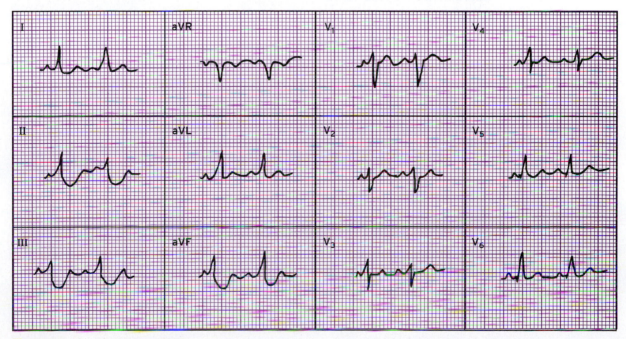

Figure 29-4   Stress test EKG.

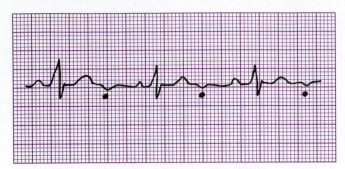

Figure 29-5 Inverted U waves.

coronary arteries to determine if there is indeed coronary artery disease. For the stress EKG to show any diagnostic changes that indicate CAD, the coronary artery in question must be at least 75% narrowed. And conditions other than CAD can result in a positive test. To better understand the reliability of the test results, it is necessary to understand the terms *sensitivity* and *specificity*.

Sensitivity refers to the percentage of patients who have a positive stress test and CAD as proven by angiogram. In other words, is the stress test sensitive enough to pick up those individuals who truly have coronary artery disease?

Specificity refers to the percentage of patients who have negative (normal) stress tests and normal coronary arteries as proven by angiogram. Is the stress test specific enough to exclude individuals who do not have CAD?

Thus the term *positive* refers to the test's sensitivity and *negative* refers to its specificity.

Categories of Stress Tests

Stress test results fall in four categories:

- *True-positive.* The stress test is positive (indicating coronary artery disease) and the angiogram is positive, confirming CAD.

- *False-positive.* The stress test is positive for CAD, but the angiogram is negative, revealing normal coronary arteries.

- *True-negative.* The stress test and angiogram are both negative for CAD.

- *False-negative.* The stress test is negative, but the angiogram is positive for CAD.

Bayes' theorem suggests that the true predictive value of any test is not just in the accuracy (sensitivity and specificity) of the test itself, but also in the patient's probability of disease, as determined before the test was done. In other words, before the stress test is done, there should be a risk assessment, based on the patient's history, heredity, and physical exam, to predict the likelihood of that patient having CAD. If this pretest risk of CAD is low, but his stress test turns out to be positive, it is likely the stress test result is a false positive. If the pretest risk is high but the stress test is negative, it's likely that the stress test is a false-negative.

After the Stress Test

What happens after the stress test? If the stress test is positive, the patient will likely be either treated with medications or scheduled for an angiogram for further diagnostic evaluation. If the test is negative, there may be no treatment indicated.

Holter Monitoring

Holter monitoring is an ambulatory EKG done to rule out intermittent arrhythmias or cardiac ischemia that might otherwise be missed on a routine EKG. The Holter monitor consists of electrodes and a small, battery-powered tape recorder onto which the rhythm is recorded in two leads. The device is small enough to be worn in a pocket or on a strap over the shoulder. It may be done as an inpatient or outpatient, though most often it is done on an outpatient basis.

Indications

- *Syncope or near-syncopal episodes.* Fainting spells could be caused by arrhythmias, which could be evident on Holter monitoring.

- *Intermittent chest pain or shortness of breath.* These could be signs of myocardial ischemia, which could be detected with a Holter monitor.

- *Suspicion of arrhythmias.* The patient who complains of palpitations, dizzy spells, or skipped beats may have arrhythmias that the Holter monitor would demonstrate.

- *Determine the effectiveness of treatment for arrhythmias.* Holter monitoring can reveal if the rhythm being treated is still occurring and can demonstrate if a newly implanted pacemaker is functioning properly.

Contraindications

- *Terminal disease state.* This is controversial. On the one hand, if a patient is terminally ill, the information obtained using the monitor would be of no long-term benefit to the patient. On the other hand, treating any newly discovered arrhythmias or ischemia might help reduce or prevent symptoms and could improve the quality of the remainder of the patient's life.
- *Severe symptoms.* Patients with severe symptoms would more appropriately be monitored in the hospital than at home.

Preparation Techniques

The patient is attached to five electrodes, which are put on the trunk instead of the arms and legs in order to prevent muscle artifact. Male patients with considerable chest hair might need the electrode sites to be shaved in order for the electrode patches to adhere properly. Female patients should have chest leads positioned beneath, not on top of, the breast. The skin is prepped prior to attaching the electrodes. This skin prep involves abrading the thin outer layer of skin so the electrodes adhere to the skin without losing contact. The electrodes are then taped to the skin to prevent dislodgment, since they will be on for 24 hours or longer. Typically, at least two leads are simultaneously recorded—either leads V_1 and V_5 or leads V_1 and II.

After being attached to the Holter monitor, the patient is given instructions, including not to remove the electrodes and not to take a bath or shower during the time the Holter is in progress, as this could cause the electrodes to become dislodged. A careful sponge bath is OK. The patient is otherwise instructed to go about normal daily activities. This includes work, hobbies, sex, and so on. The patient should not curtail activities just because the Holter is in progress. The whole purpose of the Holter monitor is to catch abnormalities that show up in the course of daily activities. Curtailing those activities defeats the purpose.

The patient is advised to document any symptoms experienced while the Holter is in progress in a small diary provided for that purpose. By pressing the marker button on the Holter monitor, the patient marks the point in the EKG at which he or she feels symptoms so that this part of the EKG can be more closely examined for changes that could cause the symptoms. For example, if at 4 P.M. the patient feels very dizzy, and the Holter reveals a short run of v-tach at that time, the arrhythmia would explain the dizziness. Treatment could then be started to prevent further ventricular arrhythmias. After the prescribed duration of Holter monitoring, the patient returns the Holter to the hospital or physician's office, whereupon it is entered into a computer and scanned for abnormalities.

Artifact Associated with Holter Monitoring

Several types of artifact can be seen on Holter monitoring. See Figure 29-6.

- *Loose electrode.* Sometimes an electrode will loosen or fall off, creating artifact that can resemble v-tach, v-fib, or asystole. The other monitored lead should prove this artifact to indeed be artifact and not the true rhythm.

- *Scratching artifact.* The patient scratches at the electrode sites, causing artifact that can resemble atrial flutter or ventricular flutter. Remember "toothbrush tachycardia"? Scratching artifact can look just like that. This type of artifact is also usually obvious in the other monitored lead. Scratching is common, as the electrode adhesive can cause skin irritation.

- *Incomplete erasure of a previously used Holter tape.* In this type of artifact, an incompletely erased Holter tape is reused, resulting in the new rhythm being recorded over the incompletely erased old one. This can make deciphering the rhythm difficult, as there will be extra P waves, QRS complexes, or T waves from the other rhythm superimposed onto this rhythm. In Figure 29-6, the arrows indicate leftover P waves and QRS complexes that were not erased.

- *Slowing of the tape during recording.* Sometimes the battery or recorder motor fails, causing the tape to slow while recording. When played back at normal speed, the rhythm will look very fast. The abnormally shortened P, QRS, and T waves and intervals will be clues to the true cause of the apparent tachycardia.

- *Slowing or sticking of the tape during playback.* If the tape sticks while being played back, the rhythm will look abnormally slow. The abnormally

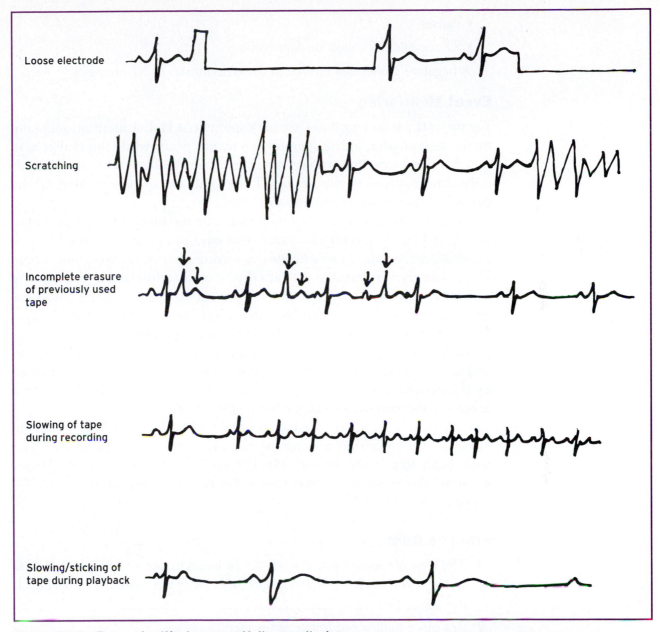

Figure 29-6   Types of artifact seen on Holter monitoring.

prolonged P, QRS, and T waves and intervals will be clues to the true cause of this apparent bradycardia.

Using modern digital recorders rather than the older tape recorders can prevent the artifact problems commonly associated with tape recorder malfunctions.

What Is a Positive Holter?

A positive Holter is one that reveals *abnormalities that could explain the patient's symptoms*. These abnormalities might include one or more of the following:

- Tachycardias
- Bradycardias

- Pauses
- ST segment elevation or depression

A negative Holter has no significant arrhythmias or ST changes.

Event Monitoring

For patients whose symptoms are very sporadic, a Holter monitor might not be the best answer, as the symptoms may not occur while the Holter is in use. An **event monitor** is a very small device the patient carries that records only abnormalities in rhythm or ST segments or that is activated by the patient whenever symptoms appear.

There are two kinds of event monitors. One monitors the rhythm continuously, but only prints out abnormalities it has been preprogrammed to find. In addition, the patient can activate this recorder whenever symptoms occur. The device then records the patient's rhythm at that time and also, by way of a built-in memory, the rhythm that was present up to five minutes before the event. The rhythm can then be transmitted via telephone or the device turned in to the physician's office for immediate interpretation.

The second type of event monitor is not programmed to recognize abnormalities, nor does it monitor the rhythm continuously. It must be activated by the patient whenever symptoms occur. It will then record the rhythm present at that time as well as just before the event.

Unlike a Holter monitor, which is usually worn for only 24 hours, event monitors can be carried or worn for extended periods of time and are thus more likely to pick up abnormalities that are only sporadic. Like the Holter monitor, the event monitor is said to be *negative* if arrhythmias or ST-T changes are not found.

Practice Quiz

1. The type of monitor that is worn for 24 hours to uncover any arrhythmias or ST segment changes that might be causing the patient's symptoms is the _____

2. List three indications for stress testing. _____

   _____

   _____

3. What does Bayes' theorem have to say about the validity of test results?

   _____

   _____

4. Is ST segment elevation of 5 mm indicative of a positive stress test or a negative stress test? _____

5. True or false: Patients on medications such as beta-blockers and nitrates might be advised to avoid taking these medications for a period of time before the stress test.

6. Target heart rate is_____

7. Event monitoring differs from Holter monitoring in what ways? _____

_____

_____

8. The most commonly used protocol for treadmill stress testing is the ____

_____

9. The protocol used most often for post-MI patients just before or following hospital discharge is the _____

10. What is a MET? _____

Practice Quiz Answers

1. The type of monitor worn for 24 hours to uncover any arrhythmias or ST segment changes that might be causing the patient's symptoms is the **Holter monitor.**

2. Indications for stress testing are the following (choose any three): **to determine the presence or absence of CAD, for post-CABG and post-PTCA evaluation, for diagnosis and treatment of exercise-induced arrhythmias, as follow-up to cardiac rehab,** and **to evaluate individuals with a family history of heart disease.**

3. Bayes' theorem says that **the validity of a test result depends not only on the test accuracy, but also on the probability that the patient in question would have the disease.**

4. ST segment elevation of 5 mm is **indicative of a positive stress test.** ST elevation that high indicates an infarction beginning.

5. **True.** Patients on beta-blockers and nitrates might be advised to avoid taking these medications for a period of time before the stress test.

6. Target heart rate is **220 minus the patient's age.**

7. Event monitoring differs from Holter monitoring in that **event monitoring can be worn or used over a prolonged period,** whereas Holter monitoring is typically used only for 24 hours. Also, Holter monitoring involves continuous recording of the rhythm, whereas **event monitoring records only abnormalities or rhythms present when activated by the patient.**

8. The most commonly used protocol for treadmill stress testing is the **Bruce protocol.**

9. The protocol used most often for post-MI patients just before or following hospital discharge is the **Naughton protocol.**

10. A MET is a **metabolic equivalent, a measurement of oxygen consumption, where 1 MET is the resting oxygen consumption of a seated adult.**

Artificial Pacemakers

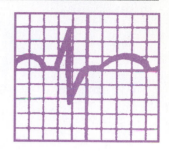

Chapter 30 Objectives

Upon completion of this chapter, the student will be able to:

- State the primary function of a pacemaker.
- Outline the indications for a pacemaker.
- Name the two components of a permanent pacemaker.
- Describe the types of temporary pacemakers.
- Define the terms *firing, capture,* and *sensing.*
- State what each letter of the pacemaker code means.
- Identify pacemaker rhythms as being either VVI or DDD.
- Identify the different kinds of pacemaker malfunctions.

Chapter 30 Outline

Chapter 30 Glossary

Capture: The depolarization of the atrium and/or ventricle as a result of a pacemaker's firing. Determined by the presence of a P wave and/or QRS after the pacemaker spike.

Demand: A pacemaker's firing only when needed. This requires that the pacemaker be able to sense the patient's intrinsic beats.

Firing: The pacemaker's generation of an electrical stimulus.

Fixed-rate pacemaker: A kind of pacemaker that fires regardless of the patient's intrinsic rhythm.

Inhibit: To prevent from performing an action.

Intrinsic: The patient's own.

Pacing catheter: A wire that is inserted into the heart for delivery of pacing stimuli.

Pacing interval: The programmed distance between consecutive pacemaker spikes. Is essentially the same as the R-R interval, but of paced beats rather than intrinsic beats.

Pulse generator: The battery pack that generates the electricity delivered to the heart through the pacing catheter.

Sensing: The pacemaker's ability to detect the patient's intrinsic beats in order to determine if it needs to fire.

Tachyarrhythmia: An arrhythmia with a heart rate greater than 100.

Transcutaneous: Through the skin.

Transvenous: Through a vein.

Trigger: To cause an action by the pacemaker.

Introduction

The primary function of an artificial pacemaker is to prevent the heart rate from going too slow. Pacemakers provide an electrical stimulus when the heart is unable to generate its own or when its own is too slow to provide adequate cardiac output. *Pacemakers do not force the heart to beat.* They simply send out an electrical signal, just as the heart's normal pacemakers do. If the heart is healthy enough, it should respond to that stimulus by depolarizing. You'll recall that pacemakers can pace the atrium, the ventricle, or both.

Indications

Indications for a pacemaker may include the following:

- Symptomatic sinus bradycardia
- Junctional rhythms
- Idioventricular rhythm
- Dying heart
- Asystole
- 2:1 AV block
- Type II second-degree AV block
- Third-degree AV block
- Sick sinus syndrome
- Overdrive suppression of tachyarrhythmias

Permanent versus Temporary Pacemakers

A **permanent pacemaker** has two components—a **pulse generator** (a battery pack), inserted surgically into a pocket made just under the right clavicle, and a **pacing catheter,** which is inserted via the subclavian vein into the

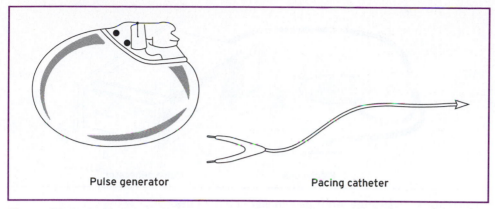

Figure 30-1   Pulse generator and pacing catheter of a permanent pacemaker.

superior vena cava and down into the right atrium or ventricle. Permanent pacemaker batteries are made of lithium and usually last between 5 and 15 years. See Figure 30-1.

Temporary pacemakers can be of various types, the two most common being the **transvenous,** in which a pacing catheter is inserted into a large vein and threaded into the right atrium and down into the right ventricle, and the **transcutaneous,** which involves large pacing electrodes attached to the chest and back that pace the heart through the chest wall. Both of these temporary pacer methods require a pulse generator at the patient's bedside. See Figures 30-2 and 30-3.

Pacemaker Terminology

Firing refers to the pacemaker's generation of an electrical stimulus. It is noted on the EKG by the presence of a **pacemaker spike.**

Capture refers to the presence of a P wave or a QRS (or both) after the pacemaker spike. This indicates that the tissue in the chamber being paced has depolarized. The pacemaker is then said to have "captured" that chamber. Paced QRS complexes are wide and bizarre and resemble PVCs.

Sensing refers to the pacemaker's ability to recognize the patient's own intrinsic rhythm or beats in order to decide if it needs to fire. Most pacemak-

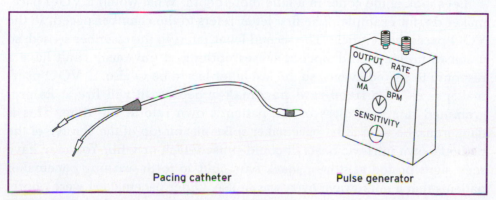

Figure 30-2   Transvenous pacemaker components.

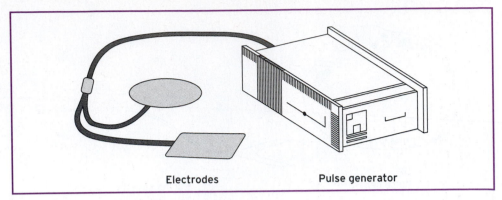

Electrodes   Pulse generator

Figure 30-3 Transcutaneous pacemaker components.

ers function on a **demand mode,** meaning they fire only when needed (only on demand).

Three-Letter Pacemaker Code

Pacemakers are referred to by a three-letter code:

- The first letter refers to the chamber paced.
  V = ventricle
  A = atrium
  D = dual (atrium and ventricle)
  O = none

- The second letter refers to the *chamber sensed.*
  V = ventricle
  A = atrium
  D = dual (atrium and ventricle)
  O = none

- The third letter refers to the *response to sensed events.*
  I = inhibited (pacemaker watches and waits, does not pace until needed)
  T = triggered (pacemaker sends out a signal in response to a sensed event)
  D = dual (inhibited and triggered)
  O = none

Let's look at the codes in a little more depth. What would a VOO pacemaker do, for example? The first letter refers to the chamber paced, so the VOO paces the ventricle. The second letter refers to the chamber sensed, so it senses nothing. And since it senses nothing, it obviously can't have a response to sensed events, so the last letter has to be O also. A VOO pacemaker is called a **fixed-rate pacemaker** because it will fire at its programmed rate regardless of the patient's own rate at the time. This is dangerous, because if the pacemaker spike hits on top of the T wave of the patient's own intrinsic beats, it could cause v-tach or v-fib. You may have seen signs posted at stores, snack bars, and so forth warning pacemaker patients that a microwave oven was in use. Older pacemakers were poorly insulated and could be turned into fixed-rate pacemakers by microwaves.

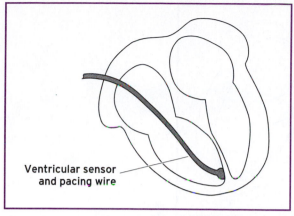

Figure 30-4   VVI pacemaker inserted into the right ventricle.

Newer pacemakers are well insulated and do not have that problem. VOO pacemakers are not used today.

VVI Pacemakers

The most common kinds of pacemakers in use today are the VVI and the DDD. The **VVI pacer,** also known as a **ventricular demand pacer,** was at one time the most commonly used permanent pacer. It's now in second place. The VVI pacer consists of a catheter with both pacing and sensing capabilities that is inserted into the right ventricle. See Figure 30-4.

The VVI pacemaker paces the ventricle, providing a spike and then a wide QRS complex. It senses the ventricle, so it looks for intrinsic QRS complexes to determine if it needs to fire. Let's say the patient is in a sinus rhythm with a heart rate of 80 and the pacemaker is set at a rate of 60. The sensor would "see" the patient's own QRS complexes and realize it does not need to fire. It will be inhibited. If the patient's heart rate falls to a rate below the pacemaker's preset heart rate, the pacer will not see QRS complexes at a fast enough rate, so it will fire and pace the heart. As with your own conduction system, whichever is the fastest pacemaker is the one in control. Since the VVI pacer senses only intrinsic QRS complexes, it ignores the P waves. Therefore, *there will be no relationship between P waves and paced QRS complexes.*

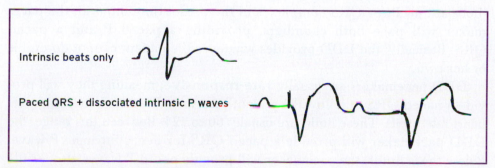

Intrinsic beats only

Paced QRS + dissociated intrinsic P waves

Figure 30-5   VVI pacemaker options.

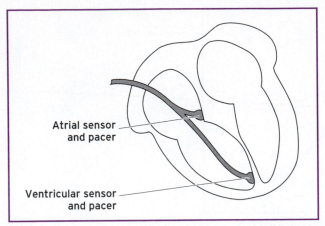

Figure 30-6 DDD pacemaker sensor and pacer wires in right atrium and ventricle.

VVI pacemakers provide two options:

- *Intrinsic beats only.* The pacemaker does not pace because it does not need to. The rhythm is fast enough, so the pacemaker is inhibited. There will be no pacemaker spikes.

- *Paced QRS, dissociated intrinsic P waves.* The pacemaker senses and paces only the ventricle. There will be pacemaker spikes preceding only the QRS complexes. Intrinsic P waves, if present, will be ignored by the pacemaker. See Figure 30-5.

DDD Pacemakers

The **DDD pacemaker** is the most modern and the most physiologic. It is known as an **AV universal pacemaker** and is now the most commonly inserted permanent pacemaker. It paces and senses both atrium and ventricle. See Figure 30-6.

The DDD pacemaker senses intrinsic atrial activity and takes advantage of the patient's own P waves. If the DDD pacemaker senses the patient's P waves within its preset rate, it will not need to give another P wave, so its atrial pacer will be inhibited. The ventricle, however, will then be triggered to give a QRS if the patient does not have his or her own QRS in the preset length of time after the P wave. *DDD pacemakers provide a constant relationship between P waves and QRS complexes.* If the pacemaker senses intrinsic P waves and QRS complexes within the appropriate time interval, it will be inhibited, and it will just watch and wait until it's needed. If there are no Ps or QRS complexes in the preset time interval, the pacemaker will pace both chambers, providing a paced P and a paced QRS. Basically, the DDD provides whatever the patient cannot do on his or her own.

DDD pacemakers are usually **rate-responsive,** meaning they will provide a paced QRS to follow the patient's intrinsic P waves between preset heart rate limits. These limits are usually 60 to 125. Between this range, the DDD pacemaker will provide a paced QRS for every intrinsic P wave. Below these limits, the pacemaker will provide paced P waves also, as the intrinsic atrial rate is too slow. Above these limits, the DDD pacemaker will not provide a paced QRS for each intrinsic P wave because that would result in a tachycardia dangerous to the patient. Are you thoroughly confused?

Let's break that down a bit. Say the patient has an underlying third-degree AV block, which means a lot of P waves compared to QRS complexes, right? If the atrial rate is between 60 and 125, the DDD pacemaker will "track the P waves." The pacemaker will provide a paced QRS complex to follow each intrinsic P wave (assuming the patient does not have his or her own QRS at the right time after the P wave). It will not provide paced P waves, as it won't need to.

If the atrial rate drops below 60, the DDD pacemaker will provide paced P waves as well as QRS complexes as needed to keep the heart rate within the range of 60 to 125.

If the atrial rate exceeds 125, the DDD pacemaker will ignore some of those P waves and track others. Therefore, there may be paced QRS complexes after only every second or third intrinsic P wave, and so forth. Why does it do this? If the atrial rate is faster than 125, and the pacemaker provides a paced QRS after each P wave, the patient ends up with a heart rate of 125. That may be so fast that cardiac output drops. If the atrial rate exceeds the upper limit, the pacemaker senses the atrial rate and decides to obey only some, rather than all, of the intrinsic P waves.

DDD pacemakers provide four options:

- *Intrinsic beats only.* The pacemaker does not fire because it does not need to. The intrinsic rate is fast enough. There will be no pacemaker spikes.

- *Paced P wave, intrinsic QRS.* The pacemaker paces the atrium, providing a pacemaker spike and a paced P wave. Following this, the patient's own QRS occurs. There is therefore a spike only before the P wave.

- *Paced P wave, paced QRS.* The pacemaker paces both chambers, providing a spike before the P wave and a spike before the QRS.

- *Intrinsic P wave, paced QRS.* The patient has his or her own P waves, so the pacemaker tracks them and provides a paced QRS to follow. There is a pacemaker spike only before the QRS. See Figure 30-7.

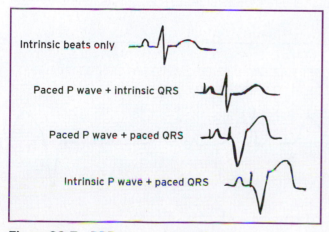

Figure 30-7 DDD pacemaker options.

DDD versus VVI Practice

On the following strips, tell whether the pacemaker is DDD or VVI (or undeterminable).

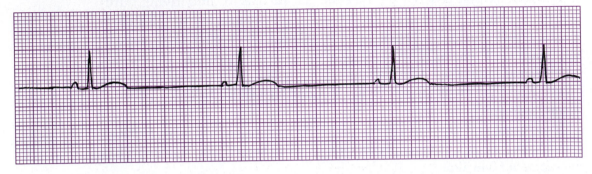

1. _____

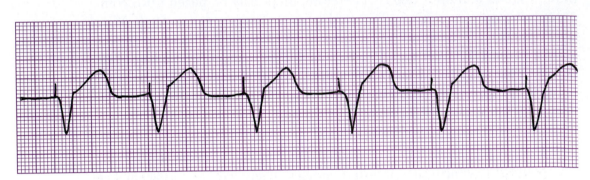

2. _____

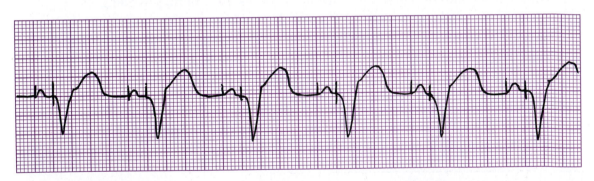

3. _____

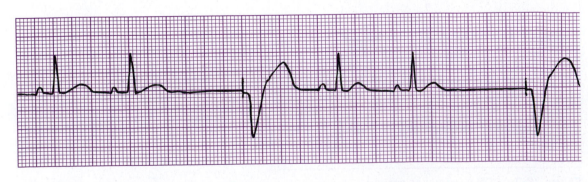

4. _____

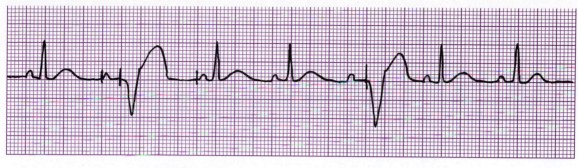

5. _____

Answers to DDD versus VVI Practice

1. **Can't tell which kind of pacemaker.** Since there are no paced beats at all, it is not possible to tell if it's a DDD or a VVI pacemaker.

2. **VVI.** There are pacemaker spikes preceding the QRS complexes, and there are no P waves in sight. Had this been a DDD pacemaker, there should have been some paced P waves also.

3. **DDD.** There are pacemaker spikes preceding the P waves and the QRS complexes.

4. **VVI.** There are four intrinsic beats and two paced beats on the strip. The paced beats pace only the ventricle. With this long a pause before a paced beat kicks in, a DDD pacemaker would have provided a paced P wave as well.

5. **DDD.** This strip has a little of everything. The first beat is all intrinsic. The second beat paces atrium and ventricle, as evidenced by the pacemaker spikes preceding the P wave and the QRS. The third beat has a paced P wave and an intrinsic QRS. The fourth, sixth, and seventh beats are all intrinsic. The fifth beat has an intrinsic P wave followed by a paced QRS.

Pacemaker Malfunctions

Like any gadget, pacemakers sometimes malfunction. The typical malfunctions follow.

Failure to Fire

Here the pacemaker fails to send out its electrical stimulus when it should. This can mean the pacemaker battery is dead or that connecting wires are interrupted. Or it can mean the pacemaker has oversensed something like extraneous muscle artifact and thinks it's not supposed to fire. Failure to fire is evidenced by the lack of pacemaker spikes where there should've been. It usually results in a pause. Figure 30-8 is an example of failure to fire.

In Figure 30-8, the patient's pacemaker rate is set at 60 and there are no pacemaker spikes anywhere. The rhythm is a very slow sinus bradycardia with a heart rate of about 28. The pacemaker should have prevented the heart rate from going this slowly, but it didn't fire.

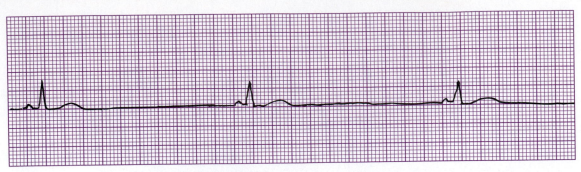

Figure 30-8 Failure to fire.

Loss of Capture

There is no P or QRS after the pacemaker spike in loss of capture. This is often simply a matter of turning up the pacemaker's voltage so that it sends out more juice to tell the heart what to do. Maybe the signal it sent out was too weak to get a response from the chamber. Another possibility is that the pacing catheter has lost contact with the wall of the chamber it's in and cannot cause depolarization. That could be corrected by a simple position change of the patient, or it could necessitate surgery to adjust the catheter placement. Loss of capture can also occur when the heart is too damaged to respond to the pacer's stimulus. See Figure 30-9 for an example of loss of capture.

In Figure 30-9 we have asystole with pacemaker spikes but no Ps or QRS complexes after the spikes. The pacemaker has fired, as evidenced by the spikes, but it has not captured the chamber it's in.

Undersensing

Here the pacemaker fires too soon after an intrinsic beat, often resulting in pacemaker spikes where there shouldn't have been, such as in a T wave, an ST segment, or right on top of another QRS. This happens when the pacemaker just doesn't see that other beat. The pacemaker's sensor needs adjusting. Another possibility is a fractured sensing wire or battery failure. In Figure 30-10, we have undersensing.

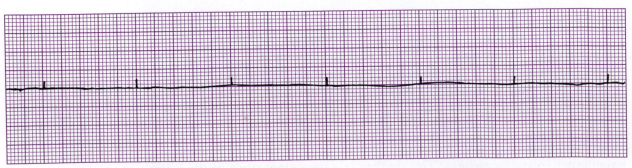

Figure 30-9 Loss of capture.

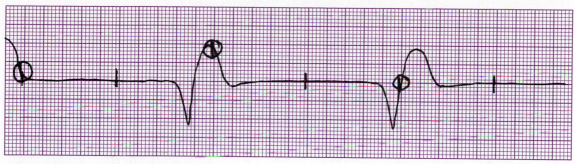

Figure 30-10 Undersensing.

In Figure 30-10, note the spikes at times when the pacer should not have fired. How do you detect undersensing? Look at the distance between two consecutive pacemaker spikes. That's the normal **pacing interval,** which will correspond to a certain paced heart rate. *There should be exactly that same distance between the patient's own intrinsic beats and the next paced beat.* If the distance is less than that, there is undersensing. In Figure 30-10, the circled pacemaker spikes indicate undersensing.

But this strip also shows another malfunction. Do you know what it is? Look it over carefully before continuing.

There is loss of capture in addition to the undersensing. All the uncircled spikes plus the first circled one did not result in a P or QRS complex at a time when they should have. The second and third circled ones would not be considered loss of capture even though they also don't result in a P or QRS. Why? Remember the refractory periods? From the beginning of the QRS to the upstroke of the T wave is the absolute refractory period. A spike that occurs during that time cannot possibly capture. That's not a pacemaker malfunction, it's just physiology.

For a summary of pacemaker malfunctions, see Table 30-1.

Table 30-1 Pacemaker Malfunctions Summary

PACEMAKER MALFUNCTIONS	EKG EVIDENCE
Failure to fire	Lack of pacemaker spikes where there should have been. Usually results in a pause.
Loss of capture	Pacemaker spikes not followed by P waves or QRS complexes.
Undersensing	Paced beats or spikes too close to previous beats. Often results in spikes inside T waves, ST segments, or QRS complexes.

Pacemaker Malfunctions Practice

On the strips that follow, indicate the pacer malfunction(s), if any.

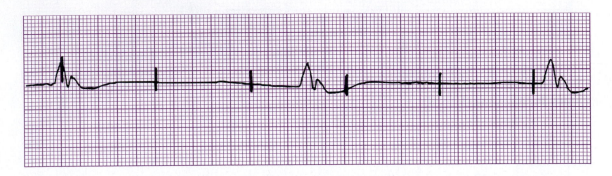

Situation: This patient passed out at home. The paramedics found him with a barely palpable, very slow pulse. His VVI pacemaker is set at 60.

1. _____

Situation: This patient had a DDD pacemaker inserted three years ago and now appears in the ER complaining of sudden onset of dizziness and syncope. The pacemaker rate is set at 68.

2. _____

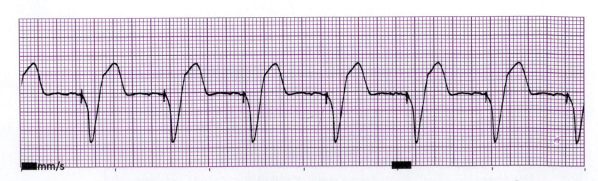

Situation: This patient has a DDD pacemaker set at 72. She's seen in her doctor's office for a routine checkup. She feels fine.

3. _____

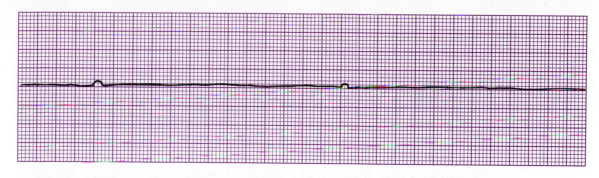

Situation: This patient is seen in the ER in cardiac arrest. His DDD pacemaker is set at 70.

4. _____

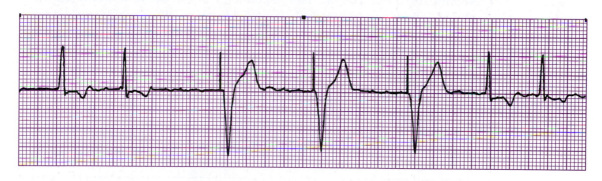

Situation: This patient had a VVI pacemaker inserted recently because of slow atrial fibrillation. It's set at 60. She feels fine.

5. _____

Answers to Pacemaker Malfunctions Practice

1. **Undersensing and loss of capture.** We have pacer spikes in inappropriate places, such as inside the first QRS complex. It is clear this pacer is not sensing the QRS complexes, since it does nothing in response to those intrinsic complexes. The pacer should have been inhibited by the patient's intrinsic QRS complexes. Also note the spikes are regular at a rate of 60. This is essentially a fixed-rate pacer now because it's not sensing anything. In addition, there is loss of capture, as evidenced by the pacer spikes not followed by Ps or QRSs at times when they should have been. The patient's underlying rhythm is idioventricular rhythm with a rate of 23.

2. **No malfunction at this time.** This strip shows a normally functioning DDD pacemaker. Note the upward atrial spikes followed by a tiny blip of a P wave, then a ventricular spike followed by a wide QRS. Though the pacemaker seems fine right now, it could be that it malfunctions intermit-

tently, causing the symptoms, so the patient will still need close observation. It is also possible that the patient's dizziness and syncope were caused by something totally unrelated to the pacemaker.

3. **No malfunction noted.** This strip shows a normally functioning DDD pacemaker. See the very small intrinsic P waves preceding each QRS? The pacemaker senses them and tracks them, providing the paced QRS to follow those Ps since the patient does not have her own QRS complexes in the programmed time.

4. **Failure to fire.** There are two intrinsic P waves on this strip. The pacemaker should have sensed them and provided a paced QRS to follow them. In addition, it should have paced the atrium and then the ventricle, as necessary, at its programmed rate of 70. It didn't. There's not a pacemaker spike in sight.

5. **No malfunction noted.** The pacemaker rate is set at 60, and it fires at 60 when the atrial fibrillation slows down. Note the pacing interval from spike to spike on the three paced beats. Now look at the interval between the second QRS and the paced beat that follows. It's exactly the same interval. The pacemaker is therefore sensing the underlying rhythm, and it's firing and capturing appropriately.

Practice Quiz

1. List five indications for an artificial pacemaker._____

   _____

   _____

   _____

   _____

2. The first letter of the pacemaker code refers to _____

3. The second letter of the pacemaker code refers to _____

4. The third letter of the pacemaker code refers to _____

5. Name the malfunction of a pacemaker that has no P wave or QRS after the pacemaker spike. _____

   _____

6. The pacemaker's ability to recognize the patient's own intrinsic rhythm in order to decide if it needs to fire is called _____

7. The pacemaker's generation of an electrical impulse is called_____

   _____

8. A DDD pacemaker paces which chamber(s)? _____

9. The DDD pacemaker senses which chamber(s)? _____

10. Failure to fire is evidenced by _____

Practice Quiz Answers

1. Five indications for an artificial pacemaker would include any of the following: **symptomatic sinus bradycardia, junctional rhythms,**

idioventricular rhythm, dying heart, asystole, 2:1 AV block, type II second-degree AV block, third-degree AV block, sick sinus syndrome, and **overdrive suppression of tachyarrhythmias.**

2. The first letter of the pacemaker code refers to the **chamber paced.**

3. The second letter of the pacemaker code refers to the **chamber sensed.**

4. The third letter of the pacemaker code refers to the **pacemaker's response to sensed events.**

5. A pacemaker that has no P wave or QRS after the pacemaker spike has **failure to capture.**

6. The pacemaker's ability to recognize the patient's own intrinsic rhythm in order to decide if it needs to fire is called **sensing.**

7. The pacemaker's generation of an electrical impulse is called **firing.**

8. A DDD pacemaker paces **dual chambers–atrium and ventricle.**

9. The DDD pacemaker senses **dual chambers–atrium and ventricle.**

10. Failure to fire is evidenced by the **lack of pacemaker spikes where there should have been.**

Scenarios

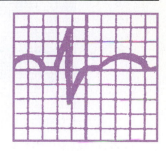

Chapter 31 Objectives

Upon completion of this chapter, the student will be able to:

- Correlate certain rhythms with their treatment.
- Display critical thinking skills.

Chapter 31 Outline

Chapter 31 Glossary

Midsternal: In the middle of the sternum.

Thrombolytics: Medications that dissolve blood clots.

Scenario A: Mr. Johnson

Mr. Johnson, age 52, was admitted to the hospital's telemetry floor complaining of mild chest discomfort that lasted two hours and was unrelieved by antacids. His parents both had a history of heart disease, so Mr. Johnson was afraid he might be having a heart attack. His initial EKG in the emergency department was completely normal, and his pain was relieved with one sublingual nitroglycerin tablet. Medical history included a two-pack-a-day cigarette habit, as well as major surgery the previous week to remove a small colon cancer. Mr. Johnson had been asleep in his room for about an hour when the nurse observed the strip shown in Figure 31-1 on his cardiac monitor.

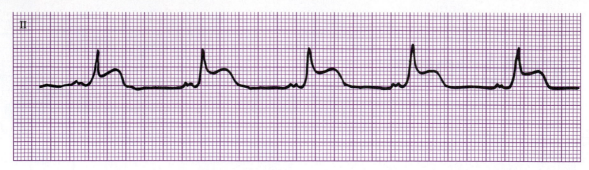

Figure 31-1 Mr. Johnson's rhythm.

1. What do you see of concern on the rhythm strip in Figure 31-1? _____

   _____

The nurse went to check on Mr. Johnson and found him just awakening and complaining of a dull ache in his chest. Per unit protocol, the nurse did a 12-lead EKG, shown in Figure 31-2.

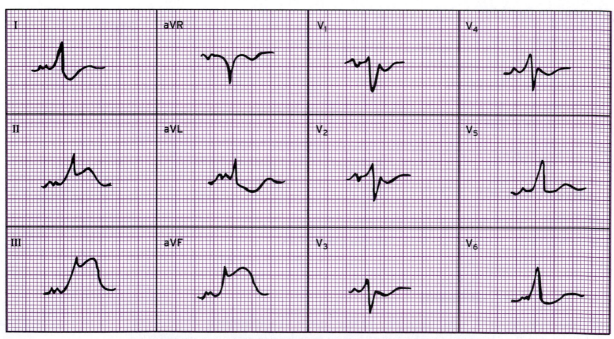

Figure 31-2 Mr. Johnson's 12-lead EKG done during chest pain.

2. What conclusion do you draw from the EKG in Figure 31-2? _____

   _____

3. Mr. Johnson was moved to the coronary care unit and was started on a nitroglycerin infusion and a heparin infusion. For what purpose were these infusions started? _____

   _____

4. Mr. Johnson was also started on oxygen by nasal prongs. What beneficial effect would the oxygen be expected to have? _____

5. The physician considered starting thrombolytic therapy, but due to Mr. Johnson's recent surgery decided he was not a candidate for thrombolytics. What is the mode of action of thrombolytic medications? _____

6. What is the danger of giving thrombolytics to someone who had recent surgery? _____

Shortly after arrival in CCU, Mr. Johnson called his nurse and told her he felt "funny." He denied pain but stated he felt "full in the head." The nurse noticed the rhythm in Figure 31-3 on the monitor in Mr. Johnson's room.

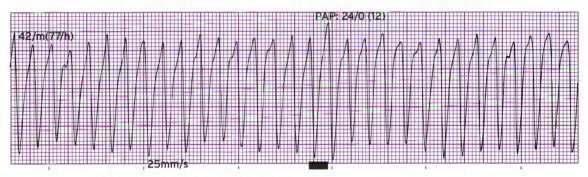

Figure 31-3 Mr. Johnson's second rhythm strip.

7. What is the rhythm shown in Figure 31-3? _____

8. Mr. Johnson's arrhythmia spontaneously converted back to sinus rhythm without treatment. The nurse notified the physician, who ordered labs to be drawn. What electrolyte abnormality can cause this rhythm? _____

9. What other blood abnormality can cause this rhythm? _____

10. What medications could have been used to treat this arrhythmia if it had continued? _____

Mr. Johnson's lab work revealed a very low potassium level. He was given supplemental potassium intravenously, and his arrhythmia did not recur. His blood oxygen level was normal.

Shortly after breakfast the next morning, Mr. Johnson developed midsternal chest pain radiating to his left arm. The pain was severe, and he broke out in a cold sweat and complained of mild nausea. His nurse gave him a sublingual nitroglycerin tablet and increased the rate of his nitroglycerin infusion.

11. What is another medication that could be given to treat Mr. Johnson's chest pain? _____

12. A 12-lead EKG was done stat (immediately) and is seen in Figure 31-4. What conclusion do you draw from this EKG? _____

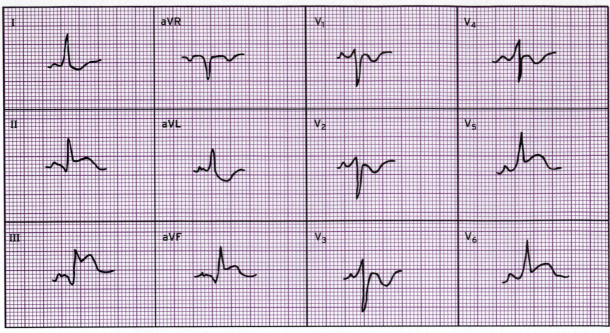

Figure 31-4 Mr. Johnson's second 12-lead EKG.

Within 15 minutes, Mr. Johnson's pain was gone but his blood pressure was very low and his rhythm had changed. See Figure 31-5 for his next rhythm.

13. What is the rhythm in Figure 31-5? _____

14. What effect does this rhythm have on cardiac output? _____

15. What medication should the nurse give now? _____

16. Where are the possible sites of the block? _____

17. If the block were at the bundle branches, what effect would atropine have? _____

_____

After the appropriate medication was given, Mr. Johnson's blood pressure returned to normal, and his rhythm was as seen in Figure 31-6.

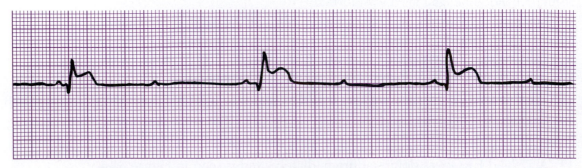

Figure 31-5 Mr. Johnson's third rhythm strip.

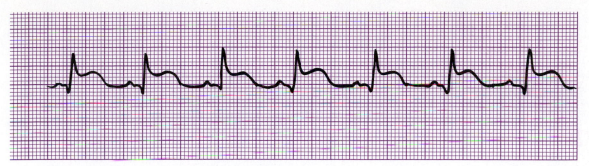

Figure 31-6 Mr. Johnson's fourth rhythm strip.

18. What rhythm is shown in Figure 3-16? _____

19. What symptoms, if any, would you expect Mr. Johnson to have with this rhythm? _____

_____

Mr. Johnson's cardiologist was concerned about the implications of the most recent EKG and his arrhythmias. He took Mr. Johnson to the cardiac catheterization lab to do an angiogram. It revealed significant blockage in two of his coronary arteries.

20. Based on the two EKGs in Figures 31-2 and 31-4, which two coronary arteries do you suspect were blocked? _____

Balloon angioplasty was attempted but was unsuccessful, so Mr. Johnson was taken to the operating room to have bypass surgery. He did well and was home in a week.

Scenario B: Ms. Capitano

Ms. Capitano was a 23-year-old woman who presented to the ER with complaints of fatigue and dizziness. She had a negative medical history and did not smoke. Aside from birth control pills, she took no medication and denied illegal drug use. She did drink five or six soft drinks daily and had two to three cups of coffee every morning. Cardiac monitor revealed the rhythm seen in Figure 31-7.

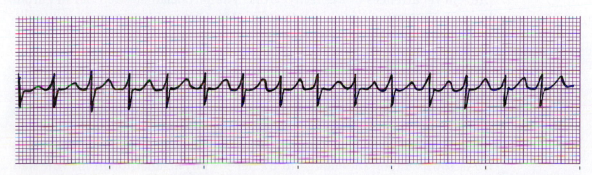

Figure 31-7 Ms. Capitano's initial rhythm in the ER.

1. What is the rhythm shown in Figure 31-7?_____

2. What is the likely cause of this rhythm in Ms. Capitano's case? _____

   _____

3. The physician ordered adenosine to be given intravenously. The rhythm strip shown in Figure 31-8 was the result. What happened?_____

   _____

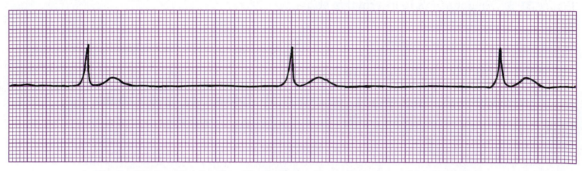

Figure 31-8   Ms. Capitano's rhythm after adenosine administration.

After a few seconds of the slow heart rate, Ms. Capitano's heart rate sped back up–to the 250s this time–and she stated that she felt as though she were going to pass out. Her blood pressure, which had been 110/60, dropped to 68/50, and she was now very pale and drenched in a cold sweat.

4. What effect was the tachycardia having on her cardiac output? _____

   _____

5. Ms. Capitano's preload would be expected to do what? Why?_____

   _____

Ms. Capitano's condition had worsened–she was now in shock. The ER physician elected to perform synchronized electrical cardioversion. After a low-voltage shock, Ms. Capitano's rhythm converted to sinus rhythm with a heart rate in the 90s and her blood pressure improved. Soon her color was back to normal and her skin was dry. She was admitted to the coronary care unit for close observation and was started on calcium channel blockers to prevent recurrences of her tachycardia. The physician advised her to curtail her caffeine intake. After a day in CCU, Ms. Capitano was transferred to the telemetry floor. She was sent home a day later, doing well.

Scenario C: Mr. Farley

A few years ago, Mr. Farley was diagnosed with chronic atrial fibrillation and was started on digitalis. He'd done well, with a heart rate running in the 70s and 80s since then. For the last few days, however, Mr. Farley had felt lousy– nothing specific, just "not right," as he would later describe it. He didn't think it was important enough to bother his physician, though his wife had fussed at him to do so. Believing his problem to be related to his atrial fibrillation, Mr. Farley doubled up on his digitalis dose. If one pill a day was good, two a day had to be better, he reasoned. After five days of this, he began suffering from violent nausea and vomiting episodes. His wife dragged the reluctant Mr. Farley to the hospital. His initial rhythm strip is shown in Figure 31-9.

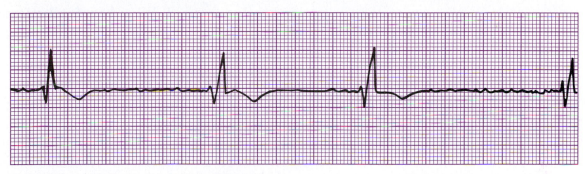

Figure 31-9   Mr. Farley's initial rhythm strip.

1. What is the rhythm in Figure 31-9?_____

2. What effect does atrial fibrillation have on the atrial kick? _____

    _____

3. Lab tests revealed that the level of digitalis in Mr. Farley's bloodstream was at toxic levels. Name three rhythms that can be caused by digitalis toxicity._____

    _____

The physician contemplated sending Mr. Farley to the CCU, but since his blood pressure was good and he looked OK, he was sent to the telemetry floor instead. His nausea was treated with medication and he was taken off digitalis. Three hours after arriving on the telemetry floor, Mr. Farley passed out in the bathroom. His wife ran to get the nurse just as the nurses, having seen his rhythm on the monitor, were running toward his room. His new rhythm is shown in Figure 31-10.

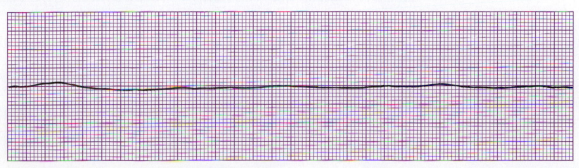

Figure 31-10   Mr. Farley's second rhythm strip.

4. What is the rhythm in Figure 31-10?_____

5. The emergency team was called and CPR was initiated. What two medications would be appropriate to give at this time? _____

_____

6. After successful resuscitation, Mr. Farley was transferred to the CCU, where a temporary pacemaker was inserted. What beneficial effect would the pacemaker have?_____

_____

7. A few hours after the pacemaker was inserted, the nurse noticed evidence of loss of capture on the monitor. On the monitor strip in Figure 31-11, what would tell her there was loss of capture? _____

_____

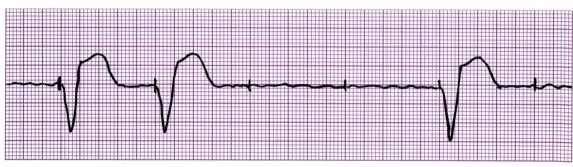

Figure 31-11 Mr. Farley's third rhythm strip.

8. What can be done to restore capture? _____

_____

Capture was restored, and Mr. Johnson rested well for the next few hours. Suddenly, he went into v-tach with a heart rate of 200. The nurses could tell the v-tach was originating in the left ventricle, so they knew it was not induced by irritation from the pacemaker wire in the right ventricle.

9. With a pacemaker in place, what can be done to terminate the tachycardia?

_____

10. With the v-tach now resolved, Mr. Farley was started on a lidocaine infusion to prevent a recurrence of the v-tach. What is lidocaine's effect on the ventricle? _____

_____

11. The rest of Mr. Farley's hospital stay was uneventful. Since his problem began with his inappropriate self-dosing of digitalis, what would you tell Mr. Farley regarding his digitalis dose in the future? _____

_____

Scenario D: Mr. Lew

Age 78, Mr. Lew had outlived his wife and most of their friends. He had never been in the hospital and had not seen his physician in seven years. By all accounts, he was unusually healthy for his age. He was not alarmed by the occasional tightness in his chest—and in fact took it as a sign that he was out of shape and needed to exercise more. One summer day, while mowing the lawn, the chest tightness came back, but this time it was much more intense, and Mr. Lew became concerned. He called his son to take him to the hospital. On the way, Mr. Lew passed out in the car and slumped over onto his son, causing an accident. Ambulances rushed the duo to the closest ER. Stephen, the son, was treated for a fractured arm and was discharged in a cast. Though not injured in the accident, Mr. Lew was in much worse shape. See his EKG in Figure 31-12.

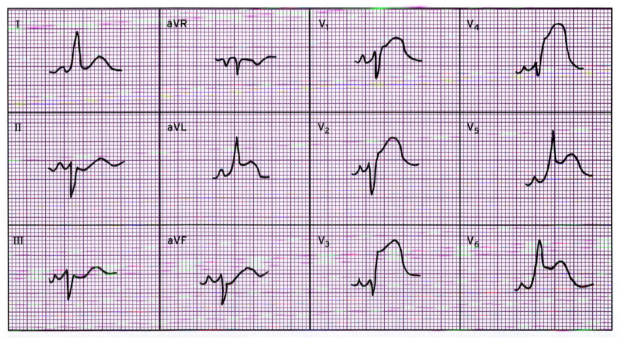

Figure 31-12   Mr. Lew's initial 12-lead EKG.

1. What conclusion do you draw from the EKG in Figure 31-12?_____

_____

Mr. Lew's condition was precarious. His blood pressure was low and he was in danger of cardiac arrest. Thrombolytic therapy was started, and within one hour Mr. Lew's blood pressure had improved. Soon he was in the rhythm shown in Figure 31-13.

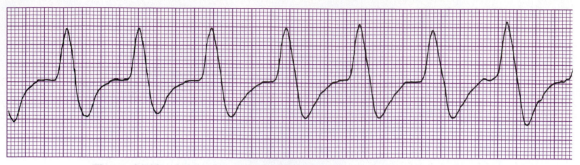

Figure 31-13 Mr. Lew's rhythm strip after thrombolytic therapy.

2. What is the rhythm in Figure 31-13? _____

3. What, if any, treatment does this rhythm require in this case? _____

   _____

4. What was the likely cause of this rhythm? _____

   This rhythm converted back to sinus rhythm within 30 minutes. Mr. Lew's condition improved over the next hour, and he was transferred to the coronary care unit, where he stabilized.

   When Stephen came by to see his dad the next day, Mr. Lew whispered to him that he was having mild chest pain again, but that it wasn't bad enough to bother the nurses. Stephen, however, alerted the nurse, who did an EKG while the pain was in progress. See the EKG in Figure 31-14.

5. What conclusion do you draw from the EKG in Figure 31-14? _____

   _____

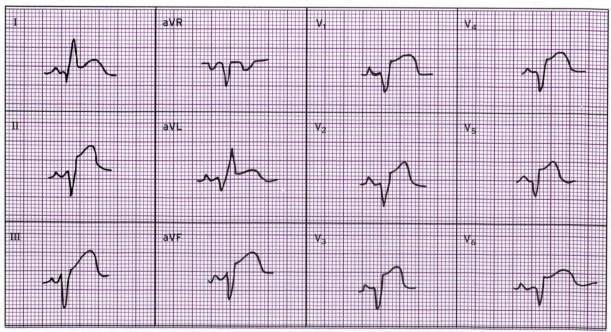

Figure 31-14 Mr. Lew's EKG done during chest pain.

Mr. Lew's nitroglycerin and heparin infusions, which had been started in the ER, were adjusted and Mr. Lew was taken for an emergency angiogram. An occlusion of the left main coronary artery was noted, along with blockage in another coronary artery.

6. Based on the two EKGs in Figures 31-12 and 31-14, which other coronary artery is involved? _____

_____

7. What is the cause of the ST segment depression noted on Mr. Lew's first EKG? _____

_____

Mr. Lew was taken to the operating room for emergency bypass surgery. Following cardiac arrest in the operating room, he returned to the CCU in critical condition. Before the surgical nurses had gotten back to the OR after having brought Mr. Lew to CCU, they heard the emergency page on the loudspeaker. Mr. Lew was cardiac arresting again. They rushed back to CCU to help. The cardiac surgeon had opened the chest sutures and was doing manual chest compressions by squeezing Mr. Lew's heart in his hands. Mr. Lew's rhythm strip is shown in Figure 31-15.

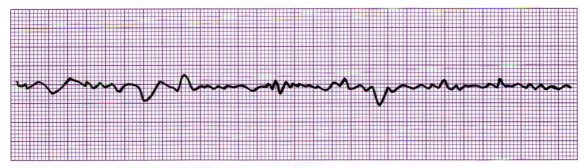

Figure 31-15 Mr. Lew's rhythm during cardiac arrest.

8. What is the rhythm in Figure 31-15?_____

Internal defibrillator paddles were inserted into the open chest cavity and placed on either side of Mr. Lew's heart. A small volt was discharged, and Mr. Lew's rhythm changed to the one shown in Figure 31-16.

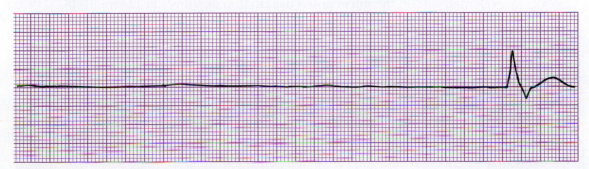

Figure 31-16 Mr. Lew's rhythm after defibrillation.

9. What is the rhythm in Figure 31-16?_____

CPR was started again, and the staff administered various medications as well as temporary pacing—all to no avail. Mr. Lew did not make it.

10. Occlusion of the left main coronary artery causes a massive heart attack sometimes known as what? _____

Scenario E: Mrs. Epstein

Mrs. Epstein had had her pacemaker implanted four years ago because of third-degree AV block. She'd been doing well until this morning, when she began to feel dizzy. She took her pulse as she'd been taught to do and found it to be 38. Her rate-responsive DDD pacemaker was set at a rate of 60 to 125. At the physician's office, the cardiologist found that the pacemaker needed a new battery. Because her heart rate was now in the 60s, he felt the battery change could wait until the next morning. He sent Mrs. Epstein to the hospital, where she was admitted to the telemetry floor.

A few hours after arrival, Mrs. Epstein complained again of dizziness, this time much worse. Her rhythm is shown in Figure 31-17.

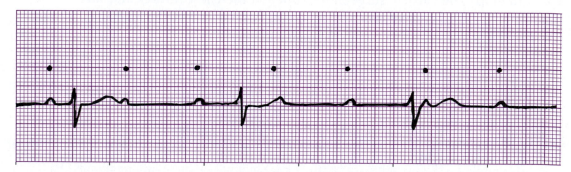

Figure 31-17 Mrs. Epstein's rhythm during a dizzy spell in the hospital.

1. What is the rhythm in Figure 31-17?_____

2. What is her pacemaker doing? _____

3. What is the likely cause of this problem?_____

The nurse, following hospital protocol, gave atropine, and Mrs. Epstein's heart rate climbed to the 60s. After notifying the cardiologist of the situation, the nurse rushed Mrs. Epstein to the cardiac catheterization lab, where an emergency pacemaker battery change was done. After her return to the telemetry floor, the nurse noted her rhythm as shown in Figure 31-18.

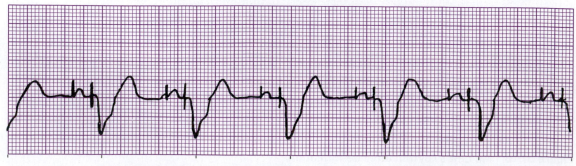

Figure 31-18 Mrs. Epstein's rhythm on return from her pacemaker battery change.

4. What is the rhythm in Figure 31-18?_____

5. Is the pacemaker functioning properly? If not, what is the problem?_____

_____

Mrs. Epstein was discharged the following day in good condition.

Answers to Scenarios

Scenario A: Mr. Johnson

1. Of concern is the ST segment elevation in lead II on this strip. The sinus bradycardia is not a concern, especially since Mr. Johnson had been asleep, but the ST elevation is worrisome.

2. Mr. Johnson is having an inferior wall MI, as evidenced by the ST elevation in leads II, III, and aVF and by the reciprocal ST depression in the anterior leads.

3. Nitroglycerin dilates coronary arteries and thus increases the flow to the tissues. Heparin is an anticoagulant that will prevent clots from forming in the coronary arteries. It will not, however, dissolve any that may already be there.

4. The oxygen will improve tissue concentration of oxygen and can help prevent arrhythmias and decrease the heart's workload.

5. Thrombolytic medications dissolve blood clots.

6. The danger of giving thrombolytics to someone who had recent surgery is that severe bleeding may occur at the surgical site.

7. The rhythm is ventricular flutter. The pattern is zigzag and the rate is about 300.

8. Potassium deficit (hypokalemia) can cause v-flutter.

9. Hypoxia is another blood abnormality that can cause v-flutter.

10. Lidocaine, procainamide, and amiodarone could be used to abolish the v-flutter.

11. Morphine is another medication that can be used to treat chest pain.

12. The MI is extending into the lateral wall now, as evidenced by the new ST elevation in leads V_5 to V_6.

13. This rhythm is 2:1 AV block. There are two P waves to every QRS on this strip.

14. This rhythm can cause the cardiac output to drop.

15. The nurse should now give atropine to speed up the heart rate.

16. The block could be at the AV node or the bundle branches.

17. If the block were at the bundle branches, atropine may have no effect on the heart rate, or it could make things worse by speeding up the sinus rate and increasing the block ratio. Atropine speeds up the rate of the sinus node and increases AV conduction, causing the impulses to come more rapidly. The impulses blast through the AV node only to arrive at the still-blocked bundle branches (atropine has no effect on the bundle

branches). Epinephrine and/or pacing would be indicated for a block at the bundle branches.

18. This rhythm is sinus rhythm.

19. Mr. Johnson should have no symptoms from this rhythm. He should in fact feel much better now that his heart rate is more normal.

20. The two coronary arteries blocked were probably the right coronary artery, which supplies the inferior wall of the left ventricle, and the circumflex, which supplies the lateral wall. It is also possible that Mr. Johnson is left-dominant, with a circumflex coronary artery that is very prominent and supplies not only the lateral wall, but the inferior wall as well. (Review Chapter 2 for a refresher on the coronary arteries.)

Scenario B: Ms. Capitano

1. The rhythm is SVT. The heart rate is about 150, the rhythm is regular, and P waves are not discernible.

2. The likely cause of this rhythm in this case is caffeine overdose.

3. The heart rate slowed dramatically to a junctional bradycardia. This is not unusual after adenosine administration. In fact, sometimes the heart completely stops for a few seconds before the sinus node kicks back in.

4. The tachycardia is dropping her cardiac output to dangerously low levels.

5. Ms. Capitano's preload would be very low, as the heart rate is too fast to allow adequate ventricular filling.

Scenario C: Mr. Farley

1. The rhythm is slow atrial fibrillation. Note the wavy, undulating baseline and the absence of P waves.

2. In atrial fibrillation, there is no atrial kick at all, thus causing a drop in cardiac output of about 15 to 30%.

3. Digitalis toxicity can cause almost any arrhythmia, such as 2:1 atrial tachycardia, junctional tachycardia; atrial tachycardia; sinus pauses, arrests, and blocks; all degrees of AV blocks; and slow junctional and ventricular rhythms.

4. The rhythm is asystole.

5. Atropine and epinephrine would be appropriate to give, as they both work to speed up the heart rate. Epinephrine also helps restore pumping function in cardiac arrest.

6. A pacemaker would prevent Mr. Farley's heart rate from going too slow.

7. Loss of capture is evidenced by the pacemaker spikes not followed by a QRS complex.

8. Capture might be restored by repositioning Mr. Farley in bed or by increasing the voltage sent out by the pacemaker.

9. A pacemaker provides the possibility of overdriving the tachycardia. The pacemaker rate is dialed up to a rate exceeding the patient's heart

rate. The pacemaker then assumes control (usurps) the underlying rhythm. The pacemaker can then be slowly turned down, allowing the sinus node to assume control.

10. Lidocaine decreases the irritability of the ventricle and makes it less responsive to ventricular impulses.

11. Mr. Farley should be instructed to follow his physician's prescription, not to add or subtract doses on his own. If he feels bad, he should contact his physician or go to the hospital ER.

Scenario D: Mr. Lew

1. This EKG reveals that Mr. Lew has suffered an extensive anterior MI, as evidenced by the ST elevation in I, aVL, and all the precordial leads, along with reciprocal ST depression in the inferior leads.

2. This rhythm is accelerated idioventricular rhythm.

3. It usually requires no treatment. AIVR is a common rhythm after thrombolytic therapy and is believed to be a sign of reperfusion of the tissue that was in jeopardy.

4. The probable cause of this rhythm is reperfusion.

5. Mr. Lew has now extended his MI into the inferior wall, as evidenced by the new ST elevation in II, III, and aVF. This is a catastrophic development.

6. The right coronary artery is also blocked. (It is possible also that Mr. Lew is left-dominant, with his inferior wall supplied by the circumflex coronary artery. In that case, occlusion of the left main coronary artery would also disrupt flow to the inferior wall.)

7. The ST depression in the first EKG was reciprocal changes.

8. The rhythm is ventricular fibrillation.

9. The rhythm is agonal rhythm (dying heart).

10. Occlusion of the left main coronary artery is sometimes referred to as the *widow-maker*.

Scenario E: Mrs. Epstein

1. The rhythm is third-degree AV block. Note that the P-P intervals are regular and the R-R intervals are also regular, but at a different rate. The PR intervals vary.

2. Her pacemaker is doing nothing. There are no pacemaker spikes anywhere.

3. The likely cause of this is a dead pacemaker battery.

4. The rhythm is dual-chamber pacing. Note the pacemaker spikes preceding the P waves and QRS complexes.

5. The pacemaker is functioning properly.

Glossary

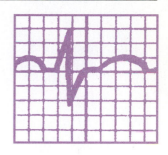

Aberration: The abnormally shaped QRS complex that results when a premature supraventricular impulse finds the conduction system only partially able to conduct its impulses.

Ablation: Destruction of an accessory conductive pathway in the heart.

Acetylcholine: A hormone released as a result of parasympathetic stimulation.

Actin: A contractile protein found in cardiac cells.

Action potential: The depolarization and repolarization events that take place at the cell membrane. Also refers to the diagram associated with these polarity events.

Adrenergic: Referring to the sympathetic nervous system fibers that release norepinephrine.

Afterload: The pressure against which the heart must pump in order to expel its blood.

Agonal rhythm: A ventricular rhythm characterized by very slow, irregular QRS complexes and absent P waves. Also called *dying heart*.

Algorithm: A flowchart.

Alpha receptors: Receptors that affect vasoconstriction.

Amplitude: The height of the waves and complexes on the EKG.

Anaerobic: Without oxygen.

Angina: Chest pain caused by a decrease in myocardial blood flow.

Angiogram: An invasive procedure in which dye is injected into blood vessels in order to determine their patency (openness).

Angioplasty: An invasive procedure in which a small balloon is used to open narrowed arteries.

Antegrade: In a forward direction.

Anterior: The front side.

Antiarrhythmic: Medications used to treat or prevent arrhythmias.

Aorta: Largest artery in the body; into which the left ventricle empties.

Aortic sinuses of Valsalva: The location of the openings to the coronary arteries. Located at the base of the aorta.

Apex: The pointy part of the heart where it rests on the diaphragm.

Arteriole: A very small artery that empties into a capillary bed.

Artery: A blood vessel that carries blood away from the heart to the tissues or the lungs.

Artifact: Unwanted jitter or interference on the EKG tracing.

Arrhythmia: Abnormal heart rhythm.

Arteriosclerosis: Hardening of the arteries caused by buildup of fatty plaque on arterial walls.

Asystole: No heart beat. Characterized by a flat line on the EKG.

Atheroma: Fatty plaque that builds up on the walls of arteries, narrowing their lumen (internal diameter).

Atrial kick: The phase of ventricular diastole in which the atria contract to propel their blood into the ventricles.

Atrium: The upper, thin-walled receiving chambers of the heart.

Augment: Increase.

Automaticity: The ability of cardiac cells to initiate an impulse without outside stimulation.

Autonomic nervous system: The nervous system controlling involuntary biological functions.

AV block (atrioventricular block): A disturbance in conduction in which some or all impulses from the sinus node are either delayed on their trip to the ventricles or do not reach the ventricle at all.

AV dissociation (atrioventricular dissociation): A condition in which the atria and ventricles depolarize and contract independently of each other.

AV node: The group of specialized cells in the conduction system that slows impulse transmission to allow atrial contraction to occur.

Axillary: Referring to the armpit.

Axis: The mean direction of the heart's current flow.

Baroreceptors: Receptors inside arterial walls that sense changes in blood pressure.

Base: The top of the heart; the area from which the great vessels emerge.

Baseline: The line from which the EKG waves and complexes take off. Also called the *isoelectric line*.

Bayes' theorem: The theorem that states that the predictive value of a test is based not only on the accuracy of the test itself but on the patient's probability of disease, as determined by a risk assessment done prior to the testing.

Beta receptors: Receptors that affect heart rate, contractility, and airway size.

Bifascicular: Referring to two of the fascicles of the bundle branch system.

Bigeminy: Every other beat is an abnormal beat.

Bipolar: Having a positive and a negative pole.

Blood pressure: The pressure exerted on the arterial walls by the circulating blood.

Bradycardia: Slow heart rate, usually less than 60.

Bundle branches: Conduction pathways extending from the bundle of His in the lower right atrium to the Purkinje fibers in the ventricles. There is a right and a left bundle branch.

Bundle of His: A confluence of conduction fibers between the AV node and the bundle branches.

Calibration: A method of verifying the correct performance of an EKG machine.

Capillaries: The smallest blood vessels in the body; nutrient and gas exchange takes place here.

Capture: The depolarization of the atrium and/or ventricle as a result of a pacemaker's firing. Determined by the presence of a P wave and/or QRS after the pacemaker spike.

Cardiac arrest: An emergency in which the heart stops beating.

Cardiac output: The amount of blood expelled by the heart each minute.

Cardioversion: Synchronized electrical shock to the heart to convert an abnormal rhythm to sinus.

Chemoreceptors: Receptors in arterial walls that sense changes in pH and oxygenation status.

Cholinergic: Pertaining to acetylcholine, or to the parasympathetic nervous system.

Chordae tendineae: Tendinous cords that attach to the AV valves and prevent them from everting.

Compliance: The ability of a heart chamber, in particular the left ventricle, to expand to accommodate the influx of blood.

Conduction system: A network of specialized cells whose job is to create and conduct the electrical impulses that control the cardiac cycle.

Conductivity: The ability of a cardiac cell to pass an impulse along to neighboring cells.

Congestive heart failure (CHF): Fluid buildup in the lungs as a result of the heart's inability to pump adequately.

Contractility: The ability of a cardiac cell to contract and do work.

Contraindications: Reasons to avoid doing a test or procedure.

Couplet: A pair of beats.

Critical rate: The rate at which a bundle branch block appears or disappears.

Defibrillation: Asynchronous electrical shock to the heart, used to treat ventricular fibrillation and pulseless v-tach.

Delta wave: The slurred upstroke to the QRS complex that is seen in Wolff-Parkinson-White (WPW) syndrome.

Depolarization: The wave of electrical current that changes the resting negatively charged cardiac cell to a positively charged one.

Diaphoresis: Sweating.

Diastasis: The phase in diastole in which the atrial and ventricular pressures are equalizing.

Diastole: The phase of the cardiac cycle in which the ventricles fill with blood.

Dissociation: The lack of relationship between two pacemaker sites in the heart.

Distal: Farther away from a body part.

Dorsal: The back side of the body.

Ectopy: Beats that arise from a pacemaker other than the sinus node. Understood to mean ventricular beats if the kind of ectopy is not specified.

Einthoven's triangle: The triangle formed by joining leads I, II, and III at the ends.

Electrocardiogram: A printout of the electrical signals generated by the heart.

Electrocardiograph: The EKG machine.

Electrodes: Adhesive patches attached to the skin to receive the electrical signals from the heart.

Electrolytes: Blood chemicals.

Embolus: Blood clot that has broken off and is traveling through a blood vessel.

Endocardium: The innermost layer of the heart.

Epicardium: Layer of the heart that is the same as the visceral pericardium.

Ergometer: An arm bicycle used in stress testing.

Escape: A safety mechanism in which a lower pacemaker fires at its slower inherent rate when the faster, predominant pacemaker fails.

Excitability: The ability of a cardiac cell to depolarize when stimulated.

External: On the outside.

Fascicle: A branch of the left bundle branch.

Fibrillation: The wiggling or twitching of the atrium or ventricle.

Firing: The pacemaker's generation of an electrical impulse.

Focus: Location.

Frank-Starling principle: States that increased stretch of myocardial fibers by increased preload will result in increased contractile force.

Frontal leads: Limb leads I, II, III, aVR, aVL, and aVF.

Fusion beat: A beat that results when a sinus beat arrives to depolarize the ventricle at the same time a PVC was activating the same tissue.

Galvanometer: A component of an EKG machine that transforms electrical energy into mechanical energy, allowing the EKG to be printed out.

Heart rate: The number of times the heart beats in one minute.

Hemiblock: A block of one of the fascicles of the left bundle branch.

Hexiaxial diagram: A diagram of the six frontal leads intersecting at the center; serves as the basis for the axis circle.

Holter monitor: A device used for 24-hour cardiac monitoring to check for arrhythmias or ST segment abnormalities.

Homeostasis: Balance. Refers to the body's ability to compensate to change.

Hypercalcemia: Elevated blood calcium level.

Hyperkalemia: Elevated blood potassium level.

Hypertension: Elevated blood pressure.

Hypertrophy: Overgrowth of myocardial tissue.

Hypocalcemia: Low blood calcium level.

Hypokalemia: Low blood potassium level.

Hypotension: Low blood pressure.

Hypoxia: Low blood oxygen level.

Indications: Reasons to perform a test or procedure.

Indicative changes: EKG changes that indicate the presence of an MI.

Infarction: Death of tissue. A myocardial infarction (MI) is a heart attack.

Inferior: Toward the foot.

Injury: Damage to tissue.

Interatrial tracts: The pathways that carry the electrical impulse from the sinus node through the atrial tissue to the AV node. Also called *internodal tracts.*

Intercostal: Between the ribs.

Intervals: Measurements of time between EKG waves and complexes.

Ischemia: Oxygen deprivation in the tissues.

Isoelectric line: The flat line between the EKG waves and complexes. Also called the baseline.

Isovolumetric: Maintaining the same volume.

J point: The point where the QRS complex and ST segment join together.

Kent bundle: The accessory pathway in WPW.

Lateral: On the side.

Lead: An electrocardiographic picture of the heart.

Macroshock: A large electrical shock caused by improper or faulty grounding of electrical equipment.

Mean arterial presure: The average pressure in the aorta during the cardiac cycle.

Medial: Toward the middle.

Mediastinum: The cavity between the lungs, in which the heart is located.

MET: Metabolic equivalent, a measurement of oxygen consumption.

Microshock: A small electrical shock made possible by a conduit, such as a pacemaker, directly in the heart.

Multifocal: Coming from more than one location.

Myocardial infarction: Heart attack.

Myocardium: The muscular layer of the heart.

Myosin: A contractile protein found in cardiac cells.

Neuropathy: Condition that causes a decrease in sensation, especially pain, in susceptible individuals.

Oxygen: An element inhaled from the atmosphere that is necessary for body function.

Pacemaker: The intrinsic or artificial focus that propagates or initiates the cardiac impulse.

Papillary muscle: The muscle to which the chordae tendineae are attached at the bottom.

Parietal: Referring to the wall of a body cavity.

Paroxysmal: Occurring suddenly and stopping just as suddenly.

Perfusion: The supplying of blood and nutrients to tissues.

Perfusion pressure: The pressure required to perfuse an organ or tissue with required nutrients.

Pericarditis: An inflammation of the pericardium.

Pericardium: The sac that encloses the heart.

Peripheral: Away from the center.

Purkinje fibers: Fibers at the terminal ends of the bundle branches. Responsible for transmitting the impulses into the ventricular myocardium.

Perpendicular: At a right angle to.

Polarized: Possessing an electrical charge.

Posterior: The back side.

Preexcitation: Depolarizing tissue earlier than normal.

Preload: The pressure in the left ventricle at the end of diastole, when its volume is greatest.

Protodiastole: The phase of systole in which ventricular, pulmonary artery, and aortic pressures equalize.

Proximal: Nearer to a body part.

Pulse pressure: The mathematical difference between the systolic and diastolic blood pressures.

P wave: The EKG wave reflecting atrial depolarization.

Quadrant: One-fourth of a circle.

QRS complex: The EKG complex representing ventricular depolarization.

Refractory: Resistant to.

Reperfusion: Supplying blood and oxygen to tissues that have been deprived for a period of time.

Repolarization: The wave of electrical current that returns the cardiac cell to its resting, electrically negative state.

Resuscitation: Returning a lifeless person to consciousness.

Retrograde: In a backward direction.

R-R interval: The distance (interval) between consecutive QRS complexes. Usually measured at the peaks of the R waves.

Sagittal: A plane of dissection that slices the body vertically into right and left.

Segment: The flat line between EKG waves and complexes.

Semilunar: Half-moon-shaped. Refers to the aortic and pulmonic valves.

Sensing: The ability of an artificial pacemaker to "see" the intrinsic rhythm in order to determine whether the pacemaker needs to fire.

Sensitivity: The ability of a test to pick out the people who are truly diseased.

Septum: The fibrous tissue that separates the heart into right and left sides.

Sinus node: The normal pacemaker of the heart.

Somatic: Referring to the body.

Specificity: The ability of a test to exclude those who are not diseased.

Standardization: Calibration of an EKG machine.

Stent: A mesh device introduced into coronary arteries to prevent their reocclusion after PTCA.

Sternum: Breastbone.

Stroke volume: The volume of blood expelled by the heart with each beat.

Stylus: The pen on the EKG machine.

Subclavian: Beneath the clavicle (collarbone).

Subendocardial: Referring to the myocardial layer just beneath the endocardium.

Subepicardium: Referring to the myocardial layer just beneath the epicardium.

Superficial: Shallow.

Superior: Up toward the head.

Supraventricular: Originating in a pacemaker above the ventricle.

Syncope: Fainting spell.

Systemic vascular resistance: The pressure the heart must overcome in order to expel its blood.

Systole: The phase of the cardiac cycle in which the heart contracts and expels its blood.

Tachycardia: Fast heart rate, greater than 100.

Telemetry: A method of monitoring a patient's rhythm remotely. The patient carries a small transmitter that relays his or her cardiac rhythm to a receiver located at another location.

Thoracic: Referring to the chest cavity.

Thrombolysis: The act of dissolving a blood clot.

Thyrotoxicosis: Also called *thyroid storm*. A condition in which the thyroid gland so overproduces thyroid hormones that the body's metabolic rate is accelerated to a catastrophic degree. The body temperature, heart rate, and blood pressure rise to extreme levels.

Transcutaneous: By way of the skin.

Transmembrane potential: The electrical charge at the cell membrane.

Transmural: Through the full thickness of the wall at that location.

Transvenous: By way of a vein.

Transverse: A plane of dissection that slices the body horizontally into top and bottom.

Triaxial diagram: The diagram of leads I, II, and III joined at the center or of aVR, aVL, and aVF joined at the center.

Tricuspid: Having three cusps.

Trifascicular: Referring to a block of three fascicles of the bundle branch system or to a block of two fascicles of the bundle branch system plus a first-degree AV block.

Trigeminy: Every third beat is abnormal.

T wave: The EKG wave that represents ventricular repolarization.

Unifocal: Coming from one location.

Unipolar: A lead consisting of only a positive pole.

Usurpation: The act of a lower pacemaker stealing control from the predominant pacemaker; results in a faster heart rate than before.

U wave: A small wave sometimes seen on the EKG. It follows the T wave and reflects late repolarization.

Vagus nerve: The nerve that is part of the parasympathetic nervous system. Causes the heart rate to slow when stimulated.

Valve: A structure in the heart that prevents backflow of blood.

Vasoconstrict: To make a blood vessel's walls squeeze down, narrowing the vessel's lumen.

Vasodilate: To make the blood vessel's walls relax, thus widening the blood vessel.

Vector: An arrow depicting the direction of electrical current flow in the heart.

Vein: A blood vessel that transports deoxygenated blood away from the tissues.

Vena cava: The largest vein in the body, returns deoxygenated blood to the heart.

Ventral: The front or stomach side of the body.

Ventricles: The lower pumping chambers of the heart.

Venule: A very small vein that drains blood away from a capillary bed.

Visceral: Referring to an organ itself.

WPW: Wolff-Parkinson-White syndrome, a preexcitation syndrome characterized by a short PR interval and a delta wave.

Index

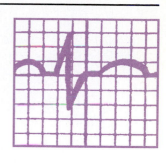